Complementary and Integrative Medicine

Editor

ROBERT B. SAPER

MEDICAL CLINICS OF NORTH AMERICA

www.medical.theclinics.com

Consulting Editor
BIMAL H. ASHAR

September 2017 • Volume 101 • Number 5

ELSEVIER

1600 John F. Kennedy Boulevard • Suite 1800 • Philadelphia, Pennsylvania, 19103-2899

http://www.theclinics.com

MEDICAL CLINICS OF NORTH AMERICA Volume 101, Number 5
September 2017 ISSN 0025-7125, ISBN-13: 978-0-323-54558-7

Editor: Jessica McCool
Developmental Editor: Alison Swety

Medical Clinics of North America (ISSN 0025-7125) is published bimonthly by Elsevier Inc., 360 Park Avenue South, New York, NY 10010-1710. Months of publication are January, March, May, July, September, and November. Business and editorial offices: 1600 John F. Kennedy Boulevard, Suite 1800, Philadelphia, PA 19103-2899. Periodicals postage paid at New York, NY, and additional mailing offices. Subscription prices are USD $268.00 per year (US individuals), $563.00 per year (US institutions), $100.00 per year (US Students), $330.00 per year (Canadian individuals), $731.00 per year (Canadian institutions), $200.00 per year (Canadian and foreign students), $402.00 per year (foreign individuals), and $731.00 per year (foreign institutions). To receive student/resident rate, orders must be accompanied by name of affiliated institution, date of term, and the signature of program/residency coordinator on institution letterhead. Orders will be billed at individual rate until proof of status is received. Foreign air speed delivery is included in all Clinics' subscription prices. All prices are subject to change without notice. **POSTMASTER:** Send address changes to *Medical Clinics of North America*, Elsevier Health Sciences Division, Subscription Customer Service, 3251 Riverport Lane, Maryland Heights, MO 63043. **Customer Service: Telephone: 1-800-654-2452** (U.S. and Canada); **1-314-447-8871** (outside U.S. and Canada). **Fax: 314-447-8029. E-mail: journalscustomerserviceusa@elsevier.com** (for print support); **journalsonlinesupport-usa@elsevier.com** (for online support).

Reprints. For copies of 100 or more of articles in this publication, please contact the Commercial Reprints Department, Elsevier Inc., 360 Park Avenue South, New York, NY 10010-1710. Tel.: 212-633-3874; Fax: 212-633-3820; E-mail: reprints@elsevier.com.

Medical Clinics of North America is also published in Spanish by McGraw-Hill Interamericana Editores S. A., P.O. Box 5-237, 06500 Mexico, D.F., Mexico.

Medical Clinics of North America is covered in *MEDLINE/PubMed (Index Medicus)*, *Current Contents*, *ASCA*, *Excerpta Medica, Science Citation Index*, and *ISI/BIOMED*.

PROGRAM OBJECTIVE
The goal of the *Medical Clinics of North America* is to keep practicing physicians up to date with current clinical practice by providing timely articles reviewing the state of the art in patient care.

TARGET AUDIENCE
All practicing physicians and other healthcare professionals.

LEARNING OBJECTIVES
Upon completion of this activity, participants will be able to:
1. Review the use of complementary and integrative therapies in neurological and mental health disorders.
2. Discuss the use of integrative medicine in respiratory and cardiovascular disorders.
3. Recognize the role of integrative and complimentary therapies in specialities such as oncology and pain management, among others.

ACCREDITATION
The Elsevier Office of Continuing Medical Education (EOCME) is accredited by the Accreditation Council for Continuing Medical Education (ACCME) to provide continuing medical education for physicians.

The EOCME designates this enduring material for a maximum of 15 *AMA PRA Category 1 Credit*(s)™. Physicians should claim only the credit commensurate with the extent of their participation in the activity.

All other healthcare professionals requesting continuing education credit for this enduring material will be issued a certificate of participation.

DISCLOSURE OF CONFLICTS OF INTEREST
The EOCME assesses conflict of interest with its instructors, faculty, planners, and other individuals who are in a position to control the content of CME activities. All relevant conflicts of interest that are identified are thoroughly vetted by EOCME for fair balance, scientific objectivity, and patient care recommendations. EOCME is committed to providing its learners with CME activities that promote improvements or quality in healthcare and not a specific proprietary business or a commercial interest.

The planning committee, staff, authors and editors listed below have identified no financial relationships or relationships to products or devices they or their spouse/life partner have with commercial interest related to the content of this CME activity:
Bimal H. Ashar, MD, MBA, FACP; Monica Aggarwal, MD; Brooke Aggarwal, EdD, MS; Gary N. Asher, MD, MPH; Vanessa Baute, MD; Suzanne M. Bertisch, MD, MPH; Stephanie Cheng, MD; Delia Chiaramonte, MD; Lorenzo Cohen, PhD; Sharon Democker, MD; Anjali Fortna; Paula Gardiner, MD, MPH; Bradley N. Gaynes, MD, MPH; Katherine A. Gergen Barnett, MD; Jonathan Gerkin, MD; Randy Horwitz, MD, PhD; Anna K. Koch, MSc(Psych); Mikhail Kogan, MD; Joshua Korzenik, MD; Amy B. Locke, MD, ABIHM; Gabriel Lopez, MD; Jun J. Mao, MD, MSCE; Jessica McCool; Mariatu Koroma Nelson, MD; Jyothi Rao, MD, FAARFM; Seema Rao, MD; Melinda Ring, MD; Robert B. Saper; Jeyanthi Surendrakumar; Halané Wahbeh, ND, MCR; Rebecca Erwin Wells, MD, MPH; Katie Widmeier; Gloria Y. Yeh, MD, MPH; Eric S. Zhou, PhD.

The planning committee, staff, authors and editors listed below have identified financial relationships or relationships to products or devices they or their spouse/life partner have with commercial interest related to the content of this CME activity:
Robert Alan Bonakdar, MD, FAAFP, FACN is a consultant/advisor for American Specialty Health Incorporated; Thorne Research Inc; and Metagenics, Inc, and receives royalties/patents from Oxford University Press and Wolters Kluwer.
Jost Langhorst, MD is on the speakers' bureau for REPHA Gmbh Biologische Arzneimittel and Dr Falk Pharma UK Ltd, and has research support from REPHA Gmbh Biologische Arzneimittel; Dr Falk Pharma UK Ltd; Dr. Willmar Schwabe Pharmaceuticals; and TECHLAB, Inc.

UNAPPROVED/OFF-LABEL USE DISCLOSURE
The EOCME requires CME faculty to disclose to the participants:
1. When products or procedures being discussed are off-label, unlabelled, experimental, and/or investigational (not US Food and Drug Administration [FDA] approved); and
2. Any limitations on the information presented, such as data that are preliminary or that represent ongoing research, interim analyses, and/or unsupported opinions. Faculty may discuss information about pharmaceutical agents that is outside of FDA-approved labelling. This information is intended solely for CME and is not intended to promote off-label use of these medications. If you have any questions, contact the medical affairs department of the manufacturer for the most recent prescribing information.

TO ENROLL

To enroll in the *Medical Clinics of North America* Continuing Medical Education program, call customer service at 1-800-654-2452 or sign up online at http://www.theclinics.com/home/cme. The CME program is available to subscribers for an additional annual fee of USD $295.

METHOD OF PARTICIPATION

In order to claim credit, participants must complete the following:

1. Complete enrolment as indicated above.
2. Read the activity.
3. Complete the CME Test and Evaluation. Participants must achieve a score of 70% on the test. All CME Tests and Evaluations must be completed online.

CME INQUIRIES/SPECIAL NEEDS

For all CME inquiries or special needs, please contact elsevierCME@elsevier.com.

MEDICAL CLINICS OF NORTH AMERICA

Contributors

CONSULTING EDITOR

BIMAL H. ASHAR, MD, MBA, FACP
Associate Professor of Medicine, Division of General Internal Medicine, The Johns Hopkins University School of Medicine, Baltimore, Maryland, USA

EDITOR

ROBERT B. SAPER, MD, MPH
Chair, Academic Consortium for Integrative Medicine & Health, McLean, Virginia, USA; Associate Professor, Department of Family Medicine, Director of Integrative Medicine, Boston Medical Center, Boston University School of Medicine, Boston, Massachusetts, USA

AUTHORS

BROOKE AGGARWAL, EdD, MS
Associate Research Scientist, Division of Cardiology, Department of Medicine, Columbia University Medical Center, New York, New York, USA

MONICA AGGARWAL, MD
Assistant Professor, Division of Cardiology, University of Florida, Gainesville, Florida, USA

GARY N. ASHER, MD, MPH
Associate Professor, Department of Family Medicine, The University of North Carolina at Chapel Hill, Chapel Hill, North Carolina, USA

VANESSA BAUTE, MD
Department of Neurology, Wake Forest Baptist Health, Winston-Salem, North Carolina, USA

SUZANNE M. BERTISCH, MD, MPH
Physician, Division of Pulmonary, Critical Care, and Sleep Medicine, Instructor, Medicine, Beth Israel Deaconess Medical Center, Harvard Medical School, Boston, Massachusetts, USA

ROBERT ALAN BONAKDAR, MD, FAAFP, FACN
Director of Pain Management, Scripps Center for Integrative Medicine, La Jolla, California, USA

STEPHANIE CHENG, MD
Assistant Professor of Clinical Medicine, Division of Geriatrics, Department of Medicine, University of California San Francisco, San Francisco, California, USA

DELIA CHIARAMONTE, MD
Assistant Professor, Departments of Family and Community Medicine and Epidemiology and Public Health, Associate Director and Director of Education, Center for Integrative Medicine, University of Maryland School of Medicine, Baltimore, Maryland, USA

LORENZO COHEN, PhD
Professor, Chief, Section of Integrative Medicine, Director, Integrative Medicine Program, Department of Palliative, Rehabilitation and Integrative Medicine, The University of Texas MD Anderson Cancer Center, Houston, Texas, USA

SHARON DEMOCKER, MD
Medical Director, War Related Illness and Injury Study Center, VA Medical Center, Washington, DC, USA

PAULA GARDINER, MD, MPH
Associate Professor, Department of Family Medicine, Boston Medical Center, Boston University School of Medicine, Boston, Massachusetts, USA

BRADLEY N. GAYNES, MD, MPH
Professor, Department of Psychiatry, The University of North Carolina at Chapel Hill, Chapel Hill, North Carolina, USA

KATHERINE A. GERGEN BARNETT, MD
Vice Chair of Primary Care Innovation and Transformation, Department of Family Medicine, Boston Medical Center, Boston, Massachusetts, USA

JONATHAN GERKIN, MD
Associate Professor, Department of Psychiatry, The University of North Carolina at Chapel Hill, Chapel Hill, North Carolina, USA

RANDY HORWITZ, MD, PhD
Medical Director, Arizona Center for Integrative Medicine, Associate Professor of Medicine, University of Arizona College of Medicine – Tucson, Tucson, Arizona, USA

ANNA K. KOCH, MSc(Psych)
Department of Integrative Gastroenterology, Alfried Krupp von Bohlen und Halbach-Stiftungsprofessur für Naturheilkunde Klinik für Naturheilkunde und Integrative Medizin, Kliniken Essen-Mitte, Knappschafts-Krankenhaus, Faculty of Medicine, University of Duisburg-Essen, Essen, Germany

MIKHAIL KOGAN, MD
Medical Director, Center for Integrative Medicine, Assistant Professor, Department of Medicine, Division of Geriatrics and Palliative Care Medicine, Associate Director, Geriatric and Integrative Medicine Fellowships, George Washington University, School of Medicine & Health Sciences, Washington, DC, USA

MARIATU KOROMA NELSON, MD
Medical Director of Goodwin House, Lead Physician, Geriatric Medicine, Virginia Hospital Center, Arlington, Virginia, USA

JOSHUA KORZENIK, MD
Division of Gastroenterology, Hepatology, and Endoscopy, Department of Medicine, Brigham and Women's Hospital, Harvard Medical School, Boston, Massachusetts, USA

JOST LANGHORST, MD
Department of Integrative Gastroenterology, Alfried Krupp von Bohlen und Halbach-Stiftungsprofessur für Naturheilkunde Klinik für Naturheilkunde und Integrative Medizin, Knappschafts-Krankenhaus, Department of Internal and Integrative Medicine, Kliniken Essen-Mitte, Faculty of Medicine, University of Duisburg-Essen, Essen, Germany

AMY B. LOCKE, MD, FAAFP
Associate Professor, Co-Director Resiliency Center, Office of Wellness and Integrative Health, Department of Family and Preventive Medicine, The University of Utah, Salt Lake City, Utah, USA

GABRIEL LOPEZ, MD
Assistant Professor, Section of Integrative Medicine, Department of Palliative, Rehabilitation and Integrative Medicine, Clinical Medical Director, Integrative Medicine Center, The University of Texas MD Anderson Cancer Center, Houston, Texas, USA

JUN J. MAO, MD, MSCE
Chief, Integrative Medicine Service, Memorial Sloan Kettering Cancer Center, New York, New York, USA

JYOTHI RAO, MD, FAARFM
Clinician, Shakthi Health and Wellness Center, Mt Airy, Maryland, USA

SEEMA RAO, MD
Geriatrician and Integrative Medicine Physician, San Diego, California, USA

MELINDA RING, MD
Executive Director, Osher Center for Integrative Medicine at Northwestern University, Drs. Pat and Carl Greer Distinguished Physician in Integrative Medicine, Clinical Associate Professor of Medicine and Medical Social Sciences, Northwestern University Feinberg School of Medicine, Chicago, Illinois, USA

HELANÉ WAHBEH, ND, MCR
Department of Neurology, Oregon Health & Science University, Portland, Oregon, USA

REBECCA ERWIN WELLS, MD, MPH, FAHS
Department of Neurology, Wake Forest Baptist Health, Winston-Salem, North Carolina, USA

GLORIA Y. YEH, MD, MPH
Associate Professor of Medicine; Division of General Medicine and Primary Care, Beth Israel Deaconess Medical Center, Harvard Medical School, Boston, Massachusetts, USA

ERIC S. ZHOU, PhD
Staff Psychologist, Department of Pediatric Oncology, Dana-Farber Cancer Institute, Boston, Massachusetts, USA

Contents

behavior modification and the use of complementary health therapies as part of conventional cancer care. Integrative approaches can provide patients relief from cancer and cancer treatment–related symptoms, leading to improvements in their physical and psychosocial health. An evidence-informed approach is important when recommending an integrative cancer plan. Efforts at enhancing communication between patients and health care providers, as well as between integrative practitioners and conventional health care teams, are critical to achieving optimal health and healing for patients with cancer.

Chronic pain is one of the most common conditions seen in the clinic, and it is often one of the most frustrating for both clinicians and patients. This condition stems from common comorbidities, including depression, insomnia, fatigue, and physical deconditioning, which often create barriers to recovery. In addition, chronic pain has had divergent approaches for treatment, including an overemphasis on analgesia and curative treatments while underemphasizing the biopsychosocial needs of those in pain. This article attempts to provide an initial framework for approaching those in pain and initiating patient-centered options to support improvements in pain, function, and self-care.

More than 80% of people in the United States who are older than 65 years have 1 or more chronic medical problems, and 50% have 2 or more. The cost of care for the elderly is at least 3 to 4 times that of younger populations and is rapidly growing, mostly because of a lack of preventive approaches and overly medicalized and fragmented care. This article summarizes the most up-to-date evidence for specific integrative modalities for common geriatric conditions, including falls, frailty, osteoporosis, and end-of-life palliative care.

In today's health care system where there are increased demands for health care provider productivity, increased pay for performance metrics, decreased reimbursements, and ever-increasing demands of electronic medical records, providers are at risk for high rates of burnout. Indeed, recent studies have indicated that more than 50% of US physicians are now experiencing burnout and that burnout is rising dramatically faster among physicians than in any other US professional field. These high rates of burnout have many downstream consequences, for both the providers and for the patients they serve.

Foreword

Enhancing the Doctor-Patient Relationship

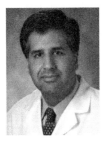

Bimal H. Ashar, MD, MBA, FACP
Consulting Editor

Over the past three decades, the use of healing modalities outside the realm of western allopathic medicine has increased dramatically. An estimated 30% to 40% of Americans use some form of complementary or alternative medicine. This use results in over $30 billion in out-of-pocket expenditures yearly. The term "integrative medicine" has recently evolved to emphasize that synergy may exist between allopathic practices and nontraditional medicine that has the potential to enhance patient care.

But why did patients look to alternatives to western medicine in the first place? There are likely a multitude of reasons. Remarkable advances in allopathic medicine over the last century have saved and extended numerous lives. Yet, many patients are afflicted by ailments for which there are limited options. To search for alternatives would be an anticipated response. In addition, we suffer from a dearth of medications designed for disease prevention. Complementary and integrative medicine may offer patients a potentially natural choice (whether proven or unproven) that allows them to try to take control of their own health.

Despite the high prevalence of complementary and integrative medicine use, most patients do not disclose such use to their providers. This may be due to the fact that patients feel that their physicians would not understand or that their physician would look down upon them. The truth is that most forms of integrative therapies are not taught in any depth in medical school, resulting in a knowledge gap for most providers. In this issue, Dr Saper has brought together experts from numerous specialties to help fill some of that gap. The goal for most providers will not be to blindly adopt all complementary and integrative therapies, but to be able to engage their patients in

Med Clin N Am 101 (2017) xv–xvi
http://dx.doi.org/10.1016/j.mcna.2017.07.003
0025-7125/17/© 2017 Published by Elsevier Inc.

medical.theclinics.com

meaningful discussions of the risks and benefits of any modality. Such engagement will likely strengthen the provider-patient relationship.

Bimal H. Ashar, MD, MBA, FACP
Division of General Internal Medicine
Johns Hopkins University School of Medicine
601 North Caroline Street
#7143
Baltimore, MD 21287, USA

E-mail address:
Bashar1@jhmi.edu

Preface

Integrative Medicine and Health

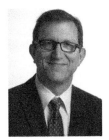

Robert B. Saper, MD, MPH
Editor

Integrative medicine and health (IMH) "reaffirms the importance of the relationship between practitioner and patient, focuses on the whole person, is informed by evidence, and makes use of all appropriate therapeutic and lifestyle approaches, healthcare professionals and disciplines to achieve optimal health and healing."[1] IMH is not a new specialty; it is a model of care that focuses on prevention and wellness and is particularly relevant given the current challenges facing US health care.

Despite spending 17% of gross domestic product on health care, the United States lags behind most western countries in many indicators of health status.[2] One reason is the morbidity, disability, cost, and mortality associated with chronic illnesses such as pain, depression, obesity, and cardiovascular disease. Simple cures for these conditions are unfortunately few and far between. Care is often fragmented, hard to access, and challenging to navigate. Patient experience, an increasingly important metric for hospitals and providers, often suffers. As health professionals try their best to care for these complex patients, burnout is common as pressures increase to see more patients in less time, to generate more revenue, and to comply with mounting administrative, regulatory, and documentation burdens.

IMH can help address these challenges. Many chronic illnesses are caused or exacerbated by poor nutrition, sedentariness, excessive stress, inadequate sleep, tobacco, alcohol, and substance use. IMH helps patients with chronic conditions adopt lifestyle behaviors such as healthy eating, physical activity, stress management, improved sleep habits, smoking cessation, and reduction in alcohol and substance use. IMH also incorporates a range of therapies that are relatively safe, effective, and inexpensive for reducing symptoms. Examples include acupuncture and yoga for low back pain (see Robert Alan Bonakdar's article, "Integrative Pain Management," in this issue), mindfulness-based stress reduction for depression (see Gary N. Asher and colleagues' article, "Complementary Therapies for Mental Health Disorders," in this issue), and lifestyle modification for heart disease (see Monica Aggarwal and colleagues' article,

Med Clin N Am 101 (2017) xvii–xviii
http://dx.doi.org/10.1016/j.mcna.2017.07.002
0025-7125/17/© 2017 Published by Elsevier Inc.

"Integrative Medicine for Cardiovascular Disease and Prevention," in this issue). IMH's whole person approach–understanding and addressing how illness impacts physical, emotional, social, and spiritual well-being–improves the patient experience.[3] IMH emphasizes the therapeutic importance of a trusting collaborative relationship between a team of health professionals, the patient, family, and caregivers. The value of these continuous healing relationships to quality health care is well established.[4] Last, being part of a collaborative interprofessional team providing IMH care can help bring meaning and purpose back to one's work, thus enhancing the "joy of practice" and countering burnout (see Katherine A. Gergen Barnett's article, "In Pursuit of the Fourth Aim in Health Care: The Joy of Practice," in this issue).

This special issue of *Medical Clinics of North America* reviews the current state of evidence for an IMH approach to many of the common problems and populations encountered by internists and family physicians. Many of the authors are affiliated with the Academic Consortium for Integrative Medicine and Health, comprising over 70 academic health centers and health systems committed to disseminating rigorous scientific research, curricula, and clinical care models.

The goals of the IMH approach are consistent with the "quadruple" aim: improved health outcomes, patient satisfaction, decreased costs, and provider well-being (see Katherine A. Gergen Barnett's article, "In Pursuit of the Fourth Aim in Health Care: The Joy of Practice," in this issue). Ultimately, as IMH research and clinical models mature and are increasingly incorporated into health care, medicine will become more patient-centered, relationship-centered, and interprofessional. Health care systems will successfully integrate lifestyle modification with medication, self-care with surgery, high tech with high touch, and curing with healing. When this occurs, hopefully the term "integrative" will be superfluous and no longer be necessary.

Robert B. Saper, MD, MPH
Chair, Academic Consortium for Integrative Medicine and Health
6728 Old McLean Village Drive
McLean, VA 22101, USA

E-mail address:
Robert.Saper@bmc.org

REFERENCES

1. Academic Consortium for Integrative Medicine and Health. Available at: http://imconsortium.org/about/about-us.cfm. Accessed June 27, 2017.
2. Osborn R, Squires D, Doty M, et al. In new survey of eleven countries, US adults still struggle with access to and affordability of health care. Health Aff (Millwood) 2016;35(12):2327–36.
3. Lis C, Rodeghier M, Gupta D. The relationship between perceived service quality and patient willingness to recommend at a national oncology hospital network. BMC Health Serv Res 2011;11:46. Available at: http://www.biomedcentral.com/1472-6963/11/46.
4. Committee on Quality Health Care in America, Institute of Medicine. Crossing the quality chiasm: a new health system for the 21st century. Washington, DC: National Academy of Sciences; 2001.

Complementary Therapies for Mental Health Disorders

Gary N. Asher, MD, MPH[a],*, Jonathan Gerkin, MD[b],
Bradley N. Gaynes, MD, MPH[b]

KEYWORDS

- Complementary medicine • Depression • Anxiety • Posttraumatic stress disorder
- Dietary supplements • Mind–body interventions

KEY POINTS

- Bright light therapy is a reasonable treatment as monotherapy or augmentation for major depressive disorder (MDD) and is well-established for seasonal depression.
- Mindfulness meditation may be considered for first or second-line treatment of MDD, especially in patients with mild to moderate depression.
- Kava, passion flower, and German chamomile can be considered for short-term, adjunctive treatment of generalized anxiety disorder (GAD).
- Mindfulness- and acceptance-based interventions may be beneficial for GAD in patients interested in these therapies.
- Acupuncture and mindfulness meditation may be beneficial as adjunctive treatments to conventional therapy for patients with posttraumatic stress disorder.

INTRODUCTION

In 2014, there were an estimated 43 million US adults with mental illness, which represents about 18% of the US adult population. Nearly one-half of those have serious mental illness, defined as a substantial functional impairment that limits at least 1 major life activity. In contrast, in the same year only 13% of US adults with mental illness received treatment, and only one-half of those with serious mental illness received any treatment.[1]

Although efficacy is well-established for many mental health interventions, treatment discontinuation of pharmacologic agents is not uncommon, especially owing

Disclosure Statement: The authors have nothing to disclose.
[a] Department of Family Medicine, University of North Carolina, 590 Manning Drive, CB# 7595, Chapel Hill, NC 27599-7595, USA; [b] Department of Psychiatry, University of North Carolina, 101 Manning Drive, Chapel Hill, NC 27759, USA
* Corresponding author.
E-mail address: gasher@med.unc.edu

Med Clin N Am 101 (2017) 847–864
http://dx.doi.org/10.1016/j.mcna.2017.04.004
0025-7125/17/© 2017 Elsevier Inc. All rights reserved.

to side effects. For example, about 60% of patients on second-generation antidepressants (eg, selective serotonin reuptake inhibitors [SSRIs]) experience adverse events, and between 7% and 15% of patients discontinue treatment because of adverse events.[2] Concerns about the "addictiveness" of antidepressants are also a common reason for patients' skepticism about prescription medications[3,4]; women and ethnic minorities, in particular, often prefer nonpharmacologic treatment options as first step therapies for depression.[5,6] Antidepressants also have a substantially higher treatment-specific stigma than, for example, dietary supplements.[7] Finally, many patients may have either poor access to or bias against psychological interventions.

Skepticism toward pharmacologic and psychological mental health treatments reflects a general trend toward "natural treatments" throughout medicine. In 2012, an estimated 59 million persons in the United States spent a combined $30.2 billion in out-of-pocket expenses on some type of complementary health approach.[8] Among self-reported uses of complementary therapies, stress reduction and improvements in emotional health and coping are commonly self-reported benefits.[9] Among those with self-reported anxiety or depressive disorders, estimates are as high as 50% who may be using a complementary therapy, most of whom may also be receiving conventional treatments.[10] Given the highly prevalent use of complementary therapies for mental health conditions, it is essential for health care providers to better understand the potential benefits and harms of these treatments.

We review the evidence for complementary therapies for treatment of major depressive disorder (MDD), generalized anxiety disorder (GAD), and posttraumatic stress disorder (PTSD). Complementary therapies are defined broadly as treatments that are not commonly taught or practiced in conventional medical settings. Although not comprehensive, each section reviews evidence for commonly used complementary therapies with reasonable likelihood of efficacy for each condition.

DEPRESSION

According to estimates from the World Health Organization, more than 350 million people worldwide suffer from depression, making it the second leading cause of disability throughout the world.[11] MDD[12] is defined as the presence of depressed mood and/or loss of interest or pleasure, along with at least 4 additional MDD diagnosis criteria or symptoms lasting at least 2 weeks. MDD is the most prevalent and disabling form of depression, affecting more than 16% of US adults at some time in their life.[13] MDD also exerts a negative impact on physical health[14–17] and adherence to medical treatment.[18]

Although second-generation antidepressants are the most common first-step treatments for acute MDD and recommended by most evidence-based guidelines,[19,20] patients with depression may choose nonpharmacologic options. A recent review of the prevalence of complementary therapy use in sufferers of depressive disorders indicates use ranging from 10% to 30%.[21] Many nonpharmacologic treatments are offered by practitioners or used by patients, independent of the strength of their evidence base. The Cochrane Depression and Neurosis Group lists 87 psychological interventions,[22] and a comprehensive summary of an Australian patient advocacy group cataloged 56 complementary therapies for the treatment of depression.[23] Commonly used complementary therapies include herbal remedies (eg, St. John's wort, Chinese herbal formulations), nonherbal supplements (eg, omega-3 fatty acids, S-adenosyl-L-methionine [SAMe]), acupuncture, yoga, or meditation. In addition, other treatment options such as physical exercise or light therapy have been used to treat depression.

For clinicians, a great challenge is to balance patient interest in the plethora of alternatives to pharmacologic interventions with the professional responsibility to choose treatments that are supported by scientific evidence. **Table 1** summarizes the evidence for select complementary therapies commonly used by depressed individuals in primary care.[24] For acupuncture, which is commonly used, 2 systematic reviews concluded there was insufficient evidence available to address its benefits and harms for treatment of depression, so it is not included in **Table 1**.[25,26]

Effective

Light therapy
Light therapy, also known as phototherapy, involves daily exposure to bright light and is typically administered at home with a fluorescent light box. Usually, light boxes filter out ultraviolet rays and require 20 to 60 minutes of exposure to 10,000 lux (light intensity) of cool-white fluorescent light, an amount that is about 20 times greater than ordinary indoor lighting.[27] The standard protocol is 10,000 lux for 30 minutes per day during the early morning for up to 6 weeks, with response usually seen within 1 to 3 weeks.[28] Most research has studied light therapy as an intervention for MDD with a seasonal pattern, also known as seasonal affective disorder. However, research has also assessed its use in non–seasonal MDD relative to inactive controls.[29] A recent systematic review by the Canadian Network for Mood and Anxiety Treatments

---

Table 1
Complementary therapies for MDD

Intervention	Recommendation	Comment
Light therapy	Effective as monotherapy or adjunctive therapy	Evidence base stronger for seasonal affective disorder than nonseasonal affective disorder.
Meditation (eg, MBCT)	Likely effective as monotherapy or adjunctive therapy	Evidence base stronger for preventing relapse or recurrence than for acute phase treatment.
Omega-3 fatty acids	Possibly effective as monotherapy or adjunctive therapy	Stronger evidence base for mild to moderate depression than for moderate to severe; high quality evidence is limited.
SAMe	Possibly effective as an adjunctive treatment	High-quality data are absent.
St. John's wort	Possibly effective as monotherapy for mild-to-moderate MDD and as adjunctive treatment for moderate-to-severe MDD	Stronger evidence for use in mild-to-moderate depression; studies comparing St. John's wort with inadequate antidepressant dosing limit conclusions for severe depression. Likely interactions with drugs metabolized by cytochrome P450 3A4.
Yoga	Possibly effective as an adjunctive therapy	Low methodological quality of data; most randomized, controlled trials rated as high risk of bias. Evidence stronger for mild-to-moderate MDD.

Abbreviations: MBCT, mindfulness based cognitive therapy; MDD, major depressive disorder; SAMe, S-adenosyl methionine.

(CANMAT) found 2 metaanalyses, 4 systematic reviews, and 3 additional randomized, controlled trials (RCTs) supporting light therapy's benefit for seasonal affective disorder, with data also emerging for its use as a treatment for non–seasonal affective disorder.[30] These benefits are apparent whether used as a monotherapy or an adjunctive therapy. Of note, nearly all of the trials compare light therapy with inactive placebo or sham control; little information exists about its comparative effectiveness to other established treatments for non–seasonal MDD.

Light therapy is well-tolerated. Common side effects reported include eye strain, headache, agitation, nausea, sedation, and very rarely hypomania or mania.[31] Recent comparative effectiveness research suggests light therapy and cognitive–behavioral therapy (CBT) seem to be equivalent in benefit for seasonal affective disorder in the acute treatment phase. However, CBT may be superior after 2 years.[32]

CANMAT guidelines recommend light therapy as a first-line treatment for seasonal affective disorder and a second-line treatment for mild to moderate non–seasonal MDD.[30] These recommendations are consistent with the American Psychiatric Association Task Force Report on Complementary and Alternative Medicine in MDD.[33] Bright light therapy is a reasonable treatment for MDD, as either a monotherapy or augmentation strategy, with particularly well-established benefit in seasonal MDD.

Likely Effective

Meditation or mindfulness

Meditation includes a heterogeneous group of techniques that involve training the mind through regulation of attention to affect physiologic function and state of mind. A recent review of mindfulness meditation indicated the most commonly studied form for depression is mindfulness-based cognitive therapy (MBCT). MBCT has been studied as both monotherapy and augmentation therapy, with the bulk of data addressing prevention of relapse or recurrence of a depressive episode (also known as maintenance treatment).[34] For acute phase adjunctive treatment, a metaanalysis of add-on MBCT showed a significant decrease in depression severity relative to inactive controls.[35] No acute phase monotherapy data were identified. CANMAT has identified MBCT as a second-line intervention for the acute phase treatment of MDD.[36]

For maintenance treatment focused on preventing relapse or recurrence, the data indicating benefit are stronger. A systematic review and metaanalysis considering trials in which MBCT could be monotherapy or an adjunctive treatment found that the average risk of developing a new episode of depression by 12 months was reduced by 21% compared with controls.[37] Two additional trials, comparing monotherapy MBCT with monotherapy antidepressants,[38,39] and 1 comparing MBCT with CBT,[40] showed equivalent benefit in reducing the risk of relapse or recurrence. Side effects of MBCT are not often reported but are likely minimal.

CANMAT guidelines have identified MBCT as a second-line intervention for the acute phase treatment of MDD, and have listed it as a first-line treatment for preventing relapse or recurrence of an episode.[36] It can be used either as monotherapy or adjunctive therapy. MBCT is an option that can be viewed as similar to a psychotherapy selection, but one that has stronger data supporting its role in preventing return of a depressive episode. Access to practitioners may be a limiting factor.

Possibly Effective

St. John's wort

Extracts of St. John's wort (*Hypericum perforatum*) have been used for centuries to treat various conditions, including depressive disorders. A Cochrane review of St. John's wort for depression documented available research studies published to

2008 and found a beneficial effect compared with both placebo and other antidepressant therapies across 29 double-blind RCTs.[41] The review concluded that the *Hypericum* extracts tested in the included trials (a) are superior to placebo in patients with major depression, (b) are similarly effective as standard antidepressants, (c) and have fewer side effects than standard antidepressants. The association of country of origin and precision with effects sizes complicates the interpretation.

A recent review analyzed 12 trials comparing second-generation antidepressants with St. John's wort from a variety of commercially available standardized extracts with dosages ranging from 300 to 1800 mg/d.[25] A metaanalysis of 9 of those trials (predominantly with severe depression) indicated similar response rates for patients treated with second-generation antidepressants or St. John's wort (52% vs 54%) after 6 to 12 weeks of treatment. A metaanalysis of 5 trials demonstrated no difference in remission rates between antidepressants and St. John's wort (30% vs 36%, respectively). Of note, all trials compared St. John's wort with moderate- or low-dose second-generation antidepressant regimens, but did not fully use the approved range of antidepressant doses. In addition, the authors noted that expectancy (what patients expected from the treatments) may play a greater role in complementary therapy studies conducted in countries where the treatment is commonly accepted, such as St. John's wort in Germany. This concern was also reflected in a reanalysis of the major US Hypericum Depression Trial showing participants' beliefs about treatment assignment were more strongly associated with clinical outcomes than the actual treatment received.[42]

Existing clinical practice guidelines vary in their recommendations to include St. John's wort as an option for treating depressive disorders.[30,43] CANMAT recommends it as first-line monotherapy in mild to moderate MDD and as a second-line adjunctive treatment for moderate to severe MDD.[30] The American College of Physicians, however, concludes that there is insufficient evidence about the applicability of studies of St. John's wort to patients in the United States, especially about the purity and potency of St. John's wort preparations available in this country.[43] US studies have not been able to replicate the positive findings found elsewhere. Another key consideration is the risk of drug–herb interactions. St. John's wort should not be recommended to patients taking any pharmaceutical medications without the advice of a medical provider or pharmacist with expertise in evaluating herb–drug interactions. It is well-documented that the extract is a strong inducer of CYP3A4, which can affect the metabolism of many drugs.[44] Accordingly, for patients with mild-to-moderate MDD who are interested in trying St. John's wort, appreciate the limitations of the current evidence base, and are not at risk for drug–herb interactions, it may be a reasonable option.

S-adenosyl-L-methionine

SAMe is a naturally occurring compound that may enhance the activity of the monoamine systems (involving norepinephrine and serotonin neurotransmitters) that are strongly associated with the etiology and treatment of depression. It has been marketed in some European countries since the mid-1980s for the treatment of depression. In the United States and Canada, SAMe is available as an over-the-counter dietary supplement, often used in the dose range of 800 to 1600 mg/d given in divided doses with meals over 4 to 12 weeks.[45] Studies have also used intravenous and intramuscular formulations of SAMe (200–400 mg/d across 2–8 weeks), which may be more effective than oral supplements.[46] SAMe seems to be relatively well-tolerated, with the most common side effects reported as gastrointestinal distress, insomnia, sweating, headache, irritability, restlessness, anxiety, tachycardia, and fatigue.[30]

A recent Cochrane systematic review considered its use in acute treatment as both a monotherapy and augmenting therapy; the review identified 8 trials comparing SAMe with either placebo or an antidepressant.[47] As monotherapy, very low-quality evidence suggests no effect on depressive symptoms compared with placebo, imipramine, or escitalopram. As an augmentation strategy to an SSRI, there was low-quality evidence that SAMe is superior to placebo. These findings mirrored those found in a comparative effectiveness systematic review comparing complementary medicine interventions to second generation antidepressants.[25] In these 2 reviews, secondary outcomes of response and remission rates were consistent with findings for change in depressive symptom severity. Both reviews highlighted the absence of high-quality evidence and the inability to draw firm conclusions based on the available data. CANMAT guidelines recommend SAMe as a second-line adjunctive treatment for use in mild to moderate MDD.[30] Its benefit as a monotherapy remains unclear. We agree with its use as a second-line agent.

Omega-3 fatty acids

Omega-3 fatty acids (also known as n-3 polyunsaturated fatty acids) are naturally found in fatty fish, some other seafood, and assorted nuts and seeds. They are important in brain development and have been associated with depression in a number of observational studies.[48,49] A recent Cochrane review[50] identified 25 RCTs for depression comparing omega-3 fatty acids to placebo. Omega-3 fatty acids could be administered either as the sole treatment or as adjunctive therapy. For the placebo comparison, there was very low-quality evidence that omega-3 fatty acid supplementation results in a small benefit for depressive symptoms, unlikely to be clinically meaningful. One small, low-quality study was identified comparing omega-3 fatty acid supplementation to an antidepressant with no differences found. Whether supplementation was monotherapy or adjunctive did not affect findings. The data suggested that the eicosapentaenoic acid or ethyl-eicosapentaenoic acid component of the formulation used was more likely to be associated with benefit, a finding consistent with other reviews.[51]

The Cochrane review concluded that there was not sufficient high-quality evidence to determine the effects of omega-3 fatty acid supplementation as a treatment for MDD. CANMAT, noting inconsistency in the evidence, recommends omega-3 fatty acid supplements as second-line monotherapy for mild to moderate MDD and as second-line adjunctive therapy to antidepressants for moderate to severe MDD. From our review of the evidence and clinical experience, omega-3 fatty acid supplements are at best a second-line adjunctive therapy for patients who have failed prior treatments and indicate a clear interest in trying this augmentation strategy.

Omega-3 fatty acid supplements are relatively well-tolerated with only mild side effects, primarily gastrointestinal (diarrhea, nausea, and a fishy aftertaste).[30] However, some concern exists over their potential to cause bleeding, especially in patients on concurrent antiplatelet or anticoagulant agents, especially if used above recommended doses of 2 to 3 g/d. Patients are strongly encouraged to discontinue omega-3 fatty acid supplements at least 1 week before surgery or major procedures.

Yoga

Yoga is a group of practices that originated in ancient India. In the West, yoga is often practiced as a series of movements and physical poses designed to focus the mind and stretch the body, often involving breathing exercises. Less common yoga practices include chanting and sitting meditation. The duration of yoga interventions in depression studies varies, ranging from 2 to 4 sessions a week over a 2- to 3-month period.[52] The evidence base is relatively limited. A recent metaanalysis of available RCTs (12 trials) reported moderate evidence for short-term medium-sized beneficial effects for yoga compared with usual care, but limited benefit compared with relaxation (eg, breathing techniques or progressive muscle relaxation alone) or aerobic exercise.[52] A comparative effectiveness review involving yoga and second generation antidepressants found insufficient evidence to reach a conclusion about their relative benefits and adverse effects.[25]

Side effects, although more rigorously evaluated in recent studies, have been infrequently reported in studies of yoga for depression, with the exception of fatigue and breathlessness in 1 study that seemed to be related to level of participant fitness.[53] However, there is an ongoing discussion over potential physical injuries owing to yoga, which may be underreported.

Noted limitations of yoga studies include the low quality of RCTs, variability in practice parameters and physical/mental health of participants, difficulties with suitable control conditions, and lack of long-term follow-up data.

CANMAT recommends yoga as a second-line adjunctive therapy in mild to moderate MDD.[30] Although the low methodological quality of available data limits how we can interpret the results and safety of yoga, it could be considered an ancillary treatment option for patients with depressive disorders.

ANXIETY

Anxiety disorders share features of excessive fear and worry. Related avoidance behavior can become a pervasive coping strategy. The key features of GAD are persistent and excessive worry as well as physical symptoms, such as muscle tension, fatigue, and restlessness. Common comorbidities include mood, substance, and personality disorders. Preexisting anxiety disorder is an independent risk factor for subsequent onset of suicidal ideation and attempts. Moreover, research demonstrates that comorbid anxiety disorders amplify the risk of suicide attempts in persons with mood disorders.[54]

The 12-month prevalence for GAD among US adults is 2.9%.[55] Importantly, 5% to 8% of primary care visits are estimated to be associated with GAD. In addition to impairments in mental health, patients with GAD often experience chronic pain, impaired physical function, and difficulty with activities of daily life. Together this accelerates the need to reconsider the management of this disorder and expand upon the traditional medical model to a more integrative approach, focusing on self-care.[56]

Treatments for anxiety, and more specifically GAD, include both psychotherapy and pharmacotherapy. Among psychotherapies, CBT has the greatest amount of evidence for the treatment of GAD.[57,58] Evidence-based pharmacotherapies for GAD include the SSRI, selective norepinephrine reuptake inhibitor, and tricyclic antidepressant medications.[59] However, as with pharmacotherapies for other psychiatric illnesses, treatment discontinuation owing to side effects often limits their effectiveness. Additionally, despite effective therapies, persistent residual symptoms in treatment responders is a problem, highlighting the need for new approaches.

Complementary therapies are commonly used by patients diagnosed with anxiety disorders. A 2012 survey found that compared with the general population, herbal therapy use in the past 12 months by those diagnosed with GAD was nearly 4 times more likely (12.7% vs 3.4%).[60] Based on a 2012 survey in a large sample of anxiety patients in US primary care settings, 43% endorsed complementary therapy use, including 21% reporting natural product use.[61] The most commonly used complementary therapies for anxiety reported by patients include relaxation, meditation, imagery, botanicals, yoga, acupuncture, massage, and spiritual healing.[61] For many of these, there is insufficient evidence to make a strong recommendation for or against their use in the treatment of GAD or anxiety symptoms. However, a few interventions are supported by at least 1 or more RCTs and are considered possibly effective (**Table 2**).

Possibly Effective

Kava
Piper methysticum is a plant that is native to western Pacific Islands, where it traditionally has been consumed as a beverage both for social and medicinal uses.[62] In Western countries, it is widely available in capsule and liquid extract formulas. In 2005, approximately 1% of the US adult population reported using kava for their own health.[63] Numerous studies and subsequent reviews, including a Cochrane review, support short-term use of kava for patients with mild to moderate anxiety disorders. However, a few reports of liver toxicity exist. Therefore, caution is advised for patients with liver disease or those taking medications metabolized by the liver.[64] Short-term kava use for anxiety may possibly be effective and is reasonable with appropriate monitoring of liver function.

Passion flower
Passiflora incarnata was used as a calming or sedating agent in 16th century Peru. More recently, oral formulations have been studied for treatment of anxiety. A 2007 Cochrane review reported 2 RCTs, totaling 198 participants, comparing passion flower extract with a benzodiazepine. In both studies, no differences between groups were found. However, the reviewers concluded there were too few RCTs to draw conclusions and that comparative trials with larger samples are needed.[65] Passion flower may possibly be effective for short-term use. Because of its sedating effects, caution should be used when combining with additional sedating agents.[66]

German chamomile
Matricaria recutita is an herbal remedy widely used as a calming agent. Amsterdam and colleagues[67] have studied short- and long-term use of chamomile extract in

Table 2
Complementary therapies for general anxiety disorder

Intervention	Recommendation	Comment
Chamomile	Possibly effective as monotherapy	Stronger evidence for short term use, did not prevent relapse, only 2 trials
Kava	Possibly effective as monotherapy	Stronger evidence for short-term benefit, monitor liver function, avoid with other liver metabolized agents
Mindfulness- and acceptance-based interventions	Possibly effective as monotherapy or adjunctive therapy for mild-moderate severity	Trained practitioner provision is recommended rather than self-guided practices
Music therapy	Possibly effective as adjunctive therapy	Evidence difficult to apply to primary care setting
Passion flower	Possibly effective as monotherapy	Short-term use advised, avoid additional agents with sedating effects

capsule form for GAD. In an 8-week, double-blind RCT that included 57 participants, chamomile was found to have a modest effect on reducing anxiety (Hamilton Anxiety Rating Scale scores) compared with placebo. In a longer term trial, open-label chamomile was provided to 179 subjects for up to 12 weeks. Nearly 60% of the participants responded (GAD 7 and Clinical Global Impression-Severity scores), although 15.6% discontinued treatment.[68,69] Responders who remained well for an additional 4 weeks of treatment were randomized to either chamomile (n = 46) or placebo (n = 47) for the ensuing 26 weeks. Participants randomized to chamomile extract maintained significantly lower GAD symptoms compared with placebo. However, there were no differences in the number of participants experiencing relapse (15.2% vs 25.5%; $P = .15$). Adverse events were no different between the placebo and treatment groups. Based on these, trials it seems that chamomile extract, dosed at 500 mg 3 times daily, is likely safe and may provide benefit as an intervention for mild to moderate GAD.

Mindfulness- and acceptance-based interventions
Mindfulness is a practice of nonjudgmental, present moment awareness. Acceptance is an active and aware "embrace" of all private experiences without unnecessary attempts to change their frequency or form.[70] A metaanalysis of 8 RCTs evaluating mindfulness-based stress reduction and MBCT on anxiety symptom severity reported moderate benefits (Hedges g = −0.52, 95% CI, -1.11 to 0.06). However, removal of low-quality studies from the analysis considerably reduced the effect size (Hedges g = −0.17; 95% CI, -0.54 to 0.21). High heterogeneity and insufficient power further reduce the strength of these findings.[35] Another metaanalysis, which focused on 5 mindfulness- and acceptance-based RCTs, including Acceptance and Commitment Therapy, found a large overall effect size (Hedges g = 1.08) for reduction of anxiety symptoms.[71] It is known that discontinuation rates can be significant for mindfulness-based interventions, but safety does not seem to be a significant concern.[72] Mindfulness- and acceptance-based interventions provided by trained practitioners may be recommended as either adjunct or primary treatment of mild to moderate GAD and anxiety symptoms, especially for patients interested in these therapies.

Music therapy
Music therapy is an application of music in the treatment of disease or injury. Music therapy generally involves therapeutic intervention by a trained music therapist in addition to creating or listening to music alone, which can be referred to as music medicine. Several Cochrane reviews have reported on music therapy for anxiety in the following conditions: perioperative, cancer, coronary heart disease, and mechanically ventilated patients.[73–75] The strength of the evidence for anxiety outcomes in each of the reviews was low largely owing to a high risk of bias in the included studies. In general, reviewers felt that listening to music may have a beneficial effect on anxiety in these populations, and self-selecting preferred music may be an important contributor to the effect. Although it is reasonable to recommend music therapy as an adjunctive treatment for anxiety, the evidence reviewed here comes from acute medical settings and involves music therapists and is, therefore, limited in generalizability.

POSTTRAUMATIC STRESS DISORDER

Each year in the United States, approximately 3% to 4% of the adult population reports having PTSD.[76] PTSD is often chronic and debilitating, and is frequently associated with a variety of medical and psychiatric conditions, for example, depression, substance abuse, suicidality, and impaired social functioning. It is also associated with decreased quality of life and increased health services use.[77,78] Although PTSD is commonly associated with combat trauma, it can also be triggered by physical or sexual abuse, and other major trauma or life-threatening incidents, such as motor vehicle crashes or natural disasters. Hallmark features of PTSD include symptoms related to reexperiencing the traumatic event (eg, intrusive daytime thoughts, nightmares), avoidance, negative mood, and hyperarousal.[12]

When it occurs, PTSD typically develops within a few months of a traumatic event. However, approximately one-fourth of cases experience a delayed onset of at least 6 months.[79] Validated screening tools, such as the PTSD checklist or Clinician-Administered PTSD Scale, are available for clinicians who suspect the diagnosis. Formal diagnosis is made using *Diagnostic and Statistical Manual of Mental Disorders, fifth edition*, criteria and is often performed along with a full psychiatric assessment to identify suicidality and comorbid psychiatric and substance abuse disorders. Although it is not uncommon for individuals who experience a traumatic event to quickly develop symptoms of PTSD, most recover completely within 30 days of the event.

Treatments for PTSD include both psychotherapy and pharmacotherapy. Among psychotherapies, the strongest evidence supports trauma-based CBT, which includes cognitive reframing, exposure, coping skills training, and relaxation techniques such as controlled breathing and deep muscle relaxation.[80] About 55% to 65% of patients who undergo any psychotherapy no longer meet *Diagnostic and Statistical Manual of Mental Disorders* criteria for PTSD at treatment completion.[81] Because psychotherapies require specialized training and frequent provider contact, accessibility limits their use. Evidence-based pharmacotherapies include SSRIs and serotonin norepinephrine reuptake inhibitors. However, as with their use for other psychiatric illnesses, side effects and treatment discontinuation owing to side effects limit their effectiveness.[82] Additionally, their use as monotherapy is often insufficient to relieve symptoms.[83]

Complementary therapies are widely used by patients with PTSD. Recent use estimates in PTSD populations range from 26% to 39%.[60,84] Although the great demand for complementary therapies drives continued interest in these treatments, the limitations of current treatments for PTSD highlights the need to consider all potential treatments for this challenging condition. Most commonly used complementary therapies for PTSD include relaxation or meditation techniques (17.5%), exercise (16.0%), botanic therapies (13%), and massage (8.3%) (**Table 3**). Other complementary therapies for which there is some evidence to support their use includes acupuncture (3.5%) and guided imagery (3%).[84] However, the evidence supporting efficacy for many other therapies (eg, guided imagery, healing touch, massage, relaxation techniques, yoga) is either of low quality or insufficient to recommend for or against them. Although some natural products have been assessed for treatment and symptom management

Table 3 Complementary therapies for posttraumatic stress disorder (PTSD)		
Intervention	**Recommendation**	**Comment**
Acupuncture	Possibly effective as adjunctive treatment	Many studies with low to moderate methodological quality
Meditation or mindfulness	Possibly effective as adjunctive treatment for those interested in self-management	Small to moderate benefit based on studies with low methodological quality
Omega-3 fatty acids	Likely not effective	Based on a single randomized, controlled trial

of a variety of mental health disorders, no such studies have focused specifically on the PTSD population.

Possibly Effective

Acupuncture

Acupuncture is the practice of inserting needles into specific body points, usually organized along acupuncture meridians. Many traditional medical systems from China, Japan, and Korea incorporate acupuncture into multimodal treatment plans. In the West, acupuncture may be used often as a stand-alone therapy. A recent systematic review identified 6 clinical trials of acupuncture for treatment of PTSD.[85] One high-quality RCT concluded that acupuncture was superior to waitlist control and no different than CBT for treatment of PTSD symptoms and PTSD-related depression and anxiety. The other trials reported superiority of acupuncture compared with SSRIs, as well as acupuncture plus CBT compared with CBT alone. However, the methodological quality of these other trials was low to moderate. Because most of these trials were conducted in China, where acupuncture is commonly practiced, these results may not be generalizable to Western populations. Acupuncture may be considered in addition to guideline-recommended treatments in individuals interested in complementary therapies.

Meditation or mindfulness

Meditation includes a heterogeneous group of techniques that involve training the mind through regulation of attention to affect physiologic function and state of mind.[86] Commonly studied meditative techniques include mindfulness-based stress reduction and mantra meditation. Occasionally, some movement practices such as Tai Chi, qigong, and yoga are also considered meditative practices. To date, several narrative and systematic reviews have been conducted to evaluate the efficacy of meditative techniques for PTSD symptoms, quality of life, and adverse events.[87–92] More than 16 clinical trials have been identified. Although most trials in these reviews support a small to moderate benefit of meditation for PTSD symptoms and health-related quality of life, low methodological quality limits their overall strength of evidence. In the few studies that reported on adverse events, there did not seem to be any association with meditative techniques. Mindfulness-based stress reduction may be considered for adjunctive treatment to those interested in self-management to decrease PTSD symptoms and improve quality of life.[34]

Possibly Ineffective

Omega-3 fatty acids

One RCT assessed the efficacy of fish oil supplementation for PTSD prevention in disaster relief workers in Japan after the tsunami in March 2011.[93] The trial randomized 172 relief workers to either psychoeducation or psychoeducation plus 2240 mg fish oil daily. Workers were followed for 12 weeks, and PTSD symptoms were measured using a validated scale (Impact of Event Scale-Revised). No significant difference was seen between groups in Impact of Event Scale-Revised scores or adverse events. Therefore, use of omega-3 fatty acids is not recommended for prevention or treatment of PTSD.

SUMMARY

Mental health conditions such as MDD, GAD, and PTSD remain common among the US adult population. Treatment discontinuation of well-established therapies often occurs due to side effects of pharmacologic agents, and poor access and bias against

Table 4
Resources for complementary therapies and mental health

Resource	Website	Comments
Complementary therapy resources		
Natural Medicines	https://naturalmedicines.therapeuticresearch.com/	Dietary supplement database with interaction checker
NIH National Center for Complementary and Integrative Health (NCCIH)	https://nccih.nih.gov/	Evidence-based information on many complementary therapies
NIH Office of Dietary Supplements (ODS)	https://ods.od.nih.gov/	Fact sheets and information on many dietary supplements
Guideline organizations		
American College of Physicians (ACP)	https://www.acponline.org/clinical-information/guidelines	Guideline on nonpharmacological treatments for MDD
American Psychiatric Association	http://psychiatryonline.org/guidelines	Treatment guidelines for MDD, Panic disorder, and PTSD. Task force reports on complementary therapies and MDD
Canadian Network for Mood and Anxiety Treatments (CANMAT)	http://www.canmat.org/disorders.html	Clinical guideline for management of MDD & GAD – CAM supplement
National Alliance on Mental Illness (NAMI)	http://www.nami.org/Learn-More/Treatment/Complementary-Health-Approaches	Summary information on complementary therapies for mental health
National Center for PTSD	http://www.ptsd.va.gov/professional/treatment/overview/complementary_alternative_for_ptsd.asp	Complementary therapy information for PTSD treatment
National Guideline Clearinghouse	https://www.guideline.gov/	Summaries of evidence-based clinical practice guidelines
National Institute for Health and Care Excellence (NICE)	https://www.nice.org.uk/	Evidence-based treatment guidelines
US Department of Veterans Affairs	http://www.research.va.gov/topics/	Research and treatment information on mental health and complementary therapies
Systematic review resources		
Agency for Healthcare Research and Quality	http://www.ahrq.gov/research/findings/evidence-based-reports/index.html	Evidence-based reports
Cochrane Library	http://www.cochrane.org/	Searchable library of systematic evidence reviews

psychological interventions prevent wider uptake of these interventions. Several complementary therapies now have sufficiently high-quality evidence to consider their use: bright light and mindfulness meditation for depression; the botanicals kava, passionflower, and chamomile, in addition to mindfulness- and acceptance-based interventions, for anxiety; and acupuncture and mindfulness meditation for PTSD. Clinicians interested in further information on complementary therapies should look to one of a variety of reliable sources (**Table 4**). Given the highly prevalent use of complementary therapies for mental health complaints among patients, clinicians should become more aware of the benefits and harms of these therapies.

REFERENCES

1. Behavioral health trends in the United States: results from the 2014 National survey on drug use and health. Center for Behavioral Health Statistics and Quality; 2015.

2. Gartlehner G, Thieda P, Hansen RA, et al. Comparative risk for harms of second-generation antidepressants: a systematic review and meta-analysis. Drug Saf 2008;31(10):851–65.

3. Churchill R, Khaira M, Gretton V, et al. Treating depression in general practice: factors affecting patients' treatment preferences. Br J Gen Pract 2000;50(460): 905–6.

4. van Schaik DJF, Klijn AFJ, van Hout HPJ, et al. Patients' preferences in the treatment of depressive disorder in primary care. Gen Hosp Psychiatry 2004;26(3): 184–9.

5. Cooper LA, Gonzales JJ, Gallo JJ, et al. The acceptability of treatment for depression among African-American, Hispanic, and white primary care patients. Med Care 2003;41(4):479–89.

6. Givens JL, Houston TK, Van Voorhees BW, et al. Ethnicity and preferences for depression treatment. Gen Hosp Psychiatry 2007;29(3):182–91.

7. Givens JL, Katz IR, Bellamy S, et al. Stigma and the acceptability of depression treatments among African Americans and whites. J Gen Intern Med 2007;22(9): 1292–7.

8. Nahin RL, Barnes PM, Strussman BJ. Expenditures on complementary health approaches: United States, 2012. Atlanta (GA): National Health Statistics Reports; 2016. Number 95.

9. Stussman BJ, Black LI, Barnes PM, et al. Wellness-related use of common complementary health approaches among adults: United States, 2012. Natl Health Stat Rep 2015;(85):1–12.

10. Kessler RC, Soukup J, Davis RB, et al. The use of complementary and alternative therapies to treat anxiety and depression in the United States. Am J Psychiatry 2001;158(2):289–94.

11. Ferrari AJ, Charlson FJ, Norman RE, et al. Burden of depressive disorders by country, sex, age, and year: findings from the global burden of disease study 2010. PLoS Med 2013;10(11):e1001547.

12. American Psychiatric Association. Diagnostic and statistical manual of mental disorders. 5th edition. Arlington (VA): American Psychiatric Publishing; 2013.

13. Kessler RC, Berglund P, Demler O, et al. The epidemiology of major depressive disorder: results from the National Comorbidity Survey Replication (NCS-R). JAMA 2003;289(23):3095–105.

14. Fendrich M, Avci O, Johnson TP, et al. Depression, substance use and HIV risk in a probability sample of men who have sex with men. Addict Behav 2013;38(3): 1715–8.

15. Silberbogen AK, Busby AK, Ulloa EW. Impact of psychological distress on prostate cancer screening in U.S. Military Veterans. Am J Mens Health 2013; 8(5):399–408.

16. McLaughlin K. The public health impact of major depression: a call for interdisciplinary prevention efforts. Prev Sci 2011;12(4):361–71.

17. Farmer A, Korszun A, Owen MJ, et al. Medical disorders in people with recurrent depression. Br J Psychiatry 2008;192(5):351–5.

18. DiMatteo MR, Lepper HS, Croghan TW. Depression is a risk factor for noncompliance with medical treatment: meta-analysis of the effects of anxiety and depression on patient adherence. Arch Intern Med 2000;160(14):2101–7.

19. Qaseem A, Barry MJ, Kansagara D. Nonpharmacologic versus pharmacologic treatment of adult patients with major depressive disorder: a clinical practice guideline from the American College of Physicians Nonpharmacologic Versus Pharmacologic Treatment of Adults With MDD. Ann Intern Med 2016;164(5): 350–9.

20. Jobst A, Brakemeier EL, Buchheim A, et al. European Psychiatric Association Guidance on psychotherapy in chronic depression across Europe. Eur Psychiatry 2016;33:18–36.

21. Solomon D, Adams J. The use of complementary and alternative medicine in adults with depressive disorders. A critical integrative review. J Affect Disord 2015;179:101–13.

22. Cochrane Depression A, and Neurosis Group. CCDAN Topic List: intervention - psychological therapies. Secondary CCDAN Topic List: intervention - psychological therapies. Available at: http://ccdan.cochrane.org/sites/ccdan.cochrane.org/files/uploads/CCDAN%20topics%20list_psychological%20therapies%20for%20website.pdf. Accessed November 15, 2016.

23. Jorm AF, Allen NB, Morgan AJ, et al. A guide to what works for depression; 2nd Edition. beyondblue: Melbourne; 2013.

24. Gartlehner G, Gaynes BN, Amick HR, et al. AHRQ comparative effectiveness reviews. Nonpharmacological versus pharmacological treatments for adult patients with major depressive disorder. Rockville (MD): Agency for Healthcare Research and Quality (US); 2015.

25. Gartlehner G, Gaynes BN, Amick HR, et al. Comparative benefits and harms of antidepressants, psychological, complementary, and exercise treatments for major depression: an evidence report for a clinical practice guideline from the American College of Physicians Benefits and harms of treatments for major depression. Ann Intern Med 2016;164:331–41.

26. Smith CA, Hay PP, MacPherson H. Acupuncture for depression. Cochrane Database Syst Rev 2010;(1):CD004046.

27. National Institute of Mental Health. Seasonal Affective Disorder. 2016. Available at: https://www.nimh.nih.gov/health/topics/seasonal-affective-disorder/index.shtml. Accessed November 6, 2016.

28. Martensson B, Pettersson A, Berglund L, et al. Bright white light therapy in depression: a critical review of the evidence. J Affect Disord 2015;182:1–7.

29. Perera S, Eisen R, Bhatt M, et al. Light therapy for non-seasonal depression: systematic review and meta-analysis. Br J Psychiatry Open 2016;2(2):116–26.

30. Ravindran AV, Balneaves LG, Faulkner G, et al. Canadian Network for Mood and Anxiety Treatments (CANMAT) 2016 clinical guidelines for the management of

adults with major depressive disorder: section 5. complementary and alternative medicine treatments. Can J Psychiatry 2016;61(9):576–87.

31. Bauer M, Pfennig A, Severus E, et al. World Federation of Societies of Biological Psychiatry (WFSBP) guidelines for biological treatment of unipolar depressive disorders, part 1: update 2013 on the acute and continuation treatment of unipolar depressive disorders. World J Biol Psychiatry 2013;14(5):334–85.

32. Rohan KJ, Meyerhoff J, Ho SY, et al. Outcomes one and two winters following cognitive-behavioral therapy or light therapy for seasonal affective disorder. Am J Psychiatry 2016;173(3):244–51.

33. Freeman MP, Fava M, Lake J, et al. Complementary and alternative medicine in major depressive disorder: the American Psychiatric Association Task Force report. J Clin Psychiatry 2010;71(6):669–81.

34. Khusid MA, Vythilingam M. The emerging role of mindfulness meditation as effective self-management strategy, Part 1: clinical implications for depression, post-traumatic stress disorder, and anxiety. Mil Med 2016;181(9):961–8.

35. Strauss C, Cavanagh K, Oliver A, et al. Mindfulness-based interventions for people diagnosed with a current episode of an anxiety or depressive disorder: a meta-analysis of randomised controlled trials. PLoS One 2014;9(4):e96110.

36. Parikh SV, Quilty LC, Ravitz P, et al. Canadian Network for Mood and Anxiety Treatments (CANMAT) 2016 clinical guidelines for the management of adults with major depressive disorder: section 2. Psychological treatments. Can J Psychiatry 2016;61(9):524–39.

37. Clarke K, Mayo-Wilson E, Kenny J, et al. Can non-pharmacological interventions prevent relapse in adults who have recovered from depression? A systematic review and meta-analysis of randomised controlled trials. Clin Psychol Rev 2015; 39:58–70.

38. Segal ZV, Bieling P, Young T, et al. Antidepressant monotherapy vs sequential pharmacotherapy and mindfulness-based cognitive therapy, or placebo, for relapse prophylaxis in recurrent depression. Arch Gen Psychiatry 2010;67(12): 1256–64.

39. Kuyken W, Hayes R, Barrett B, et al. Effectiveness and cost-effectiveness of mindfulness-based cognitive therapy compared with maintenance antidepressant treatment in the prevention of depressive relapse or recurrence (PREVENT): a randomised controlled trial. Lancet 2015;386(9988):63–73.

40. Manicavasgar V, Parker G, Perich T. Mindfulness-based cognitive therapy vs cognitive behaviour therapy as a treatment for non-melancholic depression. J Affect Disord 2011;130(1–2):138–44.

41. Linde K, Berner MM, Kriston L. St John's wort for major depression. Cochrane Database Syst Rev 2008;(4):CD000448.

42. Chen JA, Papakostas GI, Youn SJ, et al. Association between patient beliefs regarding assigned treatment and clinical response: reanalysis of data from the Hypericum Depression Trial Study Group. J Clin Psychiatry 2011;72(12): 1669–76.

43. Qaseem A, Barry MJ, Kansagara D. Nonpharmacologic versus pharmacologic treatment of adult patients with major depressive disorder: a clinical practice guideline from the American College of Physicians. Ann Intern Med 2016;164: 350–9.

44. Mueller SC, Majcher-Peszynska J, Uehleke B, et al. The extent of induction of CYP3A by St. John's wort varies among products and is linked to hyperforin dose. Eur J Clin Pharmacol 2006;62(1):29–36.

45. De Berardis D, Orsolini L, Serroni N, et al. A comprehensive review on the efficacy of S-Adenosyl-L-methionine in Major Depressive Disorder. CNS Neurol Disord Drug Targets 2016;15(1):35–44.
46. Sarris J, Kavanagh DJ, Byrne G. Adjuvant use of nutritional and herbal medicines with antidepressants, mood stabilizers and benzodiazepines. J Psychiatr Res 2010;44(1):32–41.
47. Galizia I, Oldani L, Macritchie K, et al. S-adenosyl methionine (SAMe) for depression in adults. Cochrane Database Syst Rev 2016;(10):CD011286.
48. Stahl LA, Begg DP, Weisinger RS, et al. The role of omega-3 fatty acids in mood disorders. Curr Opin Investig Drugs 2008;9(1):57–64.
49. Appleton KM, Rogers PJ, Ness AR. Updated systematic review and meta-analysis of the effects of n-3 long-chain polyunsaturated fatty acids on depressed mood. Am J Clin Nutr 2010;91(3):757–70.
50. Appleton KM, Sallis HM, Perry R, et al. Omega-3 fatty acids for depression in adults. Cochrane Database Syst Rev 2015;(11):CD004692.
51. Sarris J, Murphy J, Mischoulon D, et al. Adjunctive nutraceuticals for depression: a systematic review and meta-analyses. Am J Psychiatry 2016;173(6):575–87.
52. Cramer H, Lauche R, Langhorst J, et al. Yoga for depression: a systematic review and meta-analysis. Depress Anxiety 2013;30(11):1068–83.
53. Pilkington K, Kirkwood G, Rampes H, et al. Yoga for depression: the research evidence. J Affect Disord 2005;89(1–3):13–24.
54. Sareen J, Cox BJ, Afifi TO, et al. Anxiety disorders and risk for suicidal ideation and suicide attempts: a population-based longitudinal study of adults. Arch Gen Psychiatry 2005;62(11):1249–57.
55. Kessler RC, Petukhova M, Sampson NA, et al. Twelve-month and lifetime prevalence and lifetime morbid risk of anxiety and mood disorders in the United States. Int J Methods Psychiatr Res 2012;21(3):169–84.
56. McPherson F, McGraw L. Treating generalized anxiety disorder using complementary and alternative medicine. Altern Ther Health Med 2013;19(5):45–50.
57. Borkovec TD, Newman MG, Pincus AL, et al. A component analysis of cognitive-behavioral therapy for generalized anxiety disorder and the role of interpersonal problems. J Consult Clin Psychol 2002;70(2):288–98.
58. Borkovec TD, Ruscio AM. Psychotherapy for generalized anxiety disorder. J Clin Psychiatry 2001;62(Suppl 11):37–42 [discussion: 43–5].
59. Baldwin DS, Anderson IM, Nutt DJ, et al. Evidence-based guidelines for the pharmacological treatment of anxiety disorders: recommendations from the British Association for Psychopharmacology. J Psychopharmacol 2005;19(6):567–96.
60. Ravven SE, Zimmerman MB, Schultz SK, et al. 12-month herbal medicine use for mental health from the national Comorbidity Survey Replication (NCS-R). Ann Clin Psychiatry 2011;23(2):83–94.
61. Bystritsky A, Hovav S, Sherbourne C, et al. Use of complementary and alternative medicine in a large sample of anxiety patients. Psychosomatics 2012;53(3):266–72.
62. Singh YN. Kava: an overview. J Ethnopharmacol 1992;37(1):13–45.
63. Kennedy J. Herb and supplement use in the US adult population. Clin Ther 2005;27(11):1847–58.
64. Pittler MH, Ernst E. Kava extract for treating anxiety. Cochrane Database Syst Rev 2003;(1):CD003383.
65. Miyasaka LS, Atallah AN, Soares BG. Passiflora for anxiety disorder. Cochrane Database Syst Rev 2007;(1):CD004518.

66. Larzelere MM, Campbell JS, Robertson M. Complementary and alternative medicine usage for behavioral health indications. Prim Care 2010;37(2):213–36.
67. Amsterdam JD, Li Y, Soeller I, et al. A randomized, double-blind, placebo-controlled trial of oral Matricaria recutita (chamomile) extract therapy for generalized anxiety disorder. J Clin Psychopharmacol 2009;29(4):378–82.
68. Keefe JR, Mao JJ, Soeller I, et al. Short-term open-label chamomile (Matricaria chamomilla L.) therapy of moderate to severe generalized anxiety disorder. Phytomedicine 2016;23(14):1699–705.
69. Mao JJ, Xie SX, Keefe JR, et al. Long-term chamomile (Matricaria chamomilla L.) treatment for generalized anxiety disorder: a randomized clinical trial. Phytomedicine 2016;23(14):1735–42.
70. Hayes S. The Six Core Processes of ACT. Available at: https://contextualscience.org/the_six_core_processes_of_act. Accessed December 10, 2016.
71. Vollestad J, Nielsen MB, Nielsen GH. Mindfulness- and acceptance-based interventions for anxiety disorders: a systematic review and meta-analysis. Br J Clin Psychol 2012;51(3):239–60.
72. Williams JW, Jr., Gierisch JM, McDuffie J, et al. An overview of complementary and alternative medicine therapies for anxiety and depressive disorders: supplement to efficacy of complementary and alternative medicine therapies for posttraumatic stress disorder. Washington (DC); 2011.
73. Bradt J, Dileo C, Grocke D, et al. Music interventions for improving psychological and physical outcomes in cancer patients. Cochrane Database Syst Rev 2011;(8):CD006911.
74. Bradt J, Dileo C, Potvin N. Music for stress and anxiety reduction in coronary heart disease patients. Cochrane Database Syst Rev 2013;(12):CD006577.
75. Bradt J, Dileo C, Shim M. Music interventions for preoperative anxiety. Cochrane Database Syst Rev 2013;(6):CD006908.
76. Kessler RC, Berglund P, Demler O, et al. Lifetime prevalence and age-of-onset distributions of DSM-IV disorders in the National Comorbidity Survey Replication. Arch Gen Psychiatry 2005;62(6):593–602.
77. Amaya-Jackson L, Davidson JR, Hughes DC, et al. Functional impairment and utilization of services associated with posttraumatic stress in the community. J Trauma Stress 1999;12(4):709–24.
78. Weisberg RB, Bruce SE, Machan JT, et al. Nonpsychiatric illness among primary care patients with trauma histories and posttraumatic stress disorder. Psychiatr Serv 2002;53(7):848–54.
79. Smid GE, Mooren TT, van der Mast RC, et al. Delayed posttraumatic stress disorder: systematic review, meta-analysis, and meta-regression analysis of prospective studies. J Clin Psychiatry 2009;70(11):1572–82.
80. Foa EB, Rothbaum BO, Riggs DS, et al. Treatment of posttraumatic stress disorder in rape victims: a comparison between cognitive-behavioral procedures and counseling. J Consult Clin Psychol 1991;59:715–23.
81. Bradley R, Greene J, Russ E, et al. A multidimensional meta-analysis of psychotherapy for PTSD. Am J Psychiatry 2005;162(2):214–27.
82. Gartlehner G, Gaynes BN, Amick HR, et al. Comparative benefits and harms of antidepressant, psychological, complementary, and exercise treatments for major depression: an evidence report for a clinical practice guideline from the American College of Physicians. Ann Intern Med 2016;164(5):331–41.
83. Hageman I, Andersen HS, Jorgensen MB. Post-traumatic stress disorder: a review of psychobiology and pharmacotherapy. Acta Psychiatr Scand 2001;104(6):411–22.

84. Libby D, Pilver C, Desai R. Complementary and alternative medicine use among individuals with posttraumatic stress disorder. Psychol Trauma Theor Res Pract Policy 2013;5(3):277–85.

85. Kim YD, Heo I, Shin BC, et al. Acupuncture for posttraumatic stress disorder: a systematic review of randomized controlled trials and prospective clinical trials. Evid Based Complement Alternat Med 2013;2013:615857.

86. Nash J, Newberg A. Toward a unifying taxonomy and definition for meditation. Front Psychol 2013;4:806.

87. Hilton L, Maher AR, Colaiaco B, et al. Meditation for posttraumatic stress: systematic review and meta-analysis. Psychol Trauma 2016. [Epub ahead of print].

88. Strauss JL, Coeytaux R, McDuffie J, et al. Efficacy of Complementary and Alternative Medicine Therapies for Posttraumatic Stress Disorder. Washington (DC), 2011.

89. Banks K, Newman E, Saleem J. An overview of the research on mindfulness-based interventions for treating symptoms of posttraumatic stress disorder: a systematic review. J Clin Psychol 2015;71(10):935–63.

90. Kim SH, Schneider SM, Kravitz L, et al. Mind-body practices for posttraumatic stress disorder. J Investig Med 2013;61(5):827–34.

91. Lang AJ, Strauss JL, Bomyea J, et al. The theoretical and empirical basis for meditation as an intervention for PTSD. Behav Modif 2012;36(6):759–86.

92. Wahbeh H, Senders A, Neuendorf R, et al. Complementary and alternative medicine for posttraumatic stress disorder symptoms: a systematic review. J Evid Based Complement Altern Med 2014;19(3):161–75.

93. Nishi D, Koido Y, Nakaya N, et al. Fish oil for attenuating posttraumatic stress symptoms among rescue workers after the great east Japan earthquake: a randomized controlled trial. Psychother Psychosom 2012;81(5):315–7.

Integrative Medicine for Insomnia

Eric S. Zhou, PhD[a],*, Paula Gardiner, MD, MPH[b], Suzanne M. Bertisch, MD, MPH[c]

KEYWORDS

- Sleep disorders • Insomnia • Integrative medicine • Alternative therapy
- Complementary medicine

KEY POINTS

- Insomnia is a common sleep disorder that is associated with poorer physical and psychological health.
- The comprehensive evaluation of a patient's health status is important when diagnosing insomnia and devising a treatment plan.
- Consistent evidence has demonstrated the efficacy of cognitive-behavioral therapy (CBT) for insomnia. CBT should be considered as first-line treatment.
- There is a growing body of literature suggesting that mindfulness-based stress management, yoga, and tai chi may improve insomnia symptoms. Current data do not support routine use of dietary supplements for sleep.
- Well-designed research studies are needed to better understand the impact of other complementary treatment approaches for insomnia (eg, acupuncture).

INSOMNIA

Insomnia is characterized by difficulty initiating and/or maintaining sleep or early morning awakenings. It is a remarkably common problem across the life span. One-third of the general population experiences insomnia symptoms and 10% to 15% meet criteria for insomnia disorder. Insomnia disorder is marked by chronic sleep disturbance that causes distress or impairs daytime function. Insomnia imparts tremendous societal and economic impact, resulting from workplace absenteeism, accidents, and declines in productivity.[1–3] Chronic sleep dysfunction is also associated with a variety of deleterious health outcomes, such as cardiovascular disease,[4,5] diabetes,[6] and obesity,[7] as well as impaired mood and cognitive function.[8,9]

Disclosure Statement: The authors have nothing to disclose.
[a] Department of Pediatric Oncology, Dana-Farber Cancer Institute, 450 Brookline Avenue, Boston, MA 02215, USA; [b] Boston Medical Center, Boston University School of Medicine, 1 Boston Medical Center Place, Boston, MA 02218, USA; [c] Division of Pulmonary, Critical Care, and Sleep Medicine, Medicine, Beth Israel Deaconess Medical Center, Harvard Medical School, 330 Brookline Avenue, Boston, MA 02215, USA
* Corresponding author.
E-mail address: eric_zhou@dfci.harvard.edu

Med Clin N Am 101 (2017) 865–879
http://dx.doi.org/10.1016/j.mcna.2017.04.005
0025-7125/17/© 2017 Elsevier Inc. All rights reserved.

Despite the psychological, physical, and financial burden of insomnia, it remains an underdiagnosed and poorly understood condition. In both primary care and the hospital setting, insomnia is often inadequately discussed and actively treated.[10,11] There is a notable gap between clinical practice guidelines for evaluating and treating chronic insomnia and current clinical care. Given this gap, patients commonly self-treat with alcohol[12] or nonprescription sleep aids, with nearly 20% using either a prescribed and/or a nonprescribed sleep aid within the past month.[13] Those who do consult their physicians about their poor sleep are often treated with pharmacotherapy.[14] At least 6 million Americans (3.0%–3.5% of the population) report use of a prescription medication for insomnia within the past 30 days.[13,15] Rates of use have increased over the past decade.[13] There are concerns regarding the use of pharmacotherapy as insomnia treatment, including dependence,[16] increased risk for motor vehicle accidents,[17] falls in the elderly,[18] and psychiatric and medical conditions.[19,20] Moreover, there are limited data on long-term efficacy.[21] Given these concerns and patient preferences often for nonpharmacological treatment,[22] it is important for patients with insomnia to be offered evidence-based nonpharmacologic approaches that may improve their sleep. Integrative insomnia therapies, including complementary and alternative medicine (CAM), are treatment options that are commonly used by adults with insomnia in the United States.[23–25] Biologically based therapies (eg, herbs) and mind-body therapies (eg, meditation) are the most commonly used CAM therapies for insomnia.[24]

INSOMNIA EVALUATION

Providers should remember that insomnia symptoms are likely underreported during routine clinical care. Patients often overlook their poor sleep because they may misattribute it as a symptom of another health issue. They also may have become resigned to the condition or are not aware that effective treatment options exist.[26–28] The evaluation of insomnia requires a broad approach and starts with a thorough medical and psychiatric history. Several risk factors exist for insomnia that should alert clinicians to the increased possibility of insomnia disorder (**Box 1**).[9,29–32]

Patients should be specifically asked about the timing of their sleep habits (eg, when they go to sleep; how long it takes them to fall asleep; frequency and duration of night awakenings; wake time; naps; quality and variability of their sleep pattern). Further, the

---

Box 1
Risk factors for insomnia

- Female sex
- Older age (>60 years)
- Medication side effects
- Night/Rotating shift work
- Travel across time zones
- Psychosocial distress
- Substance use
- Pregnancy
- Poor physical health (eg, congestive heart failure, sleep-disordered breathing)
- Poor mental health (eg, depression, anxiety, schizophrenia)

provider should discuss psychological (eg, depression) and physiologic (eg, medication use, chronic pain) factors that may be directly impacting sleep. The review of systems should inquire about symptoms consistent with of other sleep disorders, such as sleep apnea and restless legs syndrome. In addition, understanding behaviors (eg, using electronic devices in bed, staying in bed when not sleeping, stress-relieving practices including exercise), occupational factors (eg, shift work), and environmental disruptors (eg, frequent time zone travel) are important. Both prescription and nonprescription medications, as well as "drugs of habit" (eg, alcohol and caffeine) should be reviewed. Last, assessment of the daytime consequences of insomnia is critical, as these may be the main outcomes that treatment targets.

Given the known variability in sleep patterns, the collection of daily sleep diaries or logs for several weeks is a critical tool in the evaluation of insomnia. In addition to providing information on sleep timing, patterns often become evident that suggest circadian rhythm disorders or other important behaviors, such as excessive time in bed not sleeping. Data supporting the validity of commercially marketed wearable devices for assessing sleep are limited and are therefore generally not recommended.[33] For patients who are unable or unwilling to keep a sleep log, actigraphy[34] (a validated device worn on the wrist) may be used to track sleep/wake activity. However, these are generally limited to the sleep specialty clinic or research setting. Polysomnography (ie, sleep study) is not routinely indicated for the evaluation of insomnia unless there is concern for other sleep disorders (eg, obstructive sleep apnea).[35]

Should insufficient information be obtained during the clinical interview or sleep logs, there are additional instruments that can be used to gain further insight on sleep-related information. Providers should consider the use of standardized measures collected before or during a medical visit. Brief measures that can be considered include the Insomnia Severity Index[36] and Pittsburgh Sleep Quality Index (PSQI).[37] These measures require relatively minimal patient burden, provide a clinician with information to initiate a conversation with the patient, and quantify changes in symptoms over time.

In the primary care setting, patients may present with subclinical levels of insomnia symptomatology. In these cases, a stepped care approach can be used whereby increasing levels of patient need and distress warrant referrals to increasing levels of specialty sleep care and resources.[38]

TREATMENT OF INSOMNIA

Positive patient outcomes may come in the form of subjective improvements to nighttime (eg, improved overall sleep quality) and/or daytime functioning (eg, less fatigue and improved concentration). Objective improvements to sleep-specific variables may include decreased sleep-onset latency, less wake after sleep onset, and improved sleep efficiency. These variables describe common challenges experienced by patients with insomnia. Specifically, sleep-onset latency refers to the time taken for a patient to fall asleep. Wake after sleep onset describes the total amount of time a patient spends awake in the middle of the night. Sleep efficiency describes the ratio of the total time spent asleep divided by the total sleep opportunity.

Integrative Therapies

Cognitive-behavioral therapy

Cognitive-behavioral therapy for insomnia (CBT-Insomnia) is composed of several primary components: sleep restriction, stimulus control, cognitive restructuring, sleep hygiene, relaxation, and relapse prevention. Sleep restriction[39] limits time in bed to increase sleep drive and regulate circadian rhythms. Stimulus control[40,41] provides patients with "rules" to retrain their minds and bodies to relearn to associate sleep with their bed and bedroom environment. Stimulus control also aims to reduce anxiety and/or conditioned arousal that individuals experience when attempting to fall asleep. Cognitive restructuring attempts to address, challenge, and reshape the negative beliefs and distorted cognitive patterns about sleep and sleep loss that further perpetuate chronic sleep difficulties. For example, patients may worry that they may not be able to function at work the next day if they are not able to fall asleep quickly enough. This can then further increase their anxiety at bedtime, creating a vicious cycle making it more difficult to fall asleep. Sleep hygiene focuses on education about factors that promote sleep and discourage behaviors that are detrimental to sleep (eg, avoiding nicotine, caffeine, and alcohol before bedtime).[42] It is noted that sleep hygiene recommendations are often provided as monotherapy, and evidence indicates that may not be an effective treatment, by itself, for insomnia disorder.[43] Relaxation therapy can incorporate various techniques, all with the goal to reduce disruptive physical and/or cognitive arousal at bedtime. A considerable body of literature supports multiple forms of relaxation for insomnia, including progressive muscle relaxation, imagery, and autogenic training.[39–41,44–46] Relapse prevention strategies integrate the behavioral, cognitive, and educational elements, promote adherence, help the patient identify high-risk situations, and incorporate steps to reduce relapse. Effective individual components of CBT-Insomnia (sleep restriction and stimulus control) can be demanding for a patient and often create a short-term exacerbation of sleep problems.[47] Consequently, adherence may be poor[48] and may explain why some patients continue to experience insomnia symptoms after treatment.[49]

Numerous randomized controlled trials (RCTs) have demonstrated that CBT-Insomnia is highly effective.[50–52] A meta-analysis of 20 RCTs showed that CBT-Insomnia effectively improves multiple sleep outcomes (eg, wake after sleep onset, sleep efficiency).[53] Direct comparisons between CBT-Insomnia and pharmacologic treatments indicate that CBT-Insomnia is equivalently efficacious, with the benefits of CBT-Insomnia maintained over a longer duration.[16,49,52,54] In addition, CBT-Insomnia also may improve outcomes for depression, anxiety, and quality of life.[55,56] CBT-Insomnia is also efficacious in multiple patient subpopulations, such cancer,[57,58] chronic pain,[59] and numerous additional comorbid medical and psychiatric disorders.[60] Given the preponderance of evidence supporting its efficacy, several professional organizations consider CBT-Insomnia as first-line therapy for insomnia.[61–63]

Barriers to treatment with CBT-Insomnia exist even when a patient is aware and motivated to change his or her behavior. One major limitation is that there are relatively few trained providers to deliver this intervention. There are estimated to be fewer than 700 behavioral sleep medicine experts in the United States,[64] mainly limited to major cities.[65] Further, CBT-Insomnia is time and resource intensive, as it was developed to be provided over 6 to 8 individual, in-person sessions.[66] This can be a prohibitive duration due to travel time to and from the provider and out-of-pocket expenses for the patient. To combat these barriers, there are ongoing efforts to train nonsleep specialists[67] to deliver CBT-Insomnia treatment via group and telehealth mechanisms.[68–72] Briefer programs are also in development.[73] Evidence is promising that these novel delivery approaches can effectively improve insomnia symptoms. Finally, it is noted that CBT-Insomnia research has been primarily conducted in adults, with different approaches required for pediatric populations.[53,74]

Mindfulness-based practices

The use of mindfulness-based practices to improve insomnia symptoms has garnered recent interest, specifically mindfulness-based stress reduction.[75,76] Mindfulness practices purposefully bring awareness to the present moment by directing attention to the breath, physical sensations, feelings and/or thoughts. These practices aspire to view the moment with a mindset that is accepting, patient, and kind.[77] Although no definitive mechanisms have been established to explain how mindfulness-based practices affect sleep, several reasonable interrelated hypotheses have been suggested. One theory postulates that mindfulness-based practices may act through the reduction of cognitive and physiologic hyperarousal,[78] which has been implicated as a contributor to the development and/or maintenance of sleep problems.[79] This explanation posits that during the day, individuals engage in functional information processing, such as making decisions or solving problems. In the evening, these processes should deactivate and therefore facilitate sleep. A mindfulness-based practice potentially allows cognitive and physiologic deactivation and a reduction in hyperarousal by encouraging the practitioner to accept and "let go" of their daily concerns. A second hypothesis is based on literature suggesting people who ruminate tend to sleep worse.[80,81] Mindfulness-based practices may facilitate sleep by helping individuals ruminate less.[82] Recent evidence supports this notion that mindfulness-based practices reduce repetitive negative thinking, which in turn improves psychological outcomes.[83] Finally, it has been suggested that mindfulness-based practices may help individuals better pay attention to the present moment, thereby reducing the focus on not being able to sleep and/or the consequences of poor sleep.[84,85]

Within the past several years, multiple efforts have been taken to advance the science evaluating mindfulness-based practices as a treatment for insomnia. Researchers have delivered mindfulness-based practices to the general adult and cancer populations, with significant improvements to sleep in general. Although sample sizes were relatively small in some studies, evidence suggests that a mindfulness-based intervention can improve insomnia symptoms (eg, reduce total wake time, improve sleep quality) in those with both insomnia symptoms and insomnia disorder,[86–88] with efficacy comparable to that of hypnotic medications.[89] When compared with CBT-Insomnia, a mindfulness-based approach developed for cancer populations was effective at improving insomnia symptoms, but inferior to CBT-Insomnia on some sleep outcomes.[90] Other efforts have used mindfulness training as adjunctive treatment to CBT-Insomnia, creating a hybrid approach.[91] Findings have been mixed with respect to whether adding mindfulness-based practices to CBT-Insomnia improves insomnia more than CBT-Insomnia alone.[92,93]

To date, mindfulness-based practices in the treatment of insomnia show potential, and should be considered as a possible second-line or adjunctive therapy to other therapeutic approaches with a stronger evidence base (eg, CBT-Insomnia). Mindfulness-based approaches may play a particularly key role in insomnia treatment for 3 categories of patients: (1) interested in acceptance and commitment-based treatments designed to increase cognitive flexibility; (2) failed or would prefer not to attempt CBT-Insomnia, and (3) have medical/psychological conditions that may be exacerbated by CBT-Insomnia (eg, bipolar disorder). Future work is important before mindfulness-based treatment of insomnia can be considered for routine integration into clinical care. Mechanistic studies, standardized mindfulness-based insomnia protocols, and trials directly comparing mindfulness-based practices with CBT-Insomnia and pharmacologic therapies are needed.

Mind-body movement practices (yoga and tai chi)

Both yoga and tai chi represent multicomponent interventions that are thought to evoke similar physiologic processes to traditional relaxation training. Both have been investigated as treatments for insomnia. Yoga is a popular mind-body practice originally derived from India. Mechanistically, yoga acutely impacts autonomic nervous system activity and may reduce gamma-aminobutyric acid (GABA) levels and inflammatory markers over time.[94,95] These are plausible neurobiological pathways by which yoga may improve sleep quality and duration. Data from small RCTs suggest yoga improves subjective[96–99] and objective[99,100] sleep quality, and reduces insomnia symptoms in adults with chronic medical conditions.[96,98,101–104] One of the largest RCTs of yoga demonstrated reduced hypnotic medication use in cancer survivors with sleep disturbance by 21% in the yoga group compared with 5% in the control group.[99] Although clinically meaningful differences in self-reported sleep quality were seen, improvements to daytime function were more modest. Few studies have evaluated yoga specifically for insomnia disorder. One of the first studies to explore yoga in patients meeting standard diagnostic criteria for insomnia was a single-arm 8-week trial exploring Kundalini yoga, a style that emphasizes breathing techniques and meditation. Among the 20 participants completing the study (of 34 entering treatment), improvements were seen in diary-reported total sleep time, sleep quality, sleep efficiency, and total wake time.[104] Another pilot RCT reported that postmenopausal women with insomnia disorder experienced a greater reduction in insomnia symptom scores with yoga compared with a control, but without differences in polysomnographic outcomes. Another small, single-arm study exploring a combination of Hatha and viniyoga for sleep difficulties in patients with osteoarthritis found reductions in insomnia symptom scores and improvements in reported sleep-onset latency and sleep efficiency. No changes were seen in actigraphy outcomes, however.[101] To date, although the emerging data on yoga are encouraging, many clinical studies have studied participants experiencing a general sleep disturbance, rather than insomnia disorder. Furthermore, yoga studies measuring sleep outcomes have suffered from common methodological limitations, such as small sample sizes, lack of clearly defined protocols, and limited use of objective outcome measures.

Similar to yoga research, there is an emerging body of work on tai chi for sleep disturbance that has focused more on sleep quality (ie, change in self-report measures such as the PSQI) rather than insomnia disorder. Several RCTs of tai chi for sleep have demonstrated improvement in reported sleep quality, particularly among older adults. Irwin and colleagues[105] demonstrated that older adults with moderate sleep complaints who practiced tai chi were more likely to achieve significant improvements in sleep quality compared with those receiving health education (63% vs 32%, respectively). Other tai chi studies evaluating sleep quality as the primary outcome found similar improvements for older adults compared with a low-impact exercise group.[106] Another study found a clinically meaningful improvement with tai chi compared with a waitlist control.[107] Similar improvements in sleep quality have been found in patients with fibromyalgia.[108,109] However, small studies in other clinical populations, such as breast cancer[110] and arthritis,[111] have not demonstrated positive results. A recent comparative effectiveness study indicated that tai chi was less effective than CBT-Insomnia for chronic insomnia disorder, but more effective in improving sleep quality than education on aging and sleep.[112] Therefore, tai chi may improve sleep quality in diverse patient populations, and in particular older adults. Its impact on objective measures of sleep as well as chronic insomnia disorder needs to be further elucidated.

Acupuncture

A Cochrane review conducted in 2009 indicated that definitive conclusions cannot be made on acupuncture's efficacy for insomnia.[113] This conclusion was reached due to the limited number of RCTs and limited sample sizes. Further, existing research is hampered by design limitations. For example, publications have provided limited information about inclusion/exclusion criteria, randomization procedures, outcomes measured, missing baseline data, and the specific acupuncture approach(es) used.[114,115] Future research efforts should improve methodological rigor to assess whether acupuncture therapy for insomnia can be recommended.

Dietary supplements

Valerian Valerian (*Valeriana officinalis*) has been one of the most rigorously evaluated supplements for sleep purposes. Valerian's effects on the central nervous system have been attributed to valepotriates, valerenic acid, and other constituents in the essential oil.[116] Valerian extracts do contain small amounts of GABA, a key sleep-promoting neurotransmitter. However, whether exogenous GABA can cross the blood-brain barrier to produce sedative effects is not known.[117] Although numerous case series and RCTs in adults have suggested valerian impacts sleep, the totality of evidence supports generally weak effects on sleep, and minimal benefit for patients with insomnia disorder. A recent meta-analysis included only studies evaluating insomnia disorder (14 RCTs, n = 1602),[118] defined by established diagnostic criteria, standardized instruments, or medical diagnosis. This study found no difference in short-term ($\leq$6 weeks) sleep outcomes between valerian and placebo. It is important to note that a wide range of dosages and preparations were tested, and the risk of bias could not be adequately assessed given the general lack of information on preparation methodology. The rate of adverse events was similar between valerian and placebo. Given these limited data on harms, and limited evidence supporting clinically meaningful change in outcomes, the American Academy of Sleep Medicine (AASM) guides practitioners to not recommend valerian for insomnia disorder.[73]

Melatonin Melatonin (N-acetyl-5-methoxytryptamine) is a hormone synthesized from tryptophan and secreted in the pineal gland. Current evidence in humans supports melatonin's roles as a chronobiotic, influencing circadian timing, and as a modest somnogen, initiating and maintaining sleep. As light is the most important environmental cue modulating endogenous melatonin release, melatonin levels peak in darkness and are low during the daytime. In the United States, exogenous melatonin is a popular over-the-counter dietary supplement recommended for disorders of the sleep cycle, such as shift work and jet lag. In Europe, it is available only by prescription. In general, data supporting exogenous melatonin for insomnia are weak. A meta-analysis included 19 melatonin trials with 1683 patients with "sleep disorders" (ie, insomnia [n = 14], delayed sleep phase syndrome [n = 4], and rapid-eye movement behavior disorder [n = 1]). Compared with placebo, melatonin reduced sleep-onset latency by about 7 minutes, prolonged subjective (but not objective) total sleep time by approximately 8 minutes, and had modest effects on sleep quality.[38] A clinical guideline put forth by the AASM suggested against the use of melatonin for treatment of sleep onset or sleep maintenance insomnia.[73]

In contrast, the AASM recommends timed oral administration of melatonin for delayed sleep-wake phase disorder in adults and children. Delayed sleep-wake phase disorder can present as sleep-onset insomnia. This disorder is most apparent when the patient's biological clock is misaligned with his or her time zone. This often results in difficulty falling asleep "when needed" and awakening at a desired time earlier than the biological wake time. This commonly leads to insufficient sleep and reports of insomnia symptoms.

In general, melatonin is well tolerated in adults with few reported adverse events in a dose range of 0.1 mg to 10 mg.[119] Caution in children/adolescents and women of reproductive age should be exercised due to limited long-term studies and potential hormonal effects.[119] Melatonin should generally not be used during daytime due to sedation. In a placebo-controlled trial, oral melatonin decreased coagulation activity within 1 hour of dosing in healthy men. Therefore caution should be used with anticoagulants.[73]

One major issue with melatonin, and other over-the-counter dietary supplements, is the relative lack of standardization and regulation. A recent study of 31 melatonin products available in Canada found that the melatonin levels in the pills ranged between 83% and 478% of the melatonin dose reported on the label. More than 70% of the products varied from the labeled dose by more than 10%. There was also lot-to-lot variability among manufacturers. Furthermore, 26% of products also contained serotonin.[113] Therefore, if melatonin is recommended in the short term for insomnia symptoms in adults, or for treatment of circadian rhythm disorders, only products that have been third-party verified (eg, US Pharmacopeial Convention) should be used.

Other supplements The data examining other dietary supplements for insomnia are sparse. German chamomile (*Matricaria recutita*) has been used for sleep for thousands of years.[120,121] Common preparations include tea (3 cups per day) or in tinctures (1–4 mL/d). Preclinical studies suggest chamomile's mechanism of action is due to the flavone, apigenin, which modulates GABA receptors.[122] Chamomile has been studied in a few short-term trials. The most rigorous study, conducted in 34 patients, examined high-grade extract chamomile (270 mg, twice a day) for primary insomnia. Modest benefits were reported for some sleep outcomes, although conclusions were limited by small sample size.[123] Chamomile is in the same plant family (Asteraceae) as ragweed, and therefore chamomile should be used with caution in patients with a history of hay fever, as allergic reactions, including rare cases of anaphylaxis, have been reported.[120] Given chamomile's relatively safe profile, it may be reasonable to use chamomile for insomnia symptoms based on patient preference and values, although rigorous evidence supporting its efficacy is generally weak.

Exogenous consumption of the amino acid L-tryptophan has also been purported to induce sleep, although data are limited. One short-term study suggested that 250 mg tryptophan resulted in significant improvement in subjective and objective measures of sleep in persons without insomnia.[124] Another small study suggested improved sleep with L-tryptophan in sleep in individuals undergoing drug detoxification.[108] Two other short-term studies suggested modest reductions in sleep-onset latency in chronic insomnia at differing dosages. Based on available evidence suggesting clinically meaningful improvements, the AASM recommends against use of L-tryptophan for chronic insomnia.[73] It should be noted that in the 1990s, L-tryptophan was recalled from the market due to safety concerns, as it was linked to more than 1500 reports of eosinophilia-myalgia syndrome.

Lavender, specifically English lavender (*Lavandula angustifolia*), usually in the form of oil or tea, has been used for sleep purposes. Several small, very short-term (<1 week) studies in healthy individuals suggest that lavender oil may improve sleep quality.[125] In recommended doses, lavender is generally considered to be well tolerated in adults,[126] although a case report of pre-pubertal gynecomastia after use of lavender and tea tree oils has been reported.[127]

SUMMARY

Insomnia symptoms and chronic insomnia disorder are very common and frequently present in the general health care setting. There is high-quality evidence for use of CBT as a primary treatment for insomnia, with emerging evidence supporting use of additional mind-body therapies, such as mindfulness meditation. Tai chi and yoga also may improve sleep quality, particularly among older adults. However, their role in treating chronic insomnia disorder is unclear. Although dietary supplements are commonly used for insomnia, the totality of data does not currently support routine use for most patients with sleep disturbance. The role of other therapies, such as acupuncture, in treating insomnia remains uncertain. Patients with insomnia do not commonly discuss their use of complementary therapies with providers. It is essential that the patient's use of such therapeutic approaches is fully assessed.

ACKNOWLEDGMENTS

Funding support for this work was provided by the National Center for Complementary and Integrative Health (5R34AT008923-02).

REFERENCES

1. Léger D, Bayon V. Societal costs of insomnia. Sleep Med Rev 2010;14(6): 379–89.
2. Kessler R, Berglund P, Coulouvrat C, et al. Insomnia and the performance of US workers: results from the America Insomnia Survey. Sleep 2011;34(11):1608.
3. Sarsour K, Kalsekar A, Swindle R, et al. The association between insomnia severity and healthcare and productivity costs in a health plan sample. Sleep 2011;34(4):443–50.
4. Suka M, Yoshida K, Sugimori H. Persistent insomnia is a predictor of hypertension in Japanese male workers. J Occup Health 2003;45(6):344–50.
5. Chien KL, Chen PC, Hsu HC, et al. Habitual sleep duration and insomnia and the risk of cardiovascular events and all-cause death: report from a community-based cohort. Sleep 2010;33(2):177–84.
6. Vgontzas AN, Liao D, Pejovic S, et al. Insomnia with objective short sleep duration is associated with type 2 diabetes: a population-based study. Diabetes care 2009;32(11):1980–5.
7. Patel SR, Blackwell T, Redline S, et al. The association between sleep duration and obesity in older adults. Int J Obes 2008;32(12):1825–34.
8. Roth T, Ancoli-Israel S. Daytime consequences and correlates of insomnia in the United States: results of the 1991 National Sleep Foundation Survey. II. Sleep 1999;22(Suppl 2):S354–8.
9. Ohayon MM, Roth T. Place of chronic insomnia in the course of depressive and anxiety disorders. J Psychiatr Res 2003;37(1):9–15.
10. Hohagen F, Rink K, Käppler C, et al. Prevalence and treatment of insomnia in general practice. Eur Arch Psychiatry Clin Neurosci 1993;242(6):329–36.
11. Zhou ES, Partridge AH, Syrjala KL, et al. Evaluation and treatment of insomnia in adult cancer survivorship programs. J Cancer Surviv 2016;11(1):1–6.
12. Ancoli-Israel S, Roth T. Characteristics of insomnia in the United States: results of the 1991 National Sleep Foundation Survey. I. Sleep 1999;22(Suppl 2): S347–53.
13. Bertisch SM, Herzig SJ, Winkelman JW, et al. National use of prescription medications for insomnia: NHANES 1999-2010. Sleep 2014;37(2):343.

14. Leger D, Poursain B, Neubauer D, et al. An international survey of sleeping problems in the general population. Curr Med Res Opin 2008;24(1):307–17.
15. Chong Y, Fryer CD, Gu Q. Prescription sleep aid use among adults: United States, 2005-2010. NCHS data brief 2013;127:1–8.
16. Smith MT, Perlis ML, Park A, et al. Comparative meta-analysis of pharmacotherapy and behavior therapy for persistent insomnia. Am J Psychiatry 2002;159(1):5–11.
17. Hansen RN, Boudreau DM, Ebel BE, et al. Sedative hypnotic medication use and the risk of motor vehicle crash. Am J Public Health 2015;105(8):e64–9.
18. Tannenbaum C, Diaby V, Singh D, et al. Sedative-hypnotic medicines and falls in community-dwelling older adults: a cost-effectiveness (decision-tree) analysis from a US Medicare perspective. Drugs Aging 2015;32(4):305–14.
19. Chung K, Li C, Kuo S, et al. Risk of psychiatric disorders in patients with chronic insomnia and sedative-hypnotic prescription: a nationwide population-based follow-up study. J Clin Sleep Med 2015;11(5):543–51.
20. Sivertsen B, Salo P, Pentti J, et al. Use of sleep medications and risk of cancer: a matched case–control study. Sleep Med 2015;16(12):1552–5.
21. Buscemi N, Vandermeer B, Friesen C, et al. The efficacy and safety of drug treatments for chronic insomnia in adults: a meta-analysis of RCTs. J Gen Intern Med 2007;22(9):1335–50.
22. Morin CM, Gaulier B, Barry T, et al. Patients' acceptance of psychological and pharmacological therapies for insomnia. Sleep 1992;15(4):302–5.
23. Bertisch SM, Wells RE, Smith MT, et al. Use of relaxation techniques and complementary and alternative medicine by American adults with insomnia symptoms: results from a national survey. J Clin Sleep Med 2012;8(6):681–91.
24. Pearson NJ, Johnson LL, Nahin RL. Insomnia, trouble sleeping, and complementary and alternative medicine: analysis of the 2002 national health interview survey data. Arch Intern Med 2006;166(16):1775–82.
25. Bertisch SM, Wee CC, Phillips RS, et al. Alternative mind-body therapies used by adults with medical conditions. J Psychosom Res 2009;66(6):511–9.
26. Morin CM, Stone J, Trinkle D, et al. Dysfunctional beliefs and attitudes about sleep among older adults with and without insomnia complaints. Psychol Aging 1993;8(3):463.
27. Espie CA, Inglis SJ, Harvey L, et al. Insomniacs' attributions: psychometric properties of the dysfunctional beliefs and attitudes about sleep scale and the sleep disturbance questionnaire. J Psychosom Res 2000;48(2):141–8.
28. Fichten CS, Creti L, Amsel R, et al. Poor sleepers who do not complain of insomnia: myths and realities about psychological and lifestyle characteristics of older good and poor sleepers. J Behav Med 1995;18(2):189–223.
29. Kamel NS, Gammack JK. Insomnia in the elderly: cause, approach, and treatment. Am J Med 2006;119(6):463–9.
30. Mindell JA, Jacobson BJ. Sleep disturbances during pregnancy. J Obstet Gynecol Neonatal Nurs 2000;29(6):590–7.
31. Taylor DJ, Mallory LJ, Lichstein KL, et al. Comorbidity of chronic insomnia with medical problems. Sleep 2007;30(2):213.
32. Brower KJ. Insomnia, alcoholism and relapse. Sleep Med Rev 2003;7(6):523–39.
33. Shelgikar AV, Anderson P, Stephens MR. Sleep tracking, wearable technology, and opportunities for research and clinical care. Chest 2016;150(3):732–43.
34. Sadeh A. The role and validity of actigraphy in sleep medicine: an update. Sleep Med Rev 2011;15(4):259–67.

35. Chesson A Jr, Hartse K, Anderson WM, et al. Practice parameters for the evaluation of chronic insomnia. An American Academy of Sleep Medicine report. Standards of Practice Committee of the American Academy of Sleep Medicine. Sleep 2000;23(2):237–41.
36. Bastien CH, Vallieres A, Morin CM. Validation of the Insomnia Severity Index as an outcome measure for insomnia research. Sleep Med 2001;2(4):297–307.
37. Buysse DJ, Reynolds CF 3rd, Monk TH, et al. The Pittsburgh Sleep Quality Index: a new instrument for psychiatric practice and research. Psychiatry Res 1989;28(2):193–213.
38. Ferracioli-Oda E, Qawasmi A, Bloch MH. Meta-analysis: melatonin for the treatment of primary sleep disorders. PLoS one 2013;8(5):e63773.
39. Means MK, Lichstein KL, Epperson MT, et al. Relaxation therapy for insomnia: nighttime and day time effects. Behav Res Ther 2000;38(7):665–78.
40. Borkovec TD, Fowles DC. Controlled investigation of the effects of progressive and hypnotic relaxation on insomnia. J Abnorm Psychol 1973;82(1):153.
41. Nicassio P, Bootzin R. A comparison of progressive relaxation and autogenic training as treatments for insomnia. J Abnorm Psychol 1974;83(3):253.
42. Irish LA, Kline CE, Gunn HE, et al. The role of sleep hygiene in promoting public health: a review of empirical evidence. Sleep Med Rev 2015;22:23–36.
43. Kelber O, Nieber K, Kraft K. Valerian: no evidence for clinically relevant interactions. Evid Based Complement Altern Med 2014;2014:879396.
44. Woolfolk RL, McNulty TF. Relaxation treatment for insomnia: a component analysis. J Consult Clin Psychol 1983;51(4):495.
45. Morin CM, Azrin NH. Stimulus control and imagery training in treating sleep-maintenance insomnia. J Consult Clin Psychol 1987;55(2):260.
46. Lichstein KL, Johnson RS. Relaxation for insomnia and hypnotic medication use in older women. Psychol Aging 1993;8(1):103.
47. Riedel BW, Lichstein KL. Strategies for evaluating adherence to sleep restriction treatment for insomnia. Behav Res Ther 2001;39(2):201–12.
48. Matthews EE, Arnedt JT, McCarthy MS, et al. Adherence to cognitive behavioral therapy for insomnia: a systematic review. Sleep Med Rev 2013;17(6):453–64.
49. Morin CM, Vallieres A, Guay B, et al. Cognitive behavioral therapy, singly and combined with medication, for persistent insomnia: a randomized controlled trial. JAMA 2009;301(19):2005–15.
50. Espie CA, Fleming L, Cassidy J, et al. Randomized controlled clinical effectiveness trial of cognitive behavior therapy compared with treatment as usual for persistent insomnia in patients with cancer. J Clin Oncol 2008;26(28):4651–8.
51. Edinger JD, Wohlgemuth WK, Radtke RA, et al. Cognitive behavioral therapy for treatment of chronic primary insomnia: a randomized controlled trial. JAMA 2001;285(14):1856–64.
52. Sivertsen B, Omvik S, Pallesen S, et al. Cognitive behavioral therapy vs zopiclone for treatment of chronic primary insomnia in older adults: a randomized controlled trial. JAMA 2006;295(24):2851–8.
53. Trauer JM, Qian MY, Doyle JS, et al. Cognitive behavioral therapy for chronic insomnia: a systematic review and meta-analysis. Ann Intern Med 2015;163(3):191–204.
54. Jacobs GD, Pace-Schott EF, Stickgold R, et al. Cognitive behavior therapy and pharmacotherapy for insomnia: a randomized controlled trial and direct comparison. Arch Intern Med 2004;164(17):1888–96.

55. Manber R, Edinger JD, Gress JL, et al. Cognitive behavioral therapy for insomnia enhances depression outcome in patients with comorbid major depressive disorder and insomnia. Sleep 2008;31(4):489–95.

56. Thorndike FP, Ritterband LM, Gonder-Frederick LA, et al. A randomized controlled trial of an Internet intervention for adults with insomnia: effects on comorbid psychological and fatigue symptoms. J Clin Psychol 2013;69(10): 1078–93.

57. Garland SN, Johnson JA, Savard J, et al. Sleeping well with cancer: a systematic review of cognitive behavioral therapy for insomnia in cancer patients. Neuropsychiatr Dis Treat 2014;10:1113–24.

58. Zhou ES, Partridge AH, Recklitis CJ. A pilot trial of brief group cognitive-behavioral treatment for insomnia in an adult cancer survivorship program. Psychooncology 2016. [Epub ahead of print].

59. Currie SR, Wilson KG, Pontefract AJ, et al. Cognitive-behavioral treatment of insomnia secondary to chronic pain. J Consult Clin Psychol 2000;68(3):407–16.

60. Smith MT, Huang MI, Manber R. Cognitive behavior therapy for chronic insomnia occurring within the context of medical and psychiatric disorders. Clin Psychol Rev 2005;25(5):559–92.

61. Morgenthaler T, Kramer M, Alessi C, et al. Practice parameters for the psychological and behavioral treatment of insomnia: an update. An American Academy of Sleep Medicine report. Sleep 2006;29(11):1415–9.

62. Schutte-Rodin S, Broch L, Buysse D, et al. Clinical guideline for the evaluation and management of chronic insomnia in adults. J Clin Sleep Med 2008;4(5): 487–504.

63. Qaseem A, Barry MJ, Kansagara D. Nonpharmacologic versus pharmacologic treatment of adult patients with major depressive disorder: a clinical practice guideline from the American College of Physicians. Ann Intern Med 2016; 164(5):350–9.

64. Thomas A, Grandner M, Nowakowski S, et al. Where are the behavioral sleep medicine providers and where are they needed? A geographic assessment. Behav Sleep Med 2016;14(6):1–12.

65. Perlis ML, Smith MT. How can we make CBT-I and other BSM services widely available. J Clin Sleep Med 2008;4(1):11–3.

66. Morin CM, Kowatch RA, Barry T, et al. Cognitive-behavior therapy for late-life insomnia. J Consult Clin Psychol 1993;61(1):137.

67. Manber R, Carney C, Edinger J, et al. Dissemination of CBTI to the non-sleep specialist: protocol development and training issues. J Clin Sleep Med 2012; 8(2):209–18.

68. Ritterband LM, Thorndike FP, Gonder-Frederick LA, et al. Efficacy of an Internet-based behavioral intervention for adults with insomnia. Arch Gen Psychiatry 2009;66(7):692–8.

69. Espie CA, Kyle SD, Williams C, et al. A randomized, placebo-controlled trial of online cognitive behavioral therapy for chronic insomnia disorder delivered via an automated media-rich web application. Sleep 2012;35(6):769–81.

70. Zhou ES, Vrooman LM, Manley PE, et al. Adapted delivery of cognitive-behavioral treatment for insomnia in adolescent and young adult cancer survivors: a pilot study. Behav Sleep Med 2016;15(4):1–14.

71. Rybarczyk B, Lopez M, Schelble K, et al. Home-based video CBT for comorbid geriatric insomnia: a pilot study using secondary data analyses. Behav Sleep Med 2005;3(3):158–75.

72. Savard J, Villa J, Simard S, et al. Feasibility of a self-help treatment for insomnia comorbid with cancer. Psychooncology 2011;20(9):1013–9.
73. Sateia MJ, Buysse DJ, Krystal AD, et al. Clinical practice guideline for the pharmacologic treatment of chronic insomnia in adults: an American Academy of Sleep Medicine clinical practice guideline. J Clin Sleep Med 2017;13(2):307–49.
74. Zhou ES, Owens J. Behavioral treatments for pediatric insomnia. Curr Sleep Med Rep 2016;2:1–9.
75. Garland SN, Zhou ES, Gonzalez BD, et al. The quest for mindful sleep: a critical synthesis of the impact of mindfulness-based interventions for insomnia. Curr Sleep Med Rep 2016;2(3):1–10.
76. Winbush NY, Gross CR, Kreitzer MJ. The effects of mindfulness-based stress reduction on sleep disturbance: a systematic review. Explore (NY) 2007;3(6):585–91.
77. Carlson LE. Mindfulness-based interventions for physical conditions: a narrative review evaluating levels of evidence. ISRN Psychiatry 2012;2012:651583.
78. Lundh L-G, Broman J-E. Insomnia as an interaction between sleep-interfering and sleep-interpreting processes. J Psychosom Res 2000;49(5):299–310.
79. Bonnet MH, Arand DL. Hyperarousal and insomnia: state of the science. Sleep Med Rev 2010;14(1):9–15.
80. Zoccola PM, Dickerson SS, Lam S. Rumination predicts longer sleep onset latency after an acute psychosocial stressor. Psychosom Med 2009;71(7):771–5.
81. Carney CE, Edinger JD, Meyer B, et al. Symptom-focused rumination and sleep disturbance. Behav Sleep Med 2006;4(4):228–41.
82. Shapiro SL, Carlson LE, Astin JA, et al. Mechanisms of mindfulness. J Clin Psychol 2006;62(3):373–86.
83. Gu J, Strauss C, Bond R, et al. How do mindfulness-based cognitive therapy and mindfulness-based stress reduction improve mental health and wellbeing? A systematic review and meta-analysis of mediation studies. Clin Psychol Rev 2015;37:1–12.
84. Harris K, Spiegelhalder K, Espie CA, et al. Sleep-related attentional bias in insomnia: a state-of-the-science review. Clin Psychol Rev 2015;42:16–27.
85. Larouche M, Cote G, Belisle D, et al. Kind attention and non-judgment in mindfulness-based cognitive therapy applied to the treatment of insomnia: state of knowledge. Pathol Biol (Paris) 2014;62(5):284–91.
86. Zhang J-X, Liu X-H, Xie X-H, et al. Mindfulness-based stress reduction for chronic insomnia in adults older than 75 years: a randomized, controlled, single-blind clinical trial. Explore (NY) 2015;11(3):180–5.
87. Larouche M, Lorrain D, Côté G, et al. Evaluation of the effectiveness of mindfulness-based cognitive therapy to treat chronic insomnia. Revue Européenne de Psychol Appliquée 2015;65(3):115–23.
88. Black DS, O'Reilly GA, Olmstead R, et al. Mindfulness meditation and improvement in sleep quality and daytime impairment among older adults with sleep disturbances: a randomized clinical trial. JAMA Intern Med 2015;175(4):494–501.
89. Gross CR, Kreitzer MJ, Reilly-Spong M, et al. Mindfulness-based stress reduction versus pharmacotherapy for chronic primary insomnia: a randomized controlled clinical trial. Explore (NY) 2011;7(2):76–87.
90. Garland SN, Carlson LE, Stephens AJ, et al. Mindfulness-based stress reduction compared with cognitive behavioral therapy for the treatment of insomnia comorbid with cancer: a randomized, partially blinded, noninferiority trial. J Clin Oncol 2014;32(5):449–57.

91. Britton WB, Bootzin RR, Cousins JC, et al. The contribution of mindfulness practice to a multicomponent behavioral sleep intervention following substance abuse treatment in adolescents: a treatment-development study. Subst Abus 2010;31(2):86–97.

92. Ong JC, Manber R, Segal Z, et al. A randomized controlled trial of mindfulness meditation for chronic insomnia. Sleep 2014;37(9):1553.

93. Wong MY, Ree MJ, Lee CW. Enhancing CBT for chronic insomnia: a randomised clinical trial of additive components of mindfulness or cognitive therapy. Clin Psychol Psychother 2015;23(5):377–85.

94. Streeter CC, Jensen JE, Perlmutter RM, et al. Yoga Asana sessions increase brain GABA levels: a pilot study. J Altern Complement Med 2007;13(4):419–26.

95. Streeter CC, Whitfield TH, Owen L, et al. Effects of yoga versus walking on mood, anxiety, and brain GABA levels: a randomized controlled MRS study. J Altern Complement Med 2010;16(11):1145–52.

96. Afonso RF, Hachul H, Kozasa EH, et al. Yoga decreases insomnia in postmenopausal women: a randomized clinical trial. Menopause 2012;19(2):186–93.

97. Chen KM, Chen MH, Lin MH, et al. Effects of yoga on sleep quality and depression in elders in assisted living facilities. J Nurs Res 2010;18(1):53–61.

98. Cohen L, Warneke C, Fouladi RT, et al. Psychological adjustment and sleep quality in a randomized trial of the effects of a Tibetan yoga intervention in patients with lymphoma. Cancer 2004;100(10):2253–60.

99. Mustian KM, Sprod LK, Janelsins M, et al. Multicenter, randomized controlled trial of yoga for sleep quality among cancer survivors. J Clin Oncol 2013; 31(26):3233–41.

100. Beddoe AE, Lee KA, Weiss SJ, et al. Effects of mindful yoga on sleep in pregnant women: a pilot study. Biol Res Nurs 2010;11(4):363–70.

101. Taibi DM, Vitiello MV. A pilot study of gentle yoga for sleep disturbance in women with osteoarthritis. Sleep Med 2011;12(5):512–7.

102. Michalsen A, Jeitler M, Brunnhuber S, et al. Iyengar yoga for distressed women: a 3-armed randomized controlled trial. Evid Based Complement Altern Med 2012;2012:408727.

103. Chen K-M, Chen M-H, Chao H-C, et al. Sleep quality, depression state, and health status of older adults after silver yoga exercises: cluster randomized trial. Int J Nurs Stud 2009;46(2):154–63.

104. Khalsa SBS. Treatment of chronic insomnia with yoga: a preliminary study with sleep–wake diaries. Appl Psychophysiol Biofeedback 2004;29(4):269–78.

105. Irwin MR, Olmstead R, Motivala SJ. Improving sleep quality in older adults with moderate sleep complaints: a randomized controlled trial of Tai Chi Chih. Sleep 2008;31(7):1001–8.

106. Li F, Fisher KJ, Harmer P, et al. Tai Chi and self-rated quality of sleep and daytime sleepiness in older adults: a randomized controlled trial. J Am Geriatr Soc 2004;52(6):892–900.

107. Nguyen MH, Kruse A. A randomized controlled trial of tai chi for balance, sleep quality and cognitive performance in elderly Vietnamese. Clin Interv Aging 2012;7:185.

108. Wang D, Li W, Xiao Y, et al. Tryptophan for the sleeping disorder and mental symptom of new-type drug dependence: a randomized, double-blind, placebo-controlled trial. Medicine 2016;95(28):e4135.

109. Jones KD, Sherman CA, Mist SD, et al. A randomized controlled trial of 8-form tai chi improves symptoms and functional mobility in fibromyalgia patients. Clin Rheumatol 2012;31(8):1205–14.

110. Larkey LK, Roe DJ, Weihs KL, et al. Randomized controlled trial of Qigong/Tai Chi easy on cancer-related fatigue in breast cancer survivors. Ann Behav Med 2015;49(2):165–76.
111. Callahan LF, Cleveland RJ, Altpeter M, et al. Evaluation of Tai Chi Program effectiveness for people with arthritis in the community: a randomized controlled trial. J Aging Phys Act 2016;24(1):101–10.
112. Irwin MR, Olmstead R, Carrillo C, et al. Cognitive behavioral therapy vs. Tai Chi for late life insomnia and inflammatory risk: a randomized controlled comparative efficacy trial. Sleep 2014;37(9):1543–52.
113. Erland L, Saxena P. Melatonin natural health products and supplements: presence of serotonin and significant variability of melatonin content. J Clin Sleep Med 2016;13(2):275–81.
114. Chen HY, Shi Y, Ng CS, et al. Auricular acupuncture treatment for insomnia: a systematic review. J Altern Complement Med 2007;13(6):669–76.
115. Cao H, Pan X, Li H, et al. Acupuncture for treatment of insomnia: a systematic review of randomized controlled trials. J Altern Complement Med 2009;15(11):1171–86.
116. Kennedy DO, Wightman EL. Herbal extracts and phytochemicals: plant secondary metabolites and the enhancement of human brain function. Adv Nutr An Int Rev J 2011;2(1):32–50.
117. Cavadas C, Araujo I, Cotrim M, et al. In vitro study on the interaction of *Valeriana officinalis* L. extracts and their amino acids on GABAA receptor in rat brain. Arzneimittelforschung 1995;45(7):753–5.
118. Leach MJ, Page AT. Herbal medicine for insomnia: a systematic review and meta-analysis. Sleep Med Rev 2015;24:1–12.
119. Supplements CFESD, Medicine I, Council NR. Dietary supplements: a framework for evaluating safety. Washington (DC): National Academies Press (US); 2005.
120. NCCIH. Chamomile. 2016. Available at: https://nccih.nih.gov/health/chamomile/ataglance.htm. Accessed November 22, 2016.
121. Introduction to Chamomile. Available at: http://abc.herbalgram.org/site/DocServer/CRCPRESSChamomile-Section_1.5978-1-4665-7759-6.pdf?docID=6362. Accessed November, 2016.
122. Zanoli P, Avallone R, Baraldi M. Behavioral characterisation of the flavonoids apigenin and chrysin. Fitoterapia 2000;71(Suppl 1):S117–23.
123. Zick SM, Wright BD, Sen A, et al. Preliminary examination of the efficacy and safety of a standardized chamomile extract for chronic primary insomnia: a randomized placebo-controlled pilot study. BMC Complement Altern Med 2011;11(1):1.
124. Hudson C, Hudson SP, Hecht T, et al. Protein source tryptophan versus pharmaceutical grade tryptophan as an efficacious treatment for chronic insomnia. Nutr Neurosci 2013;8(2):121–7.
125. Lillehei AS, Halcon LL. A systematic review of the effect of inhaled essential oils on sleep. J Altern Complement Med 2014;20(6):441–51.
126. Moss M, Cook J, Wesnes K, et al. Aromas of rosemary and lavender essential oils differentially affect cognition and mood in healthy adults. Int J Neurosci 2003;113(1):15–38.
127. Henley DV, Lipson N, Korach KS, et al. Prepubertal gynecomastia linked to lavender and tea tree oils. N Engl J Med 2007;356(5):479–85.

Complementary and Integrative Medicine for Neurologic Conditions

Rebecca Erwin Wells, MD, MPH[a],*, Vanessa Baute, MD[a],
Helané Wahbeh, ND, MCR[b]

KEYWORDS

- Integrative medicine • Complementary medicine • Alternative medicine • Migraine
- Carpal tunnel syndrome • Headache • Dementia

KEY POINTS

- Patients are increasingly turning to complementary and alternative medicine (CAM) for neurologic conditions.
- Evidence is growing for CAM therapies, including lifestyle factors, mind-body practices, acupuncture, and supplements, in preventing and treatment migraine, carpal tunnel syndrome, and dementia.
- Clinicians are encouraged to be aware of these modalities and prepared to counsel their patients on their use.

INTRODUCTION

Although many neurologic conditions are common, cures are rare and conventional treatments are often limited. Many patients turn to complementary and alternative medicine (CAM) to find relief. CAM is defined as a group of diverse medical and health care systems, practices, and products that are not presently considered conventional medicine.[1] Although more than half of adults with common neurologic conditions use CAM, most have not discussed this use with their health care provider,[2,3] highlighting the need to make CAM use a routine part of the history and an important subject to understand as a provider. Patients are searching for additional treatments and having

The authors have nothing to disclose.
Dr R.E. Wells' research was supported by the National Center for Complementary & Integrative Health of the National Institutes of Health under Award Number 1K23AT008406-01A1. The content is solely the responsibility of the authors and does not necessarily represent the official views of the National Institutes of Health.
[a] Department of Neurology, Wake Forest Baptist Health, Medical Center Boulevard, Winston–Salem, NC 27157, USA; [b] Department of Neurology, Oregon Health and Science University, 3181 SW Sam Jackson Park Road, Portland, OR 97239, USA
* Corresponding author.
E-mail address: rewells@wakehealth.edu

http://dx.doi.org/10.1016/j.mcna.2017.04.006
0025-7125/17/© 2017 Elsevier Inc. All rights reserved.
medical.theclinics.com

an informed provider discuss and advise on CAM can clarify what modalities may have the most benefit. Devising an effective treatment plan for these conditions should include a discussion of CAM options. An integrative approach is especially important in improving self-efficacy and empowering the patient to make healthy changes that could provide significant benefit. Adherence to all treatments improves when patients believe they are actively involved in determining their plan of care. Treatments that belong within the CAM category change over time as treatments that were once considered alternative gain enough evidence to become accepted as mainstream. Lifestyle factors, mind-body practices, acupuncture, supplements, and therapeutic touch are modalities currently considered CAM and their use for migraine, carpal tunnel syndrome (CTS), and dementia are discussed in this article (**Table 1**).

MIGRAINE

Migraine is a recurrent disorder that manifests as severe, unilateral, pulsating headaches that worsen with activity, last 4 to 72 hours, and are associated with photophobia, phonophobia, nausea, and/or vomiting. Migraine is a clinical diagnosis made by history and examination, although red flags may warrant additional testing to rule out secondary headache disorders. This common and disabling condition affects 36 million Americans and costs $13 billion per year due to lost workdays, diminished productivity, and increased health care utilization.[4] Although the genetic predisposition to migraine gives rise to the condition for many individuals, effective preventive and treatment strategies can significantly diminish the frequency and disability. Pharmaceutical options have many limitations, such as patient preference, side effects, limited efficacy, comorbidities, pregnancy, and breastfeeding. These limitations may explain why up to 82% of migraineurs seek CAM options.[5] Lifestyle factors may trigger or influence the presence of individual migraine attacks, so nonpharmaceutical approaches become a key component to effective migraine prevention and management.

Nonpharmacological Treatment Options

Lifestyle
Unhealthy and irregular lifestyle factors may lower the headache threshold or even trigger individual migraine attacks. Targeting and treating lifestyle factors seems quite

Table 1
Potential nonpharmacological treatment options to consider with the strongest evidence for use for treatment and/or symptomatic relief of migraine, carpal tunnel syndrome, and dementia

Nonpharmacological Treatment Option	Neurologic Condition		
	Migraine	CTS	Dementia
Lifestyle (sleep, diet, exercise, stress)	✔	—	✔
Mind-body practices	✔	✔	✔
Acupuncture	✔	✔	—
Supplements[a]	✔	—	✔
Hand therapy[b]	—	✔	—
Therapeutic touch, music therapy	—	—	✔

[a] See **Table 2** for supplements for migraine; *Ginkgo biloba* and *Bacopa monnieri* have good evidence of benefit for dementia.
[b] Hand therapy treatment may include ultrasound; exercises to stretch the nerve, referred to as nerve gliding; myofascial release (an osteopathic manipulation technique); and/or iontophoresis.

simple but when done effectively can have profound positive effects on migraine frequency. Consistent meals, hydration, and appropriate sleep hygiene can provide the stability needed to decrease the likelihood of migraines. Lifestyle factors important in migraine prevention include

- Regularly scheduled meals; avoiding missing or delaying meal-time
- Routine hydration with noncaffeinated beverages throughout the day
- Consistent sleep schedule every night of the week, including weekends.

Certain foods, diets, and exercise may trigger or improve migraines for some individuals.[6,7] Obesity increases the risk of migraine converting from episodic to chronic. In addition, migraine and obesity are highly comorbid. Therefore, healthy diet and exercise interventions may be especially beneficial for migraineurs. Historically, long lists of foods to avoid are provided to migraine patients (eg, foods with tyramine, aspartame, monosodium glutamate, chocolate, and certain alcohols). However, the role of dietary triggers in migraine is complex because only some migraineurs may have food sensitivities and, even then, ingestion of a precipitant does not always trigger an attack. Only a few small studies with elimination diets have been conducted and evidence is promising but limited by methodological concerns. Further, broad lists of foods to avoid may be too restrictive, create undue anxiety, and limit otherwise healthy options. Carefully completed headache diaries may help patients self-identify certain triggers that can then be avoided (using the list of potential trigger foods as a guide in this process). Universal recommendations for elimination of all possible migraine food triggers in all migraine patients is not recommended, but a well-balanced diet with avoidance of fasting and skipping meals is recommended. Current research is ongoing that may help identify optimum diet and exercise programs for migraineurs.[8]

Mind-body practices

Stress is the number 1 reported trigger for migraines.[9] Treatments that target stress may be particularly beneficial in decreasing migraine frequency and in building additional coping behaviors. These behavioral interventions have grade A evidence for migraine prevention[10]:

- Cognitive behavioral therapy, including stress management and coping skills
- Biofeedback (electromyographic and thermal with relaxation)
- Relaxation training.

Evidence is beginning to emerge for treatment of migraine with mind-body practices.[11] For example, yoga[12] and mindfulness meditation[13] may be beneficial for migraines. An improvement in cardiac autonomic balance (eg, enhancement of vagal tone and drop in sympathetic drive) may be involved in the mechanism underlying these changes. Additional cognitive and affective mechanisms may be playing a role in the modulation of pain by these mind-body practices.[14] Despite American Headache Society recommendations against opioids for treatment of migraines, many patients may turn to opioids,[15] and mind-body practices may be a nonnarcotic option to achieve pain relief.[16]

Massage, chiropractic, and acupuncture

Although tension-type headaches have historically been considered a condition of muscular tension, many migraineurs also have concurrent neck pain with their migraines and find symptom relief with massage or chiropractic manipulation. Methodological shortcomings limit the interpretation of studies evaluating these treatment options[17] and more rigorous studies may suggest no additional benefit beyond placebo.[18,19] Chiropractic manipulation has been associated with rare life-threatening events, such as cervical artery dissection, although there is debate as to whether the association is causal.[20] Financial concerns often limit the widespread use of massage. Given the limited evidence, massage is not a treatment typically recommended for use in migraine. For those patients who can afford it and find symptomatic relief, it may be helpful. Future research could also further investigate the potential indirect effects of massage on migraine through its relaxation properties and resulting improvements in anxiety and/or stress. The lack of well-conducted research for chiropractic treatment, along with the potential risks of cervical manipulation, limits its recommendation for use for migraine.

Evidence suggests that acupuncture may be a helpful treatment of adults with migraines, even if the effect is similar to sham acupuncture.[21] Acupuncture also results in significantly fewer side effects compared with traditional pharmacologic treatments for migraine (6% with 24 sessions of acupuncture vs 66% with daily topiramate).[22] Given the potential benefits with minimal side effects, acupuncture may have a potential role in the treatment of migraine. Unfortunately, many patients find acupuncture cost-prohibitive, especially because it is not covered by most insurance companies in the United States. Group-based acupuncture sessions may be an affordable option if available.

Supplements

Herbs, vitamins, and minerals may help prevent headaches. Although considered natural, side effects can occur. Supplement quality and drug-supplement interactions also need to be considered. **Table 2** lists the supplements with American Academy of Neurology level A to C evidence (A, strongest; C, least strong) for use in the prevention of episodic migraine.[25] MIG-99 (an extract of the herb feverfew [*Tanacetum parthenium*]), magnesium, and riboflavin (vitamin B2) have level B evidence for migraine prevention, and coenzyme Q10 has level C evidence. Although *Petasites hybridus* (butterbur) was categorized as level A, recent concerns over hepatotoxicity have limited recommendations for its use so it is not included in the table.

Oral magnesium has historically been used for migraine during pregnancy. However, the US Food and Drug Administration (FDA) recently reclassified magnesium sulfate injections as pregnancy category D from A, based on potential teratogenic effects on fetal bone growth. Because magnesium is typically administered orally for migraine prevention, the safety of oral magnesium for migraine during pregnancy is currently under debate.[24] Given magnesium's current classification as category D, and the lack of research on the impact of daily oral magnesium on the fetus, precaution is advised for use in pregnancy.

A few studies suggest pyridoxine (vitamin B6), melatonin, omega-3 fish oil, vitamin D3, and supplement combinations (eg, folic acid/B6/B12) may have potential benefits for migraine, but evidence is preliminary and recommendations cannot be made at this time. As with daily prophylactic medications, supplements need to be used at the goal dose for 2 to 3 months before determining effectiveness.

New devices and treatment options

There are several new FDA-approved devices for treatment of migraine (eg, transcranial magnetic stimulation and transcutaneous electrical nerve stimulation) and more under investigation. Although these are an option for those seeking nondrug treatment options, they are not discussed here. However, research is promising[26,27] and further clinical use will help determine their role in clinical care.

Table 2
Supplements for migraine prevention

Oral Supplement	AAN Grade of Evidence for Migraine Treatment[a]	Typical Recommended Dose or Frequency for Migraine	Potential Side Effects[23]	Comments
MIG-99 (feverfew extract)	B	6.25 mg 3 times/d	Arthralgias, oral ulcers	• Avoid in pregnancy (can cause uterine contractions)
Magnesium citrate[b]	B	400–600 mg daily	Soft stools, diarrhea, flushing	• May be more beneficial for migraine with aura or menstrual migraine • Gastrointestinal side effects may be helpful for those with constipation • Safety during pregnancy is debated (see article for details)[24] • Renal failure should prohibit the use of magnesium
Riboflavin (vitamin B2)	B	400 mg daily	Diarrhea, polyuria, bright yellow urine	—
Coenzyme Q10 (CoQ10)	C	100 mg 3 times/d	Anorexia, dyspepsia, nausea, diarrhea, rash	—

[a] American Academy of Neurology (AAN) Guidelines: A, strongest evidence; C, least strong evidence.[25]
[b] If problems with diarrhea while on magnesium citrate, magnesium glycinate formulation may be better tolerated.

CARPAL TUNNEL SYNDROME

CTS is an entrapment of the median nerve at the wrist that causes painful paresthesias, numbness, and occasional weakness of selected hand muscles. It is the most common nerve entrapment syndrome, affecting 10 million individuals in the United States alone. Four percent of the general population, 10% of the working population, and over 30% of pregnant women have CTS.[28] Risk factors for CTS include repetitive hand use, obesity, pregnancy (progressively worse in later terms), diabetes, thyroid dysfunction, and other medical conditions.[28] The debilitating symptoms can lead to significant disability at work and in daily activities. CTS is diagnosed by history; physical examination; electrodiagnostic studies, including nerve conduction studies and electromyography; and neuromuscular ultrasound.[29]

The conventional treatment of CTS has historically been divided into surgical (ie, transection of the transverse carpal ligament) and nonsurgical options, such as splinting, oral anti-inflammatories, and steroid injections. The recurrence rate, potential complications of surgical intervention, need for less invasive treatment during pregnancy, and patient preference make integrative therapies important options to consider when developing treatment plans for CTS. Up to one-third of patients already request alternative therapies for CTS.[30] Further, these therapies can be used in an integrative approach in conjunction with traditional approaches.

Nonpharmacological Treatment Options

A variety of studies assess integrative therapies for CTS.[30] Those with limited investigative research include yoga, acupuncture, hand physical therapy, and magnet therapy. Although research evidence is limited, these options may be reasonable noninvasive considerations to try before surgical referral in select patients requesting a trial of less invasive therapy. It is reasonable to move on to another therapy if there is no improvement in symptoms after a 4 to 8 week trial.

Mind-body practices

Yoga has been explored as a treatment of CTS. In a well-designed *Journal of the American Medical Association* study, 8 weeks of yoga was compared with standard of care wrist splint use.[31] Those in the yoga-based intervention experienced increased grip strength and decreased pain when compared with the wrist splint, although no physiologic changes were seen on nerve conduction studies. Patients need to be counseled on the importance of gentle yoga, typically found in a restorative or hatha style yoga class. Patients should avoid any poses that cause discomfort in the wrist area and should inform their instructors of their condition.

Acupuncture

The 1997 National Institutes of Health consensus statement concluded that acupuncture may be useful adjunct therapy or as an acceptable alternative treatment of CTS.[32] A more recent systematic review from 2016 also confirms these findings.[33] Acupuncture treatment has been shown to be as effective as oral steroids for CTS over a 4 week period and this effect seems to be sustained over a 1-year follow-up period.[34,35] When compared with wrist splinting, patients treated with acupuncture report fewer symptoms and improved physiologic measures with improved nerve conduction velocities.[36]

Manual treatments

Hand therapy is a well-established, although underutilized, modality typically performed by physical or occupational therapists.[37] It is included here as a reminder of an effective, less invasive integrative therapy that can be used alone or as an adjunct. A hand therapy treatment session may include ultrasound; exercises to stretch the nerve, referred to as nerve gliding; myofascial release, an osteopathic manipulation technique; and/or iontophoresis. Nerve gliding was found to reduce pain and increase active range of motion of wrist extension and flexion.[37] Ultrasound is a brief, well-tolerated technique that exposes injured tissue to varying frequencies of sound waves either continuously or in a pulsed manner. When compared with superficial and continuous exposure, deep pulsed ultrasound is more effective in reducing pain, paresthesia, and sensory loss, and in improving median nerve conduction and strength.[38] This is the ultrasound modality used in most hand therapy clinics for CTS treatment.

Magnet therapy

Patients with CTS may seek treatment with magnetic wristbands and often inquire to their physicians about this treatment. The proposed mechanism of action involves increased local vascularity, vascular tone, alterations in the sodium potassium pump, and decreases in histamine and carrageenan.[39,40] Several small studies have shown improvements in electrodiagnostic testing and pain scales with the use of magnetized wristbands.[41–43] However, the research is preliminary, has methodological concerns, and only provides limited clinical information for treatment recommendations. Although magnet therapy cannot be recommended as treatment at this time for CTS, further research is important to better understand efficacy, dose, and duration.

DEMENTIA

Dementia refers to a loss of cognitive function, resulting in decreased understanding, perception, or awareness of one's thoughts and ideas. Some risk factors for dementia include age, atherosclerosis, genetics, head trauma, and various infections of the brain and body, such as syphilis or human immunodeficiency virus. Dementia may occur gradually or quickly and can be caused by brain changes associated with disease or trauma. An estimated 2 million Americans suffer from severe dementia; 1 to 5 million experience mild to moderate dementia.[44] Some causes of dementia are preventable; however, many causes of dementia, such as Alzheimer disease, have no cure. Standard of care pharmaceutical treatments attempt to, at best, slow symptom progression. Integrative therapeutics may offer complementary options to patients interested in such modalities. Due to increased popularity, research and evidence for the benefit of some of these treatments are growing, especially for memory loss.[2] With the limited options for treatment or cure, and the devastation of dementia sequelae, many are desperate to find additional options. Patients with cognitive impairment may be additionally susceptible to poor judgment, given their condition, so appropriate counseling about treatment and recommendations becomes critically important.[45]

Nonpharmacological Treatment Options

Diet and lifestyle
Nutrition, exercise, sleep, and stress all play a part in the pathophysiology of memory loss. Studies have examined prevention and treatment of age-related cognitive decline, mild cognitive impairment (MCI), and people with dementia. Often the recommendations for prevention and treatment overlap.

Nutrition One relevant and preventable risk factor is nutritional deficiencies.[46] Deficiencies of certain nutrients, especially the B vitamins, may lead to dementia. Homocysteine levels in the body are increased with deficiencies of folic acid, vitamin B1 (thiamine), and vitamin B12 (cyanocobalamin). An elevated homocysteine level is thought to be a risk factor for developing dementia and heart disease. Iron deficiency may lead to anemia, which can lead to brain cell death and eventually dementia.[47] These vitamin deficiencies may be driven by the challenges many elderly patients have in eating high-quality, fresh fruits, vegetables, whole grains, and good quality protein sources. The International Conference on Nutrition and the Brain recently developed recommendations on diet and lifestyle recommendations for the prevention of Alzheimer disease.[48] Briefly, they recommend, reducing saturated fats and trans fats intake; increasing vegetables, legumes, fruits, and whole grains; vitamin E from foods rather than supplements (15 mg/d); a reliable source of B12 (2.4 mg/d); choosing multivitamins without iron and copper unless anemia is a concern; and minimizing aluminum exposure.

Exercise Evidence from well-designed meta-analyses consistently support that physical activity and exercise, especially aerobic exercise such as walking, jogging, and bicycling, improve cognitive outcomes in older adults and individuals with dementia.[49]

Interestingly, physical activity that requires memory for muscle movement, such as tai chi and dance, also improve cognitive outcomes.[49] Exercise may affect dementia by increasing hippocampus size.[50] A current exercise recommendation for the prevention of Alzheimer disease is 40 minutes of aerobic exercise 3 times per week at an intensity equivalent to brisk walking.[48]

Sleep Approximately 25% of adults are not satisfied with their sleep: 10% to 15% have insomnia symptoms with negative daytime consequences and 6% to 10% meet diagnostic criteria for insomnia. A clear association exists between sleep impairment and cognitive impairment or Alzheimer disease.[51] Approximately 7 to 8 hours of sleep is recommended for most individuals. Evaluating and treating any underlying sleep disorders, such as obstructive sleep apnea, is also very important.[48]

Stress Psychological stress and reactivity to stress affects brain health. Chronic psychological stress contributes to cognitive decline, hippocampal injury, and neurodegenerative diseases, either directly or through stress mediators.[52] Stress clearly has an influence on cognitive function. Any intervention that could support a reduction in stress or stress reactivity would support the prevention of stress impairing cognition. Mind-body medicine is the therapy of choice for stress reduction in patients because of its great evidence for improving stress markers.

Mind-body medicine
Meditation, among most common mind-body medicine therapies, has moderate support for effectiveness for improving cognition in nonimpaired adults and older adults.[49] Evidence for meditation's mechanism of action on cognition has been evaluated directly through various pathways in meditators versus controls. For example, brain structure changes have been observed in meditators in areas associated with self-regulation, self-control, focused problem-solving, adaptive behavioral responses under changing conditions, visuospatial imagery, episodic memory retrieval, and self-processing operations.[53] A systematic review of 12 studies found evidence that meditation for older adults is feasible and may offset age-related cognitive decline.[54] Indirect mechanisms may also be at play because meditation may target other mediating factors that affect cognition, such as sleep. A systematic review found positive evidence to suggest benefit of mind-body therapies for sleep, especially in the elderly.[55] Research is limited on meditation's impact in those with MCI or dementia; however, 1 small study showed that in adults with MCI meditation positively affected the regions of the brain most related to dementia.[56] Tai chi, a form of moving meditation, also has evidence for enhancing cognitive function, especially executive functioning, in older adults.[57]

Cognitive training or stimulation has evidence from well-designed meta-analyses that consistently supports improved cognitive outcomes in people with dementia. The affected outcomes include improved memory and mental ability; making fewer errors when learning; verbal and visual learning; improved executive functioning, language, and attention; improved functioning in activities of daily living; and lower depression. Remarkably, the effects of cognitive training seem to last as long as 5 years after therapy.[49]

Supplements
Ginkgo biloba and Bacopa monnieri have good evidence of benefit for dementia. In a rigorous meta-analysis, 240 mg/d of G biloba extract was found to be effective and safe in the treatment of dementia.[58] B monnieri, otherwise known as water hyssop, also has evidence from a meta-analysis demonstrating improved cognition, especially

speed of attention.[59] Omega-3 fatty acid therapy has positive but conflicting results on dosage and benefit, so more rigorous research is recommended.[60] Other natural products, such as phosphatidylserine, huperzine-A, coenzyme Q10, and caprylic acid, are often used but still need further research to evaluate efficacy for dementia and related symptoms.

Other

Therapies such as reiki, therapeutic touch, and healing touch have moderate evidence to decrease agitation and salivary cortisol, and improve cognitive function and mood in adults with dementia.[49] Therapeutic touch reduced physical nonaggressive behaviors in 1 study with Alzheimer patients.[61] Multiple randomized controlled trials consistently demonstrate the benefit of music therapy for dementia. Taught individually or in a group setting, music therapy aims to improve quality of life and is based on music's influence on nonmusical brain and behavior functions.[49]

SUMMARY AND FUTURE CONSIDERATIONS

Complementary treatments with the best evidence for migraine include lifestyle factors, mind-body therapies, acupuncture, and supplements (MIG-99 or feverfew, magnesium, riboflavin, and CoQ10). Complementary therapies with the best evidence for CTS include yoga, acupuncture, and hand therapy. The complementary treatments with the best evidence for dementia include nutrition, exercise, cognitive training, meditation, *G biloba*, and *B monnieri*. **Table 1** summarizes which treatments to consider for each condition.

Complementary and integrative approaches may provide additional benefit in the prevention and/or treatment of migraines, CTS, and dementia. These treatments may be used concurrently with conventional therapies. The refractory and persistent nature of these conditions makes many patients seek such additional treatment options. The evidence is growing for many complementary modalities and they warrant consideration for inclusion into treatment plans. However, many complementary treatments may have adverse effects, and even ones considered safe involve time, cost, energy, and effort, all valuable resources. Although some research suggests that nonpharmacologic treatments may take longer to see benefit, their effect may be more durable over time, better tolerated, and may confer other benefits to overall wellness, such as improvements in stress, quality of life, pain, anxiety, and depression.[62]

A small (N = 10) pilot integrative program that created personalized recommendations on a combination of CAM interventions, such as diet, exercise, stress, brain stimulation, supplements, and so forth, shows promise for dementia treatment and the need for future expansion and testing.[63,64] Although multimodal treatment interventions make it difficult to tease out active ingredients, such treatment approaches demonstrate the possibility of both personalized plans and combination interventions as treatment options.

Questions persist about complementary treatments regarding optimal dose, frequency, duration, efficacy, and mechanisms. Further research with long-term data, larger sample sizes, and optimal control groups are needed. In addition, more research is needed on additional integrative therapies for neurologic conditions because current therapies still leave many patients with chronic pain and/or impaired function. It is hoped that future research will help elucidate which nonpharmacological treatments are most efficacious for which neurologic patient. Until then, providers can guide patients on the best treatment options based on evidence, interests, adherence, cost, and access.

ACKNOWLEDGMENTS

Dr V. Baute would like to acknowledge Edina Wang and Vahakn Keskinyan (3rd year medical students) for assistance with literature review, and Dr Michael Cartwright for editing and mentorship.

REFERENCES

1. Complementary, alternative, or integrative health: what's in a name? 2016; Available at: https://nccih.nih.gov/health/integrative-health. Accessed January 9, 2017.
2. Wells RE, Phillips RS, Schachter SC, et al. Complementary and alternative medicine use among US adults with common neurological conditions. J Neurol 2010; 257(11):1822–31.
3. Wells RE, Bertisch SM, Buettner C, et al. Complementary and alternative medicine use among adults with migraines/severe headaches. Headache 2011; 51(7):1087–97.
4. Hu XH, Markson LE, Lipton RB, et al. Burden of migraine in the United States: disability and economic costs. Arch Intern Med 1999;159(8):813–8.
5. Adams J, Barbery G, Lui CW. Complementary and alternative medicine use for headache and migraine: a critical review of the literature. Headache 2013; 53(3):459–73.
6. Irby MB, Bond DS, Lipton RB, et al. Aerobic exercise for reducing migraine burden: mechanisms, markers, and models of change processes. Headache 2016;56(2):357–69.
7. Orr SL. Diet and nutraceutical interventions for headache management: A review of the evidence. Cephalalgia 2016;36(12):1112–33.
8. Bond DS, O'Leary KC, Thomas JG, et al. Can weight loss improve migraine headaches in obese women? Rationale and design of the women's health and migraine (WHAM) randomized controlled trial. Contemp Clin Trials 2013;35(1): 133–44.
9. Peroutka SJ. What turns on a migraine? A systematic review of migraine precipitating factors. Curr Pain Headache Rep 2014;18(10):454.
10. Campbell JK, Penzien DB, Wall EM. Evidence-based guidelines for migraine headache: behavioral and physical treatments. US Headache Consortium 2000. Available at: http://www.neurology.org/content/55/6/754.full.pdf. Accessed July 14, 2009.
11. Wells RE, Smitherman TA, Seng EK, et al. Behavioral and mind/body interventions in headache: unanswered questions and future research directions. Headache 2014;54(6):1107–13.
12. Kisan R, Sujan M, Adoor M, et al. Effect of yoga on migraine: a comprehensive study using clinical profile and cardiac autonomic functions. Int J Yoga 2014; 7(2):126–32.
13. Wells RE, Burch R, Paulsen RH, et al. Meditation for migraines: a pilot randomized controlled trial. Headache 2014;54(9):1484–95.
14. Bushnell MC, Ceko M, Low LA. Cognitive and emotional control of pain and its disruption in chronic pain. Nat Rev Neurosci 2013;14(7):502–11.
15. Loder E, Weizenbaum E, Frishberg B, et al. Choosing wisely in headache medicine: the American Headache Society's list of five things physicians and patients should question. Headache 2013;53(10):1651–9.
16. Zeidan F, Vago DR. Mindfulness meditation-based pain relief: a mechanistic account. Ann N Y Acad Sci 2016;1373(1):114–27.

17. Chaibi A, Tuchin PJ, Russell MB. Manual therapies for migraine: a systematic review. J Headache Pain 2011;12(2):127–33.
18. Posadzki P, Ernst E. Spinal manipulations for the treatment of migraine: a systematic review of randomized clinical trials. Cephalalgia 2011;31(8):964–70.
19. Chaibi A, Benth JS, Tuchin PJ, et al. Chiropractic spinal manipulative therapy for migraine: a three-armed, single-blinded, placebo, randomized controlled trial. Eur J Neurol 2017;24(1):143–53.
20. Gouveia LO, Castanho P, Ferreira JJ. Safety of chiropractic interventions: a systematic review. Spine 2009;34(11):E405–13.
21. Coeytaux RR, Befus D. Role of acupuncture in the treatment or prevention of migraine, tension-type headache, or chronic headache disorders. Headache 2016;56(7):1238–40.
22. Yang CP, Chang MH, Liu PE, et al. Acupuncture versus topiramate in chronic migraine prophylaxis: a randomized clinical trial. Cephalalgia 2011;31(15): 1510–21.
23. Tepper SJ. Nutraceutical and other modalities for the treatment of headache. Continuum (Minneap Minn) 2015;21(4 Headache):1018–31.
24. Wells RE, Turner DP, Lee M, et al. Managing migraine during pregnancy and lactation. Curr Neurol Neurosci Rep 2016;16(4):40.
25. Holland S, Silberstein SD, Freitag F, et al. Evidence-based guideline update: NSAIDs and other complementary treatments for episodic migraine prevention in adults: report of the quality standards subcommittee of the American Academy of Neurology and the American Headache Society. Neurology 2012;78(17): 1346–53.
26. Puledda F, Goadsby PJ. An update on non-pharmacological neuromodulation for the acute and preventive treatment of migraine. Headache 2017;57(4):685–91.
27. Robbins MS, Lipton RB. Transcutaneous and Percutaneous Neurostimulation for Headache Disorders. Headache 2017;57(Suppl 1):4–13.
28. Meems M, Truijens S, Spek V, et al. Prevalence, course and determinants of carpal tunnel syndrome symptoms during pregnancy: a prospective study. BJOG 2015;122(8):1112–8.
29. Cartwright MS, Hobson-Webb LD, Boon AJ, et al. Evidence-based guideline: neuromuscular ultrasound for the diagnosis of carpal tunnel syndrome. Muscle Nerve 2012;46(2):287–93.
30. Huisstede BM, Hoogvliet P, Randsdorp MS, et al. Carpal tunnel syndrome. Part I: effectiveness of nonsurgical treatments–a systematic review. Arch Phys Med Rehabil 2010;91(7):981–1004.
31. Garfinkel MS, Singhal A, Katz WA, et al. Yoga-based intervention for carpal tunnel syndrome: a randomized trial. JAMA 1998;280(18):1601–3.
32. Acupuncture. NIH Consens Statement 1997;15(5):1–34.
33. Cox J, Varatharajan S, Cote P, et al. Effectiveness of acupuncture therapies to manage musculoskeletal disorders of the extremities: a systematic review. J Orthop Sports Phys Ther 2016;46(6):409–29.
34. Yang CP, Hsieh CL, Wang NH, et al. Acupuncture in patients with carpal tunnel syndrome: a randomized controlled trial. Clin J Pain 2009;25(4):327–33.
35. Yang CP, Wang NH, Li TC, et al. A randomized clinical trial of acupuncture versus oral steroids for carpal tunnel syndrome: a long-term follow-up. J Pain 2011;12(2): 272–9.
36. Khosrawi S, Moghtaderi A, Haghighat S. Acupuncture in treatment of carpal tunnel syndrome: a randomized controlled trial study. J Res Med Sci 2012;17(1):1–7.

37. Muller M, Tsui D, Schnurr R, et al. Effectiveness of hand therapy interventions in primary management of carpal tunnel syndrome: a systematic review. J Hand Ther 2004;17(2):210–28.

38. Ebenbichler GR, Resch KL, Nicolakis P, et al. Ultrasound treatment for treating the carpal tunnel syndrome: randomised "sham" controlled trial. BMJ 1998; 316(7133):731–5.

39. Morris CE, Skalak TC. Acute exposure to a moderate strength static magnetic field reduces edema formation in rats. Am J Physiol Heart Circ Physiol 2008; 294(1):H50–7.

40. Nikolic L, Bataveljic D, Andjus PR, et al. Changes in the expression and current of the Na+/K+ pump in the snail nervous system after exposure to a static magnetic field. J Exp Biol 2013;216(Pt 18):3531–41.

41. Kamel DM, Hamed NS, Abdel Raoof NA, et al. Pulsed magnetic field versus ultrasound in the treatment of postnatal carpal tunnel syndrome: a randomized controlled trial in the women of an Egyptian population. J Adv Res 2017;8(1): 45–53.

42. Weintraub MI, Cole SP. Neuromagnetic treatment of pain in refractory carpal tunnel syndrome: An electrophysiological and placebo analysis. J Back Musculoskelet Rehabil 2000;15(2):77–81.

43. Weintraub MI, Cole SP. A randomized controlled trial of the effects of a combination of static and dynamic magnetic fields on carpal tunnel syndrome. Pain Med 2008;9(5):493–504.

44. Plassman BL, Langa KM, McCammon RJ, et al. Incidence of dementia and cognitive impairment, not dementia in the United States. Ann Neurol 2011; 70(3):418–26.

45. Robillard JM. The online environment: a key variable in the ethical response to complementary and alternative medicine for Alzheimer's disease. J Alzheimers Dis 2016;51(1):11–3.

46. Bowman GL, Silbert LC, Howieson D, et al. Nutrient biomarker patterns, cognitive function, and MRI measures of brain aging. Neurology 2012;78(4):241–9.

47. Bhatti AB, Usman M, Ali F, et al. Vitamin Supplementation as an Adjuvant Treatment for Alzheimer's Disease. J Clin Diagn Res 2016;10(8):OE07–11.

48. Barnard ND, Bush AI, Ceccarelli A, et al. Dietary and lifestyle guidelines for the prevention of Alzheimer's disease. Neurobiol Aging 2014;35(Suppl 2):S74–8.

49. Burgener SC, Jao YL, Anderson JG, et al. Mechanism of action for nonpharmacological therapies for individuals with dementia: implications for practice and research. Res Gerontol Nurs 2015;8(5):240–59.

50. Erickson KI, Voss MW, Prakash RS, et al. Exercise training increases size of hippocampus and improves memory. Proc Natl Acad Sci U S A 2011;108(7): 3017–22.

51. Bubu OM, Brannick M, Mortimer J, et al. Sleep, cognitive impairment and Alzheimer's disease: a systematic review and meta-analysis. Sleep 2017;40(1):1–18.

52. Oken BS, Fonareva I, Wahbeh H. Stress-related cognitive dysfunction in dementia caregivers. J Geriatr Psychiatry Neurol 2011;24(4):191–8.

53. Boccia M, Piccardi L, Guariglia P. The meditative mind: a comprehensive meta-analysis of MRI studies. Biomed Res Int 2015;2015:419808.

54. Gard T, Holzel BK, Lazar SW. The potential effects of meditation on age-related cognitive decline: a systematic review. Ann N Y Acad Sci 2014;1307:89–103.

55. Neuendorf R, Wahbeh H, Chamine I, et al. The effects of mind-body interventions on sleep quality: a systematic review. Evid Based Complement Alternat Med 2015;2015:902708.

56. Wells RE, Yeh GY, Kerr CE, et al. Meditation's impact on default mode network and hippocampus in mild cognitive impairment: a pilot study. Neurosci Lett 2013;556:15–9.

57. Wayne PM, Walsh JN, Taylor-Piliae RE, et al. Effect of tai chi on cognitive performance in older adults: systematic review and meta-analysis. J Am Geriatr Soc 2014;62(1):25–39.

58. Hashiguchi M, Ohta Y, Shimizu M, et al. Meta-analysis of the efficacy and safety of *Ginkgo biloba* extract for the treatment of dementia. J Pharm Health Care Sci 2015;1:14.

59. Kongkeaw C, Dilokthornsakul P, Thanarangsarit P, et al. Meta-analysis of randomized controlled trials on cognitive effects of *Bacopa monnieri* extract. J Ethnopharmacol 2014;151(1):528–35.

60. Knochel C, Voss M, Gruter F, et al. Omega-3 fatty acids: repurposing opportunities for cognition and biobehavioral disturbances in MCI and Dementia. Curr Alzheimer Res 2017;14(3):240–54.

61. Millan-Calenti JC, Lorenzo-Lopez L, Alonso-Bua B, et al. Optimal nonpharmacological management of agitation in Alzheimer's disease: challenges and solutions. Clin Interv Aging 2016;11:175–84.

62. Khoury B, Sharma M, Rush SE, et al. Mindfulness-based stress reduction for healthy individuals: a meta-analysis. J Psychosom Res 2015;78(6):519–28.

63. Bredesen DE, Amos EC, Canick J, et al. Reversal of cognitive decline in Alzheimer's disease. Aging (Albany NY) 2016;8(6):1250–8.

64. Bredesen DE. Reversal of cognitive decline: a novel therapeutic program. Aging (Albany NY) 2014;6(9):707–17.

Integrative Medicine for Cardiovascular Disease and Prevention

Monica Aggarwal, MD[a],*, Brooke Aggarwal, EdD, MS[b],
Jyothi Rao, MD, FAARFM[c]

KEYWORDS

- Cardiovascular disease • Prevention • Integrative medicine • Nutrition
- Hypertension • Supplements • Alternative therapies • Stress

KEY POINTS

- Cardiovascular disease is traditionally treated through medications and lifestyle modifications, yet adherence to these treatments is often poor.
- The use of complementary therapies, such as nonprescription vitamins and herbs, is increasing, and patients are seeking information from their physicians about the safety and effectiveness of these therapies.
- When considering integrative therapies for cardiovascular disease, it is important to understand the underlying pathogenesis of the disease, which may be linked to chronic stress, inflammation, and altered gut microbiota.
- There is evidence for several promising integrative therapies for the treatment and prevention of cardiovascular disease, including specific nutritional approaches, meditation, yoga, acupuncture, and select supplements and herbal therapies.
- Physicians should be diligent in asking patients about any alternative therapies for cardiovascular disease that they may be using, and be capable of discussing the risk/benefit ratio of these options.

Cardiovascular disease (CVD) remains the number 1 cause of morbidity and mortality globally.[1] Early intervention with angiography and broad-based pharmaceutical therapies has contributed to a decline in deaths from CVD in the United States, yet the prevalence of risk factors and economic burden of CVD remain exceedingly high.

Disclosure Statement: M. Aggarwal and J. Rao have nothing to disclose. Dr B. Aggarwal receives research funding from an American Heart Association (grant no: AHA 16SFRN27960011) Go Red for Women Research Network award. No conflicts of interest to report.
[a] Division of Cardiology, University of Florida, 1600 Southwest Archer Road, PO Box 100288, Gainesville, FL 32610, USA; [b] Division of Cardiology, Department of Medicine, Columbia University Medical Center, 51 Audubon Avenue, Suite 505, New York, NY 10032, USA; [c] Shakthi Health and Wellness Center, 2702 Back Acre Circle Suite 290C, Mt. Airy, MD 21771, USA
* Corresponding author.
E-mail address: monica.aggarwal@medicine.ufl.edu

Commonly, patients are placed on a minimum of 4 to 6 medications at any given time, which increases financial burden, worsens compliance rates, and increases rates of side effects and medication interactions. Expenditures on medications per capita in the United States in 2014 increased 10.3% to $373.9 billion from the year prior.[2] This increase is driven primarily by new treatment options, rising prices, and increased usage of medications.[3]

Traditional lifestyle measures for prevention of CVD include smoking cessation, maintaining a healthy body weight, regular exercise, and dietary changes involving reducing saturated fats, increasing fruits and vegetables, and limiting sugar intake. However, physicians are often unaware of what specific lifestyle changes to make, such as types of exercise regimens and targeted changes in the diet.[4]

The demand for integrative medicine is fueled by, among many things, patients' desires for nonpharmacologic options. However, guidelines and regulations of these therapies are not optimal, and there are issues with contamination of supplements and different potencies in different varieties. In addition, herb-drug interactions are often not fully recognized. It is imperative for physicians to start a discussion of complementary practices with patients to ensure safety and effective use of both traditional and integrative practices.

PATHOGENESIS OF CHRONIC DISEASE STATES, INCLUDING CARDIOVASCULAR DISEASE

Cardiovascular disease has been associated with an imbalance in the autonomic nervous system.[5] The sympathetic or "fight or flight" nervous system is activated in times of stress. As a result, cortisol and epinephrine levels are heightened. These hormones allow our blood pressures and heart rates to rise so we have adequate blood flow to essential organs for flight and allow the body to be alert. Our immune system also triggers an inflammatory cascade. The parasympathetic or "rest and digest" nervous system offsets the sympathetic nervous system. It brings the cortisol levels and epinephrine levels down. Blood flow goes back to nonessential processes, such as eating and bladder and bowel movements.

Often, our bodies are heavily shifted toward sympathetic overdrive, which leads to burnout. With this imbalance, there are chronically elevated hormone levels, which result in elevated blood pressures and heart rates on a long-term basis. In times of burnout, there is significant imbalance in the immune response and there is evidence of increased inflammatory markers, decreased wound healing, and poorer response to infection.[6] With chronic stress, there is overactivation of the hormonal systems and subsequent formation of disease-causing free radicals causing oxidative stress.[7] Inflammation and oxidative stress can then cause chronic fatigue, depression, and excessive weight gain. In addition, persistent elevation of cortisol can lead to insulin resistance, which can cause diabetes and CVD, such as hypertension, ischemic heart disease, congestive heart failure, and arrhythmias.[5]

The integrative treatment approach in cardiology focuses on bringing the "rest and digest" system into balance with the "fight or flight" system. Boosting the "rest and digest" nervous system often requires learning the art of meditation, yoga, and movement. It also involves understanding the impact of food on our bodies and putting healthful foods into our system to aid in proper digestion. It also requires us to understand about environmental exposures, such as pollution and heavy metal exposures.

HYPERTENSION

Hypertension affects almost one-third of our population, with 75% of those patients taking antihypertensive medication. However, only approximately half of this group is considered well controlled. Often known as the "silent killer," hypertension is the culprit associated with end-organ damage in terms of stroke, kidney dysfunction, and vascular disease. Although hypertension is familial, obesity, smoking, and alcohol intake are well-known precipitating risk factors. Dietary changes are also essential for managing hypertension. The pioneer trial that examined the role of diet in the management of hypertension was the Dietary Approaches to Stop Hypertension (DASH) trial in 1997.

DASH was a large, prospective, multicenter trial that looked at lifestyle changes to affect blood pressure. The diet assigned to the intervention group was composed of fruits, vegetables, and low-fat dairy: a diet low in fat and cholesterol. Seventy-five percent of the US-recommended allowance of magnesium and potassium was advocated. The sodium consumption between the control and the intervention group was no different at approximately 3 g sodium per day. Within 2 weeks of the intervention, blood pressures reduced and the results sustained for another 6 weeks. Systolic blood pressure (SBP) reduced by 5.5 mm Hg and diastolic blood pressure (DBP) by 3.0 mm Hg more than the control diet.[8] This was a pivotal trial that demonstrated the effectiveness of dietary interventions in the treatment of hypertension.

Role of Sodium in the Diet for Hypertensive Patients

The role of sodium in the diet has come under controversy. For centuries, there has been a concern that excessive sodium intake triggers hypertension. The early Intersalt study[9] showed across various populations that those with a higher sodium urinary excretion rate had a higher blood pressure. Subsequently, the DASH study[8] gave patients a low-fat vegetarian diet that was high in fruits and vegetables with no sodium adjustment. Those who ate this diet were noted to have improved blood pressure. A DASH follow-up study[10] used the same diet randomizing to 3 different levels of sodium (high, medium, and low). After 30 days, patients on the lowest-sodium diet had the most significant blood pressure reduction. Thus, for a decade, the low-sodium diet was advocated. More recently, the Prospective Urban and Rural Epidemiological (PURE)[11] study evaluated more than 150,000 people and found a more moderate sodium intake was associated with the lowest overall mortality. That same year, a large meta-analysis was done corroborating this U-shaped relationship between salt intake and mortality; that is, too little and too much sodium was associated with higher mortality than usual sodium intake.[12] The Centers for Disease Control and Prevention and American Heart Association (AHA) continue to advocate a lower-sodium diet for the management of hypertension, recommending most Americans eat less than 1500 mg/d of sodium for "ideal" cardiovascular health. This recommendation continues to be controversial. We believe the most impact of sodium restriction is on patients with hypertension. Most Americans eat excessive sodium in their diet, 75% of which comes from processed, prepackaged, and restaurant foods.[13] Dietary changes, such as the DASH diet and the addition of potassium-rich foods, can counterbalance the deleterious effects of excess sodium, and should therefore be recommended.

Endothelial Dysfunction and Hypertension

One of the pathways associated with generation of essential hypertension is impaired endothelium-dependent vasodilation.[14] Healthy endothelium releases potent vasodilators in response to blood flow, which can lower vascular resistance directly. Nitric oxide (NO) is essential to causing vasodilatation of the arteries and is associated with antithrombotic and atheroresistant effects of the arterial wall.[15] Decreases in NO and increased vascular tone trigger sympathetic tone and increase sodium retention.[14] Impaired endothelium is a well-established response to cardiovascular risk factors and is a precursor to CVD.

Nitrates

Dietary nitrates and their ability to increase NO levels has been studied and shown beneficial effects in clinical settings (**Table 1**). Data suggest fruits and vegetables provide a substrate for reduction of nitrate to nitrite and NO. This production leads to vasodilatation and a decrease in blood pressure.[16] Other studies have shown the production of NO has the ability to inhibit endothelial inflammatory cell recruitment and platelet aggregation.[17] By aiding in healthy endothelial function, NO production can aid in prevention of CVD, hypertension, atherosclerosis, and stroke.[18]

Although studies on intake of nitrate and nitrite through foods have shown cardiovascular benefits,[19] nitrates have also come under criticism as toxic and associated with increased gastric cancer.[20,21] Current data, however, suggest that there is an increased risk of gastric cancer with nitrate/nitrite ingestion from nitrate-preserved meats, whereas nitrites from vegetables are associated with reduced gastric cancer risk.[22] The most recent guidelines from The International Agency for Research for Cancer stated that processed meat does indeed cause cancer (level I evidence) and that red meat was probably carcinogenic (group IIa).

L-arginine In addition to functional foods, precursors to NO, such as L-arginine, have been studied. L-arginine uses the family of enzymes called NO synthases to convert to NO. Clinical trials have yielded mixed results.[23] Early studies on humans showed improved brachial artery flow-mediated dilation in patients with essential hypertension, but this effect did not translate into lower blood pressure.[24] A recent meta-analysis, however, looked at 11 randomized controlled trials (RCTs) and concluded that L-arginine supplementation did indeed lower both SBP and DBP.[25] Response to L-arginine may differ by subset of population. One study looked at 153 patients who had experienced myocardial infarction (MI) 6 months after their event and randomized them to either 3 g L-arginine 3 times per day versus placebo. No improvement in vascular stiffness or ejection fraction was noted in those who took L-arginine. Due to increased mortality in the post-MI group, the study was discontinued. Therefore, at this time, L-arginine is not advised for patients post MI but can be considered in hypertension.[26]

Nutrients/supplements Several nutrients are listed in the following sections with their supplement doses reported in the studies. However, following an AHA-recommended

Table 1 Vegetables according nitrate concentration	
Nitrate Content (mg/100 g) of Fresh Food	**Vegetables**
Very low, <20 mg	Asparagus, garlic, onion, green bean, pepper, potato, sweet potato, tomato, and watermelon
Low, 20 to <50 mg	Broccoli, carrot, cauliflower, and chicory
Regular, 50 to <100 mg	Cabbage, turnip, and dill
High, 100 to <250 mg	Endive, sweet leaf, parsley, and leek
Very high, >250 mg	Celery, chard, lettuce, beetroot, spinach, arugula, and watercress

From d'El-Rei J, Cunha AR, Trindade M, et al. Beneficial effects of dietary nitrate on endothelial function and blood pressure levels. Int J Hypertens 2016;2016:6791519; with permission.

diet rich in fruits and vegetables, whole grains, low-fat dairy, and lean protein sources can allow for adequate sources of these nutrients often without supplementation.

Vitamin C
Vitamin C has been evaluated in many studies for its endothelium-dependent response. Several studies looking at humans have shown that blood pressure is inversely correlated with plasma ascorbate levels in epidemiologic, observational, cross-sectional, and controlled prospective clinical trials.[27] A recent meta-analysis in 2012 showed short-term benefits of reduced blood pressure with vitamin C at a median dose of 500 mg for 8 weeks, but long-term studies are needed.[28]

Flavonoids
Flavonoids are a group of more than 4000 antioxidants and are found in abundance in fruits, vegetables, wine, tea, and grains. Popular sources of flavonoids are in apples, cherries, onions, raspberries, citrus, broccoli, celery, and green tea. Many feel the benefits from the DASH diet are due to its increased fruits and vegetables, which would provide increased flavonoid content. Flavonoids have been shown to have anti-inflammatory and antiatherogenic properties.[29]

Tea
Black tea has been studied in patients with coronary artery disease (CAD) and was shown to reverse endothelial flow-mediated dysfunction.[30] A meta-analysis done in 2014 showed that there was a small but significant reduction in both SBP and DBP when black tea or green tea was ingested long-term for more than 12 weeks.[31] It is reasonable to recommend 450 to 900 mL of black tea or green tea per day.

Lycopene
Lycopene is one of the most powerful antioxidants and is found in abundance in tomatoes. It exerts its role by inhibiting oxidative stress, improving vascular function, and preventing CVD. A 2013 meta-analysis showed lycopene has potential to reduce SBP but was not conclusive for DBP.[32] Adding tomatoes and unprocessed tomato products is recommended for blood pressure reduction.

Coenzyme Q10
Coenzyme Q_{10} (CoQ10), also called ubiquinone because of its ubiquitous distribution in nature, is an antioxidant and an integral component of the mitochondrial respiratory chain for energy production. It is found in all tissues and organs of the body, but in highest concentration in the heart. With aging and CVD, CoQ10 levels decrease. There is evidence of CoQ10 deficiency in hypertension and heart failure, and in individuals on statins for hypercholesterolemia.[33,34] CoQ10 has been shown in many studies as early as 1975 to lower blood pressure in hypertensive patients. A meta-analysis in 2007 showed that CoQ10 can lower the SBP (-17 mm Hg) and DBP (-10 mm Hg) without causing side effects.[33] Although CoQ10 supplementation appears to be promising, a recent Cochrane review concluded there are no significant blood pressure reductions with the antioxidant.[35]

Magnesium
Magnesium is an essential nutrient that has a role in more than 300 reactions in the body. Magnesium lowers blood pressure by acting as a natural calcium channel blocker, competes with sodium for binding sites on vascular smooth muscle cells, and has been shown to induce endothelial-dependent vasodilation.[36] In a recent meta-analysis of 34 RCTs, magnesium at dosages of approximately 300 mg per day for 1 month helped raised intracellular levels of magnesium and helped reduce

both SBP (−2.0 mm Hg) and DBP (−1.98 mm Hg).[37] Although supplement doses may not be clear at this time, it is very reasonable to discuss food sources of magnesium with patients. Those foods with the highest levels are the dark, green leafy vegetables, unrefined grains, and legumes.

Potassium

Potassium is a critical nutrient needed to maintain total body fluid volume, electrolyte and acid balance, and many cellular functions. Although the recommended daily allowance is 4700 mg per day (120 mmol) for adults, most countries around the world report consumption of less than 70 to 80 mmol per day.[9] Processing foods lowers potassium content. Diets high in processed foods and low in fruits and vegetables contribute to low intakes.[38] Consumption of lower potassium is associated with elevated blood pressure, hypertension, and stroke.[39,40] In addition, potassium is often depleted with diuretic use for treatment of hypertension and congestive heart failure and therefore often needs to be supplemented. A meta-analysis looked at 22 RCTs and 11 cohort studies and found that increased potassium intake reduced SBP by 3.5 mm Hg (95% confidence interval 1.8–5.2) and DBP by 2.0 mm Hg (0.9–3.1) in adults, an effect seen in people with hypertension but not in those without hypertension. Most benefit in blood pressure was seen when potassium intake was up to 90 to 120 mmol per day. Higher potassium intake was associated with a 24% reduction in risk of stroke. No adverse effects on renal function, blood lipids, or catecholamine concentrations were found with higher potassium consumption.[41]

Zinc

Low zinc levels are implicated in hypertension.[42] The US Department of Agriculture lists animal proteins, nuts, whole grains, legumes, and yeast to be high in zinc. Zinc deficiency can be exacerbated by certain medications, poor intake, alcoholism, and digestive diseases such as inflammatory bowel disease. Higher dietary zinc intake results in a better taste acuity for salt. Thus, people with zinc deficiency tend to increase salt intake, which can lead to an increase in blood pressure. Although the exact mechanism is not clear, there is a correlation between zinc and the renin-angiotensin system with respect to its influence on blood pressure. Serum zinc level is the best way to assess zinc levels. Recommendations are to increase zinc through diet and supplement when needed.

Vitamin D

Vitamin D is a steroid prohormone, generated when skin is exposed to UV exposure, but also can be taken in through diet and supplements. Cross-sectional studies have shown vitamin D deficiency and increased risk of CVD: hypertension, heart failure, and ischemic heart disease.[43] Notable reasons for deficiencies are nonfortified products in the diet and obesity, which causes fat cells to bind to vitamin D and prevents the vitamin D from circulating. Due to the American Academy of Dermatology's view regarding excess UV radiation risk and premature aging and skin cancer, a safe amount of UV exposure to increase vitamin D without increasing cancer risk cannot be recommended. Therefore, due to lack of dietary sources fortified with vitamin D, supplementation is the preferred way to get levels into normal range. Findings from randomized trials of vitamin D supplementation are inconsistent. A meta-analysis in *JAMA* of 46 trials showed no effect of vitamin D supplementation on blood pressure.[44] Although vitamin D deficiency is associated with CVD and hypertension, using vitamin D for hypertension cannot be advocated at this time.

Calcium

Homeostasis of calcium has been associated with blood pressure regulation.[45] Dietary calcium appears to exert its benefits by lowering the activity of the renin-angiotensin system,[46] improve sodium-potassium balance,[47] and inhibit vascular smooth muscle cell constriction.[48] Earlier studies showed that calcium through dietary intake of whole foods showed blood pressure–lowering effects.[49] Most recently, the Multi-Ethnic Study of Atherosclerosis was a 10-year longitudinal cohort study to assess the role of calcium intake through diet and supplements and presence of atherosclerosis. Coronary artery calcification (CAC) using computed tomography was used. Using 5448 patients who had no evidence of heart disease, they found high calcium intake (average 1081 mg for women and 900 mg for men) was associated with reduced risk for CAC. However, the patients who used supplemental calcium instead of dietary calcium had a 22% increased risk of CAC. This study suggests that following the Recommended Dietary Allowance with dietary calcium may be cardioprotective, but supplements may not be the right option.[50]

Omega-3 fatty acids

Extensive literature has examined the benefit of eicosapentaenoic and docosahexaenoic acids (EPA + DHA) on blood pressure. A meta-analysis of food sources of EPA and DHA showed EPA + DHA reduced SBP (−1.5 mm Hg) and DBP (−1.0 mm Hg). The most profound effects of EPA + DHA were noted among untreated hypertensive subjects in whom SBP decreased by 4.5 mm Hg and DBP by 3.1 mm Hg. Blood pressure also decreased among normotensive subjects but to a smaller degree. Overall evidence from 70 RCTs showed doses of EPA + DHA from 1 to 5 g were associated with SBP reduction in hypertensive adults whereas greater than 2 g were needed for diastolic reduction.[51]

Amino acids

Taurine is a conditionally essential amino acid found in high concentrations in the brain, heart, and skeletal muscles. In animal and human models, taurine lowered blood pressure. Dietary sources of taurine are generally high in meat and fish and low in plant-based foods. A recent RCT with 120 patients with prehypertension showed taurine treatment upregulated the expression of enzymes associated with endothelium vasodilatation. Taurine supplementation at a dose of 1.6 g per day for 12 weeks showed a decrease in blood pressures, especially in those with high normal blood pressure. Mean SBP and DBP reduction for taurine was 7.2 and 4.7 mm Hg, respectively.[52] More studies are needed to further clarify its role in hypertension.

Apple cider vinegar

Although touted through data from animal studies, there is no evidence that vinegar reduces blood pressure in humans.

Herbs

Hawthorn

Current research suggests hawthorn may represent a safe, effective agent in the treatment of CVD and ischemic heart disease. One of the larger human studies looked at 80 patients with type 2 diabetes who had hypertension. They were randomized to receive a daily dose of either hawthorn extract (6 g dried flowering tops) or placebo. The study noted no significant change in SBP, but DBP was reduced significantly by 3.6 mm Hg over 16 weeks. No herb-drug interaction was noted.[53] Hawthorn extract appears to be a promising treatment for management of blood pressure. However, the exact dosage and formulation is not clear.

Pomegranate

Pomegranate also plays a role in reducing blood pressure, likely due to its polyphenol content. Hypertensive patients who drank pomegranate juice for as few as 2 weeks had a 36% decrease in angiotensin-converting enzyme activity and 5% reduction in SBP.[54] Although this effect was not noted in all studies, the transient increase in blood pressure after a meal high in fat was curtailed with the use of pomegranate juice.[55] It is reasonable to recommend drinking 300 mL pomegranate juice to aid in blood pressure.

Cocoa

Cocoa is a flavonoid that has been extensively studied for its blood pressure and cardiovascular benefits. The mechanism for its effects has been attributed to an increase in NO production. These effects are markedly reduced when cocoa is consumed with milk or ingested as milk chocolate.[56] High calorie load of commercially available chocolate may induce weight gain, but raw cocoa has low levels of sugar, which makes it reasonable to recommend.

Although herbs and spices may have benefits, many plants may potentially increase blood pressure, including arnica, bitter orange, ephedra, gingko, ginseng, licorice, senna, St John wort, capsicum, and yohimbine.

Exercise

Recommendations from the American College of Sports Medicine for exercise and hypertension are dynamic aerobic endurance training for at least 30 minutes per day supplemented by dynamic resistance exercise. Exact recommendations for types of exercise and reduction of blood pressure were examined in a recent meta-analysis showing that isometric resistance training showed the highest reductions in SBP.[57] The AHA recommends an average of 40 minutes of moderate to vigorous-intensity aerobic exercise 3 to 4 times per week for lowering blood pressure and cholesterol. They also define exercise as any activity that burns calories, such as walking, jogging, running, biking, playing sports, climbing stairs, weight training, and stretching.[58]

Stress and Its Role in Hypertension

Meditation has been shown to lower blood pressure and cortisol. Specifically, the AHA has deemed that behavioral therapies, such as transcendental meditation (TM), can be used in managing blood pressure (Class IIb level of evidence).[59] TM uses a mantra or chant to focus attention. It is a meditative practice recommended 20 minutes twice a day. The most recent meta-analysis in 2008 showed reduction in SBP (-4.7 mm Hg) and DBP (-3.2 mm Hg) over a median of 15 weeks. The mechanism may be associated with balancing the autonomic nervous system.[60] It is reasonable to advise patients to start a meditative practice to assist with blood pressure reduction without any potential side effects.

HYPERLIPIDEMIA

High cholesterol increases the risk of CVD and has been attributed to one-third of CAD around the world. Reduction of total cholesterol has been associated with decreased CVD and stroke.[61] Along with a large breadth of medication options, lifestyle changes, including proper diet and exercise, are important for management of hyperlipidemia.

Exercise

Studies show that there is some difference in the effect of exercise on lipids based on type of exercise. It appears that aerobic exercise decreases triglycerides and low-density lipoprotein (LDL) cholesterol. Resistance training is more commonly associated with decreases in total cholesterol and LDL cholesterol. Notably, there is a dose-dependent relationship between amount of exercise and increases in high-density lipoprotein (HDL) cholesterol.[62] The AHA recommends 30 minutes of moderate to high-intensity exercise 5 times per week for overall cardiovascular health or 25 minutes of vigorous aerobic activity with moderate to high-intensity muscle strengthening exercise at least 2 days per week.[58]

Nutrition

Food preparation over the past several decades has shifted away from fresh food and cooking daily to more frequently ordering fast food and microwaving precooked and instant meals. Foods are filled with more oil, butter, and preservatives to increase their shelf life and refined products to increase speed of cooking. We have shifted away from eating fruits and vegetables and have become a heavy meat-eating society. Recent research has focused on the impact of the food we eat on the microbiome, and consequent effects on development of inflammation and CVD. Foods high in phosphatidyl choline, such as eggs, liver, beef, and pork, are processed in the gut and the metabolites trimethylamine and trimethylamine-N-oxide (TMAO) are formed. Recent studies show that people with high production of TMAO have increased risk of CVD.[63] In animal studies, a vegetarian and/or high-fiber diet has been shown to lower the amount of choline and therefore less TMAO production. Probiotics and antibiotics also are associated with reduced amounts of TMAO and will be the source of ongoing study. Although TMAO appears to be associated with CVD, it is also possible that it is a biomarker for gut microbiome differences rather than an independent risk factor or trigger.[64] Excess salt in meat serves as a preservative and may lead to high blood pressure. Nitrates, which are used as preservatives in meat, have been associated with endothelial dysfunction[65] and insulin resistance.[66] Studies show eating just 1 fatty meal can create endothelial dysfunction within 4 hours.[67]

The role of nutrition and its impact on heart disease has always been appreciated. In the early work by Dean Ornish and colleagues,[68] they directed 48 patients with moderate-severe CAD to eat a 10% fat vegetarian diet, do moderate aerobic exercise, undergo stress management training and smoking cessation counseling, and provided support groups. Over 1.5 years, plaque regression occurred in the treatment group and progression was observed in the control group.[68] Early studies on the Mediterranean diet, featuring an abundance of vegetables, fruit, and fiber, suggested this diet reduced heart disease risk. The large PREDIMED (Prevención con Dieta Mediterránea) study is the most recent study completed and is a primary prevention study. In this study, men (55–80 years) and women (60–80 years) either had diabetes mellitus or 3 other cardiovascular risk factors. A Mediterranean diet with olive oil or nuts was compared with a standard low-fat diet. The Mediterranean diet showed a 30% relative risk reduction of MI, stroke, or death from CVDs in both the olive oil and walnut groups. Importantly, the Mediterranean diet decreased TMAO production as well.[69] This was a significant study showing that dietary changes toward a plant-based diet with fruits, vegetables, legumes, nuts, fish, and white meat is effective in reducing CVD.

Regarding whole grains, the Iowa Women's Health Study showed higher consumption led to fewer cardiovascular events.[70] In the Nurses' Health Study, a 25% decrease in cardiovascular events was noted in women who ate more than 3 servings of whole grains per day versus those who ate less than 1 serving per day.[71] Hu and Colleagues[72] recommended the optimal diet for lowering risk of CAD was a diet with non-hydrogenated fats, whole grains, and an abundance of fruits and vegetables.

Saturated and Trans-fats

Saturated fats have long been associated with risk of CVD, and reduction is advocated as part of the American College of Cardiology (ACC)/AHA guidelines. Controlled studies have shown that trans-fats increase LDL and lower HDL cholesterol, compared with nonhydrogenated unsaturated fatty acids.[73] They also increase lipoprotein [a],[74] which is a proinflammatory marker that increases triglycerides,[75] may reduce the blood vessel's ability to dilate, and increases the risk of diabetes.[76] Clinical trials show the negative impact of trans-fats on the risk of coronary heart disease.[77] The Nurses' Health Study looked at 80,082 women and found that higher trans-fats (and, to a smaller extent, saturated fats) were associated with higher risk of heart disease compared with the polyunsaturated nonhydrogenated diet.[78]

Unsaturated Fats: Polyunsaturated and Monounsaturated Fats

Unsaturated fats are categorized into monounsaturated and polyunsaturated fats (MUFAs and PUFAs, respectively). Oleic acid is the most commonly consumed monounsaturated fat, found in canola and olive oil.[79] MUFAs are almost completely absorbed by the intestine and oxidized for energy production, converted into other fatty acids, or incorporated into tissue lipids. Polyunsaturated fats (PUFAs) include omega-3 and omega-6 essential fatty acids.

Omega-3 fatty acids, mostly from marine sources, have been studied extensively. Higher consumption has been associated with decreasing mortality associated with coronary heart disease.[72] Greater consumption also correlates with improved mood, greater insulin sensitivity, increased muscle growth, and better sleep. The mechanism for reducing CVD is likely multifactorial.[80] They may reduce triglycerides, aid in blood thinning, and cause vasodilation.[81] People consuming 2 or more servings of fish per week have increased lifespan during 20-year follow-up.[82] In the US Physicians Health Study, 1 serving of fish per week was inversely related to the risk of sudden cardiac death. However, there was no association between fish consumption and MI.[83] The GISSI-Prevenzione trial included 11,324 patients with a recent (≤3 months) MI. At 3.5 years, participants taking 1 g per day of n-3 PUFA supplement had significantly less combined death, nonfatal MI, and stroke compared with the control group. This benefit resulted largely from a 45% reduction in sudden cardiac death.[84] Thus, the benefit of omega-3 fatty acids is likely related to decreased risk of sudden cardiac death rather than a reduction in MI.

Supplements of EPA and DHA widely vary in their potency. Using Web sites such as consumerlabs.com can be beneficial to find reliable supplement sources. The World Health Organization advocates 0.3 to 0.5 g of both DHA and EPA and 0.8 to 1.1 g of alpha linoleic acid (an omega-3 fatty acid primarily from seed sources) per day for all-comers.[85] For management of heart disease, doses of 1 to 4 g of omega-3 fatty acids are recommended. The proportion of EPA to DHA are variable. Overall, the ratio likely should be higher in EPA than DHA. The AHA focuses on eating fatty fish at least 2 times per week (3.5 oz) as the best source for omega-3 fatty acids.

Omega-6 fatty acids

The main omega-6 fatty acid is linoleic acid, found in corn, soy, sunflower, and safflower. Linoleic acid breaks down into eicosanoids, some of which promote inflammation,[86] platelet aggregation, and vasoconstriction. There are no clinical trials that specifically look at outcomes from adding omega-6 fatty acids to the diet. Overall, the AHA now suggests that 5% to 10% of our total energy intake should come from omega-6 fatty acids, which may bring about a decrease in coronary heart disease relative to lower intakes.[87] However, the average American diet has 14 to 25 times more omega-6 than omega-3.[88] We recommend a 1:1 or 1:2 balance of omega-6 to omega-3 fats. Common oils used in cooking and their omega-6:3 ratios are shown in **Fig. 1**.

Monounsaturated fats

Analysis of food oils used in the Mediterranean diet led to the focus on olive oil as the "golden oil" and targeted its abundance of MUFAs. Olive oil is 72% monounsaturated fat. The remainder is linoleic acid. MUFAs lower triglycerides and LDL levels and elevate HDL compared with saturated fats. In some studies, they improve cardiovascular outcomes,[89] ease oxidative stress, and improve diabetes control. Olive oil is also rich in polyphenols, which may decrease oxidative stress.[79] In 2001, the Lyon Diet Heart Study prospectively investigated the effects of a Mediterranean diet. A benefit of increased MUFA intake in survivors of first-time MI was found.[90] The PREDIMED data discussed previously also shows compelling evidence for the benefit of olive oil consumption, with the Mediterranean diet significantly predicting reduced CVD and mortality when compared with a standard low-fat diet. The dose of extra-virgin olive oil needed to create maximum benefit versus risk is unclear and requires further study.[91]

Plant-Based Supplements for Hyperlipidemia

Red yeast rice

Red yeast rice is a traditional Chinese herbal supplement that can be used as a food additive and for its cholesterol-lowering benefits. The essential ingredient is monacolin K, which is chemically identical to the active ingredient in lovastatin. One study looked at 74 patients with high cholesterol and randomized them to statin versus red yeast rice and fish oil. After 12 weeks, there was a 42.4% reduction in the red yeast rice/fish oil group compared with 39.6% reduction in the statin group. Despite these data, variability in quality and potency of red yeast rice on the market limits clinical utility. By-products in production of red yeast rice, such as citrinin, have been shown in animal studies to cause renal failure.[92,93] Although the risk of red yeast rice for muscle and liver toxicity may be lower than equivalent-dosed statins, the risk persists. Ultimately, we suggest that patients and clinicians use Internet Web sources, such as

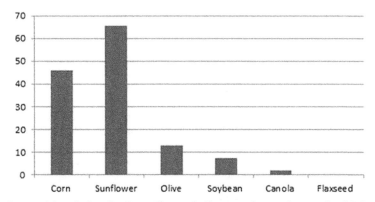

Fig. 1. Omega 6:3 ratio in oils. Note: Flaxseed oil cannot be used to cook with because it is potentially harmful when warmed. (*Data from* US Department of Agriculture, Agricultural Research Service. USDA National nutrient database for standard reference, release 28. Available at: https://www.ars.usda.gov/northeast-area/beltsville-md/beltsville-human-nutrition-research-center/nutrient-data-laboratory/docs/usda-national-nutrient-database-for-standard-reference/. Accessed April 26, 2017.)

Consumer Labs, to check efficacy and potency of nutritional supplements, for example, levels of monacolin A and citrinin content.

Plant sterols (phytosterols) and stanols

Plant sterols block intestinal cholesterol absorption by competitively binding to cholesterol receptors. They are poorly absorbed and therefore result in overall reduction in cholesterol levels. Plant sterols are found in nuts, seeds, fruits, and legumes. In studies since the 1950s, plant sterols have been shown to reduce LDL cholesterol and therefore have long been added to foods and margarines to decrease cholesterol.[94] Although studies continued to show that plant sterols reduce cholesterol, it was unclear if this translated to reduction in CVD. Sitosterolemia, an inherited disorder characterized by increased absorption of plant sterols, is also associated with xanthomas and accelerated atherosclerosis.[95] This generated concern that plant sterols, at least in high doses, could increase risk of CVD. A meta-analysis of patients with moderate levels of plant sterol intake, however, did not show an association with increased CVD.[96]

Despite the meta-analysis, scientists continue to search for the lowest plant sterol dose that seemed to reduce cholesterol without doing any harm. They started experimenting with esterified plant stanols (the saturated form of sterols) that can be incorporated into other food sources without altering the taste or texture of the food. Plant stanol esters at the dosage of 2 to 3 g per day have been shown to decrease LDL cholesterol by 10% to 20% in many population subsets, such as elderly individuals, men, patients with CAD, and patients with diabetes. Notably, this benefit is in addition to statin medications.[97] Due to this trial data, many foods advertise added plant stanols, such as plant-based margarine, marketed as Benecol.

The ACC currently acknowledges that 1 to 3 g of plant sterols per day have a benefit in reducing cholesterol and can be obtained from natural food sources, such as legumes, nuts, and seeds. The benefit plateaus at 3 g per day.[98] Regarding plant stanol esters, using plant-based margarines, such as Benecol, are good options for bringing cholesterol down. A dosage of 1.7 g serving twice daily with a heart healthy diet is reasonable.

Fiber

Many experimental and observational studies have shown that increased fiber intake reduces cardiovascular risk factors.[99] Besides the phytosterol component of plant-based foods, soluble fibers and resistant starches (ie, insoluble fibers) are hypothesized to sit longer in the colon to form gels and allow the fiber to ferment. The formation of gels allows for satiety and decreases blood sugar and lipid levels.[100] The fermentation creates healthy short-chain fatty acids, which appear to also lower cholesterol levels.[101] An extensive meta-analysis showed an additional 7 g per day of dietary fiber decreased cardiovascular risk by 9%. Seven grams can be obtained from 1 serving of whole grains with beans or lentils. Alternatively, 2 to 4 servings of fruits and vegetables provide 7 g.[102] The consensus statement from the ACC, however, states that although there is a reduction in LDL cholesterol with 3 to 12 g of fiber per day, that improvement does not clearly translate into reduction in CVD.[98]

Polyphenols/phytonutrients/phytochemicals

These terms are often used interchangeably. They are naturally occurring nutrients in plants that possess antioxidant potential. Polyphenols can be broken down into carotenoids (beta-carotene, lycopene, lutein, and zeaxanthin), flavonoids (isoflavones, anthocyanidins, flavanols, quercetin), lignans, tannins, stilbenes (reservatrol), and others. Carotenoids and flavonoids are responsible for the color in our fruits and vegetables. Much research is being devoted to clarify the biological activities of polyphenols. One study looked at older women's use of flavonoids retrospectively. Women with the most flavonoid-rich food intake had the lowest mortality.[103] One of the most impactful studies is the PREDIMED study subset analysis, which looked at polyphenol intake independently from omega-3 fatty acids and monounsaturated fats. Those with the highest polyphenol intake had the lowest cardiovascular mortality. Within the subsets of the polyphenols, the stilbenes and lignans had an inverse relationship with mortality.[104]

Stilbenes

The most common stilbene is resveratrol, found in grapes and red wine, and often attributed to the "French Paradox." One suggested mechanism of benefit is through increased NO levels in the vascular endothelium, thereby exerting a vasodilating effect.[105] Studies have also shown resveratrol to have beneficial effects to vascular aging by its effects of reducing inflammation, lowering oxidative stress, lowering platelet oxidation, and reducing thrombus formation.[106] In the Copenhagen City Heart Study[107] and the copenhagen city heart study and others,[108] 1 to 2 drinks of wine or other spirits significantly decreased cardiovascular mortality. There are insufficient data to recommend resveratrol supplements in clinical practice. However, the AHA does condone moderate alcohol intake but cautions against risks of abuse and alcoholism.[109]

Lignans

Lignans are phytoestrogens found in high quantities in flax, sesame seeds, and linseed. Benefits include lowering blood pressure, cholesterol, and C-reactive protein.[110] Supplementation at this time is not recommended, but food sources are reasonable.[111]

Coffee

Coffee beans contain polyphenols, namely lignans, caffeine, and vitamins. There appears to be a slight increase in blood pressure in coffee drinkers.[112] Coffee consumption, however, also appears to increase insulin sensitivity and decreases diabetes.[113] A meta-analysis done in 2013 found a U-shaped relationship between coffee intake and CVD. Moderate coffee consumption (3–5 cups of coffee per day) was associated with decreased CVD, whereas higher consumption was not associated with any effect.[114]

Tea

In a meta-analysis, tea consumption appeared to have a dose-dependent benefit in terms of decreasing stroke rate.[115] Results suggest a moderate improvement in LDL and total cholesterol with the addition of green tea catechins to the diet.[116] Although tea has potential, it cannot clearly be advocated for its benefits in lipid-lowering or cardiovascular benefit. It does not appear to cause harm, however, and therefore is a reasonable addition to a cardiovascular diet.

Soy

Soy has received substantial publicity because Asian countries that consume large amounts of soy have lower incidence of heart disease. Soy contains phytoestrogens called isoflavones. In early meta-analyses, when isolated soy protein with isoflavones was substituted for milk or animal fats, there was a notable decrease in LDL cholesterol concentrations. Fifty grams of soy seemed to potentiate the effect.[117] In 1999, the Food and Drug Administration approved labeling of soy proteins as cholesterol lowering and beneficial in reduction of CVD. The AHA issued a statement in 2000 that soy protein was beneficial in management of heart disease.[117] However, further studies and meta-analyses were reviewed and results were inconsistent. The AHA then put out a scientific advisory clarifying it is the soy itself and not necessarily the soy isoflavones that have showed benefit in reducing LDL cholesterol. No clear benefit of soy for improvement of HDL, triglycerides, or blood pressure was observed. Soy products in general have many potential benefits due to their high content of PUFAs, fiber, vitamins, and minerals, and low amount of saturated fat. Although soy is an es-trogen mimetic, studies have not shown increased risk of breast cancer, a common concern among patients and clinicians.[118] Currently, a diet rich in plant-based foods and soy products is reasonable for all cardiovascular patients. Isoflavone supple-ments are not recommended, as their benefit is not clear and role in promoting cancer is unknown.

Pomegranate
In small human studies, patients who drank pomegranate juice for 3 months had decreased stress-induced ischemia compared with placebo.[119] Pomegranate juice may also decrease lipid oxidation (a precursor to atherosclerosis) and oxidative stress.[120] Benefits have been noted in patients with diabetes and patients with CAD, as well.[120,121]

Beta-carotene
Beta-carotene, a carotenoid polyphenol, has long been touted for its antioxidant ef-fects. In 2 major RCTs, this claim was definitively refuted. Patients were given vitamin E, beta-carotene, both, or neither. With the addition of beta-carotene, there was not only no improvement, but rather an increase in cancer and ischemic heart dis-ease.[122,123] Therefore, beta-carotene supplementation is not recommended for pre-vention of CVD.

Vitamin E
In a clinical trial, there was an increase in death from hemorrhagic stroke with vitamin E supplementation.[122] Subsequent studies did not show benefit from the addition of vitamin E into the diet in high-risk patients or for primary prevention. Therefore, vitamin E supplementation is not recommended for prevention of CVD. Some secondary pre-vention studies show a potential role for vitamin E that needs to be clarified.[124,125] The authors currently do not recommend vitamin E supplementation in CVD.

Vitamin D
Low vitamin D levels do appear associated with an increased incidence of CVD.[126] There is a potential U-shaped relationship between vitamin D and CVD in which high vitamin D levels in women were also associated with increased CVD.[127] Meta-analyses of the small trials available have not shown a benefit of supplementation in terms of a more favorable lipid profile.[128] The largest ongoing randomized trial of vitamin D in heart disease and cancer is The Vitamin D and Omega-3 Trial (VITAL). VI-TAL will look at differences in heart disease and cancer outcomes with the use of 2000 IU vitamin D per day with more than 25,000 participants.[129]

Chelation
Chelation to treat heavy metal burden is performed through intravenous administration of ethylene diamine tetraacetic acid (disodium EDTA) into the blood stream. Disodium EDTA then binds to heavy metals, such as cadmium and lead, and divalent minerals, such as calcium. The EDTA-metal/mineral complex is then excreted into the urine. Due to the notable calcium in CAD, interest by some investigators shifted to deter-mining if chelation can be helpful for patients with CAD. The Trial to Assess Chelation

Therapy (TACT) trial in 2001 recruited patients older than 50 years, with a history of acute MI at least 6 weeks before enrollment and creatinine levels less than 2 mg/ dL. The primary composite endpoint was all-cause mortality, MI, stroke, coronary revascularization, and hospitalization for angina. Chelation therapy showed an 18% reduction in the primary composite endpoint.[130] The reduction was sustained suggesting a long-term benefit to chelation. A multivitamin and a multimineral also were given in conjunction with chelation in a subset of patients and they demonstrated even more positive, powerful results. The most profound impact was seen in the diabetes subgroup and patients with previous history of an anterior wall MI subgroup in which hazard ratios were 0.61 and 0.63 favoring chelation, respectively.[131] Currently, TACT2 is enrolling specifically diabetic patients post MI and assessing chelation's effect on primary outcomes of all-cause mortality and other cardiovascular endpoints.[132] Chelation, therefore, has potential, but recommendations are deferred until further study.

Meditation and cardiovascular disease
In an RCT of African American men and women with CAD randomized to TM versus health education, TM showed a notable 48% relative risk reduction in the primary endpoint of all-cause mortality, stroke, or MI. These changes were associated with lower blood pressure and decreased stress.[133] In response to this pivotal article, the AHA advocates TM as part of secondary prevention. Although studies are not available, it is likely that moving meditation practices, such as tai-chi, yoga, and qi gong, have similar benefits. We believe that mind-body awareness exercises are important for decreasing stress with health benefits and should be advocated to our patients, along with other lifestyle changes.[58]

HEART FAILURE

Approximately 5 million Americans are currently living with heart failure and nearly 700,000 new cases are diagnosed each year.[134] Morbidity and mortality from heart failure remains high: 50% of patients newly diagnosed with heart failure will die within 5 years.[134] Hospital readmission rates have also been shown to be as high as 50% within 6 months after initial hospitalization.[135] Heart failure is also known to adversely affect quality of life and negatively impact day-to-day activities.[136] A potential strategy to reduce the burden of heart failure and improve symptom management is to leverage the use of evidence-based complementary and integrative therapies alongside traditional medical care.

Management of heart failure often necessitates a complex, coordinated care plan unique from other patients with a CVD diagnosis, including monitoring patients' limbs for signs of fluid retention, daily weight, and salt, alcohol, and fluid intake.[137] Adherence to lifestyle recommendations among patients with heart failure conspicuously low, despite well-established medical guidelines.[138] Dietary adherence in particular, including sodium restriction, is an important target because high sodium intake can often be a precipitating factor for hospitalizations.[139] This is an area in which primary care physicians may have substantial influence.

Sodium Intake in Patients with Heart Failure

Data on sodium restriction and outcomes among patients with heart failure is inconsistent. Sodium restriction has been associated with lower rates of symptom burden, readmission, and mortality in patients with heart failure in several studies.[140,141] However, in other larger studies, including RCTs, sodium restriction has been associated with higher mortality and readmission rates.[142–144] The current recommendation of the

AHA and ACC Foundation (ACCF) is 2000 mg of dietary sodium per day for patients with heart failure, which is notably higher than the AHA's proposed limit of 1500 mg per day for the general population.[145] The recommendation for sodium intake for patients with heart failure is based on level C evidence (expert consensus).

Translation of this recommendation is difficult in practice. Among a subsample of patients with heart failure participating in The Coordinating study evaluating Outcomes of Advising and Counseling in Heart failure (COACH) trial, only 31% of those prescribed a sodium restriction of 2000 mg were compliant with the restriction.[146] Lack of adherence to prescribed levels of sodium is one reason that results are confounded in clinical trials attempting to discern the association between sodium intake and outcomes among patients with heart failure. In addition, the effects of sodium may significantly vary among patients with heart failure according to gender, race, or ethnicity.

The potential mechanism of action for the adverse effect of excess sodium in heart failure is decreased renal perfusion from decreased cardiac output, elevated systemic venous pressure, and/or shunting of blood from the kidney. This decreased perfusion leads to an increased sympathetic response and activation of the renin-angiotensin-aldosterone system, resulting in sodium and water retention even in the context of fluid overload.

Despite the conflicting evidence to date, sodium restriction to less than 2000 mg dietary sodium per day still should be recommended for most patients, consistent with AHA/ACCF guidelines for heart failure.[147] Diet education for patients with heart failure should include information specific to reading sodium values on food labels, high sodium foods to avoid, and suggested substitutions. Patients' personal sodium needs and fluid intake goals should be discussed and tailored to any coexisting conditions, such as diabetes.

Exercise

Walking capacity has been shown to be strongly associated with 10-year mortality and risk of heart failure among 2935 participants in the Health, Aging, and Body Composition Study.[148] Long-term RCTs have documented exercise training (ie, primarily walking) is associated with better functional capacity and improved quality of life. In turn, this improvement has resulted in a reduction in major cardiovascular events, hospitalizations, and cardiac mortality.[149] Supervised exercise training is generally recommended, provided patients are stable and without contraindications.[150] As an alternative to walking, a recent meta-analysis of 10 studies including 240 patients with heart failure found resistance training to increase muscle strength, aerobic capacity, and quality of life.[151] Resistance training may serve as a different approach to improve fitness among patients who are unable or unwilling to participate in aerobic activities. Although there is no AHA/ACC recommendation; studies typically used 45 to 60 minutes of aerobic exercise and resistance training 2 to 3 times per week.

Tai-chi exercise also may benefit patients with heart failure through improvements in their quality of life and capacity to exercise. Yeh and colleagues conducted a study in which 100 patients with systolic heart failure were randomized to either a tai-chi intervention for 60 minutes, twice per week, or an education-only control.[152] After 12 weeks, the tai-chi group experienced improved quality of life, exercise self-efficacy, and mood, with no observed adverse effects due to the intervention. There were no differential effects between groups in distance walked in 6 minutes or peak oxygen intake.

Mindfulness

The Support, Education, and Research in Chronic Heart Failure (SEARCH) study tested an 8-week mindfulness-based psychoeducational intervention on clinical outcomes, depression, and quality of life in patients with heart failure. Results showed that the mindfulness-based intervention compared with control subjects reduced anxiety and depression and led to significantly fewer symptoms of heart failure after 1 year.[153] Proof of concept was demonstrated for the feasibility of a new 8-week program of integrative group medical care plus mindfulness training among patients with heart failure.[154] Patients participating in the Compassionate Approach to Lifestyle and Mind-Body (CALM) Skills for Patients with CHF, experienced improvements in depression, fatigue, and satisfaction with life. This intervention should be further evaluated in a controlled trial.

Meditation

A growing body of evidence is pointing toward the positive effects of meditation for patients with heart failure; however, it is somewhat limited by small sample sizes and studies of varying quality. Curiati and colleagues[155] randomly assigned 19 patients with heart failure to either usual care or usual care plus weekly meetings including meditation. The meditation component of the intervention consisted of a 30-minute audiotape for patients to listen to at their homes, twice a day for 12 weeks. At the end of 12 weeks, the meditation group showed improved measures of exercise performance, improved quality-of-life scores, and reduction in plasma norepinephrine.

Supplements

Dietary supplements are fairly common in patients with heart failure, with use ranging from 40% to 82%.[156] In contrast, physician awareness of patients' use of herbal or dietary supplements is approximately 60%.[157] The most common reasons for lack of awareness of use are the physician not asking or patient beliefs that the physician will be judgmental.[158] These data highlight the importance of systematically asking patients about any supplements, herbs, or other forms of treatment they may be using.

Coenzyme Q10
CoQ10 may reduce the toxic effects of reactive oxygen species that are seen in patients with heart failure. A systematic Cochrane review of 7 studies with 914 participants compared CoQ10 versus placebo. The investigators were unable to make a definitive conclusion regarding use of CoQ10 for heart failure.[159] Studies included in the Cochrane analysis led the ACC and the AHA to not recommend CoQ10 for management of heart failure. Following this statement, the Q-SYMBIO study, a 2-year prospective, randomized double-blind trial including 420 patients randomly assigned to either CoQ10 100 mg 3 times daily or placebo, showed short-term endpoints of New York Heart Association (NYHA) functional classification, 6-minute walk test, and levels of N-terminal pro-B type natriuretic peptide were not significantly different.[34] However, long-term endpoints of 2-year cardiovascular and all-cause mortality and heart failure hospitalizations were significantly decreased in the CoQ10 group. Additionally, there was a significant improvement in NYHA class after 2 years. Supplementation of CoQ10 may be considered as an adjunctive treatment in dosages of 100 mg, 2 to 3 times per day.

ʟ-carnitine
A meta-analysis examining the role of ʟ-carnitine in secondary prevention of CVD included 13 trials and concluded there were no protective effects for heart failure or myocardial reinfarction, despite reductions in all-cause mortality, ventricular arrhythmias, and angina attacks.[160] A large randomized multicenter trial is recommended

to confirm these results before suggesting supplementation specifically for patients with heart failure.

Selenium

Selenium deficiency is rare among individuals in United States and Canada, and limited clinical trial data do not support recommending supplementation for prevention or treatment of heart failure.[161]

Hawthorn

Although the mechanism of action is unclear, this herb may have vasodilatory properties, antioxidant activity, inotropic action, and lipid-lowering effects. A meta-analysis of hawthorn extract in 10 double-blind, placebo-controlled trials including 855 patients with heart failure showed symptomatic as well as functional benefits.[162] However, a randomized trial limited to patients with heart failure with reduced ejection fraction did not demonstrate any benefit.[163] Hawthorn extract may be considered as an adjunctive treatment for heart failure, at 900 to 1800 mg, divided over 2 to 3 doses per day. However, the potential for hawthorn to deleteriously interact with digoxin should be noted.[164]

ARRHYTHMIAS

Sudden cardiac death affects 180,000 to 450,000 persons per year in the United States, and accounts for more than 50% of all cardiovascular-related deaths. Most sudden cardiac deaths are attributable to arrhythmias.[165,166] Traditional medical treatment includes antiarrhythmic drugs, radiofrequency ablation, and implantable cardiac defibrillators. Potential downsides to traditional antiarrhythmic drugs may include cost and possible side effects, including triggering arrhythmias themselves in some cases.[167] Complementary and integrative medical treatments for arrhythmia with promising evidence for antiarrhythmic behavior or effectiveness with limited side effects include certain supplements, yoga, and acupuncture.[168]

Omega-3 Fatty Acids (See Also Hypertension Section)

Omega-3 PUFAs, such as EPA and DHA, may be effective in preventing and treating some types of arrhythmias.[169] The results of a 2013 meta-analysis (8 RCTs of 2967 patients) showed that preoperative supplementation with omega-3 PUFAs provided significant protection against atrial fibrillation in patients undergoing cardiac surgery.[170] Among patients who underwent coronary artery bypass graft (CABG) or valvular surgery, there was a 16% lower risk of atrial fibrillation for patients receiving omega-3 PUFAs compared with placebo. Among patients with CABG only, the risk reduction for atrial fibrillation was 34%. A different meta-analysis of a general population of 32,919 randomized patients (16,465 in the treatment group and 16,454 in the control group) found supplementation with omega-3 PUFAs compared with placebo did not affect the risk of sudden cardiac death or ventricular arrhythmias.[171] Thus, it appears that preoperative supplementation of PUFAs may decrease rates of atrial fibrillation, whereas PUFAs in the overall population may not affect incidence of ventricular arrhythmias. The AHA currently recommends 2 servings of oily fish per week for cardiac (including arrhythmic) benefits.

Magnesium and Potassium

Low concentrations of magnesium and potassium may increase risk of arrhythmia.[172] Magnesium supplementation has been shown to prevent arrhythmias after cardiac surgery. In a meta-analysis of 17 RCTs, the administration of magnesium postoperatively reduced the risk of supraventricular arrhythmias by 23% (atrial fibrillation by 29%) and ventricular arrhythmias by 48%.[173] Oral administration of potassium with magnesium also was shown to be effective in reducing arrhythmias in a randomized, double-blind study of 232 patients with frequent ventricular arrhythmias.[174] Results showed that a 50% increase in the recommended minimum daily dietary intake of the 2 minerals for 3 weeks led to a moderate but significant antiarrhythmic effect. Supplementation of magnesium and potassium could be considered at 300 to 400 mg per day of magnesium and 2000 to 4700 mg of potassium per day. Usage of medications that could alter potassium levels, such as diuretics, should be taken into account before potassium administration. Good natural sources of magnesium are green leafy vegetables, nuts, legumes, and whole grains. Good sources of potassium include avocado, bananas, nuts, potatoes, citrus fruits, and green leafy vegetables.

Yoga

Yoga training could be beneficial for patients with arrhythmia because it incorporates breathing and relaxation exercises that significantly increase cardiac vagal modulation. In addition, it is easily implemented without serious adverse effects.[175] The YOGA My Heart Study examined the impact of twice-weekly, 60-minute yoga sessions for 3 months among patients with symptomatic paroxysmal atrial fibrillation on measures of arrhythmia burden, quality of life, depression, and anxiety scores.[176] The patients participated in an initial 3-month noninterventional observation period to serve as their own controls. Each yoga session consisted of 10 minutes of *pranayama* (breathing exercises), 10 minutes of warm-up exercises, 30 minutes of *asanas* (poses), and 10 minutes of relaxation exercises. After 3 months, yoga therapy significantly reduced symptomatic and asymptomatic atrial fibrillation burden. Further, patients had improvement in their heart rate, blood pressure, anxiety, and overall quality of life.

Acupuncture

A review synthesizing the evidence for acupuncture and cardiac arrhythmias concluded that 87% to 100% of participants converted to normal sinus rhythm after acupuncture. However, the review included case series or case studies, with only 1 RCT.[177] A 2011 controlled trial of 80 patients with atrial fibrillation found recurrence rates of atrial fibrillation lower in acupuncture compared with acupuncture-sham and control patients. Further studies are needed to better define the role of acupuncture in arrhythmia treatment.[178]

SUMMARY

Cardiovascular patients often desire an integrated approach, do not comply well with medical therapies, and complain of medication side effects. Thus, treating physicians need to be knowledgeable about the evidence for and against interventions such as diet, exercise, supplements, herbs, and mind/body techniques. A patient-centered evidence-based approach of discussing the risk/benefit profile of these complementary approaches will allow for a more open dialogue with our patients and hopefully improved compliance and outcomes.

REFERENCES

1. World Health Organization. Available at: www.who.int/mediacentre/factsheets. Accessed April 25, 2017.
2. Medicine use and spending shifts: a review of the use of medicines in the U.S. in 2014. Qunitiles IMS Institute; 2015.

3. Prescription drug costs [Internet] KFF. Menlo Park (CA): Kaiser Family Foundation; 2010 [December 26, 2011].

4. Haynes RB, McDonald HP, Garg AX. Helping patients follow prescribed treatment: clinical applications. JAMA 2002;288(22):2880–3.

5. Bairey Merz CN, Elboudwarej O, Mehta P. The autonomic nervous system and cardiovascular health and disease. JACC Heart Fail 2015;3(5):383–5.

6. Schneiderman N, Ironson G, Siegal SD. Stress and health: psychological, behavioral and biological determinants. Annu Rev Clin Psychol 2005;1:607–28.

7. Aschbacher K, O'Donovan A, Wolkowitz OM, et al. Good stress, bad stress and oxidative stress: insights from anticipatory cortisol reactivity. Psychoneuroendocrinology 2013;38(9):1698–708.

8. Appel LJ, Moore TJ, Obarzanek E, et al. A clinical trial of the effects of dietary patterns on blood pressure. DASH Collaborative Research Group. N Engl J Med 1997;336(16):1117–24.

9. Intersalt: an international study of electrolyte excretion and blood pressure. Results for 24 hour urinary sodium and potassium excretion. Intersalt Cooperative Research Group. BMJ 1988;297(6644):319–28.

10. Sacks FM, Svetkey LP, Vollmer WM, et al. Effects on blood pressure of reduced dietary sodium and the dietary approaches to stop hypertension (DASH) diet. N Engl J Med 2001;344(1):3–10.

11. O'donnell M, Mente A, Rangarajan S, et al. Urinary sodium and potassium excretion, mortality, and cardiovascular events. N Engl J Med 2014; 2014(371):612–23.

12. Graudal N, Jurgens G, Baslund B, et al. Compared with usual sodium intake, low-and excessive-sodium diets are associated with increased mortality: a meta-analysis. Am J Hypertens 2014;27(9):1129–37.

13. American Heart Association. Available at: https://sodiumbreakup.heart.org/sodium_and_your_health. Accessed April 25, 2017.

14. Brandes RP. Endothelial dysfunction and hypertension. Hypertension 2014; 64(5):924–8.

15. Martina V, Masha A, Gigliardi VR, et al. Long-term N-acetylcysteine and L-arginine administration reduces endothelial activation and systolic blood pressure in hypertensive patients with type 2 diabetes. Diabetes Care 2008;31(5):940–4.

16. Hord NG, Tang Y, Bryan NS. Food sources of nitrates and nitrites: the physiologic context for potential health benefits. Am J Clin Nutr 2009;90(1):1–10.

17. Lundberg JO, Weitzberg E, Gladwin MT. The nitrate–nitrite–nitric oxide pathway in physiology and therapeutics. Nat Rev Drug Discov 2008;7(2):156–67.

18. Bryan NS. Nitrite in nitric oxide biology: cause or consequence? A systems-based review. Free Radic Biol Med 2006;41(5):691–701.

19. D'El-Rei J, Cunha AR, Trindade M, et al. Beneficial effects of dietary nitrate on endothelial function and blood pressure levels. Int J Hypertens 2016;2016: 6791519.

20. Kapil V, Khambata RS, Robertson A, et al. Dietary nitrate provides sustained blood pressure lowering in hypertensive patients: a randomized, phase 2, double-blind, placebo-controlled study. Hypertension 2014;65(2):320–7.

21. Mcnally B, Griffin JL, Roberts LD. Dietary inorganic nitrate: from villain to hero in metabolic disease? Mol Nutr Food Res 2015;60(1):67–78.

22. Terry P, Terry JB, Wolk A. Fruit and vegetable consumption in the prevention of cancer: an update. J Intern Med 2001;250(4):280–90.

23. Gokce J. L-arginine and hypertension. J Nutr 2004;134(10 Suppl):2807S–11S.

24. Lekakis JP, Papathanassiou S, Papaioannou TG, et al. Oral l-arginine improves endothelial dysfunction in patients with essential hypertension. Int J Cardiol 2002;86(2–3):317–23.

25. Dong JY, Qin LQ, Zhang Z, et al. Effect of oral l-arginine supplementation on blood pressure: a meta-analysis of randomized, double-blind, placebo-controlled trials. Am Heart J 2011;162(6):959–65.

26. Schulman SP, Becker LC, Kass DA, et al. L-arginine therapy in acute myocardial infarction. JAMA 2006;295(1):58.

27. Houston MC, Fox B, Taylor N. What your doctor may not tell you about hypertension: the revolutionary nutrition and lifestyle program to help fight high blood pressure. New York: Warner Books; 2003.

28. Juraschek SP, Guallar E, Appel LJ, et al. Effects of vitamin C supplementation on blood pressure: a meta-analysis of randomized controlled trials. Am J Clin Nutr 2012;95(5):1079–88.

29. Salvamani S, Gunasekaran B, Azmi Shaharuddin NA, et al. Antiartherosclerotic effects of plant flavonoids. Biomed Res Int 2014;2014:1–11.

30. Duffy S, Keaney J, Holbrook M, et al. Short- and long-term black tea consumption reverses endothelial dysfunction in patients with coronary artery disease. ACC Curr J Rev 2002;11(1):28.

31. Gang L, Xiaohong H. GW25-e0837 effects of tea intake on blood pressure: a meta-analysis of 21 randomized controlled trials. J Am Coll Cardiol 2014; 64(16). C112.

32. Li X, Xu J. Lycopene supplement and blood pressure: an updated meta-analysis of intervention trials. Nutrients 2013;5(9):3696–712.

33. Rosenfeldt FL, Haas SJ, Krum H, et al. Coenzyme Q10 in the treatment of hypertension: a meta-analysis of the clinical trials. J Hum Hypertens 2007;21(4): 297–306.

34. Mortensen SA, Rosenfeldt F, Kumar A, et al, Q-SYMBIO Study Investigators. The effect of coenzyme Q10 on morbidity and mortality in chronic heart failure: results from Q-SYMBIO: a randomized double-blind trial. JACC Heart Fail 2014; 2(6):641–9.

35. Ho MJ, Li EC, Wright JM. Blood pressure lowering efficacy of coenzyme Q10 for primary hypertension. Cochrane Database Syst Rev 2016;(3):CD007435.

36. Houston M. The role of magnesium in hypertension and cardiovascular disease. J Clin Hypertens 2011;13(11):843–7.

37. Zhang X, Li Y, Del Gobbo LC, et al. Effects of magnesium supplementation on blood pressure novelty and significance. Hypertension 2016;68(2):324–33.

38. Cordain L, Eaton SB, Sebastian A, et al. Origins and evolution of the Western diet: health implications for the 21st century. Am J Clin Nutr 2005;81:341–54.

39. Dyer AR, Elliott P, Shipley M. Urinary electrolyte excretion in 24 hours and blood pressure in the Intersalt study. II. Estimates of electrolyte blood pressure associations corrected for regression dilution bias. Am J Epidemiol 1994;139(9): 940–51.

40. D'elia L, Barba G, Cappuccio FP, et al. Potassium intake, stroke, and cardiovascular disease. J Am Coll Cardiol 2011;57(10):1210–9.

41. Aburto NJ, Hanson S, Gutierrez H, et al. Effect of increased potassium intake on cardiovascular risk factors and disease: systematic review and meta-analyses. BMJ 2013;346:f1378.

42. Saltman P. Trace elements and blood pressure. Ann Intern Med 1983;98(5 Part 2):823–7.

43. Judd SE, Tangpricha V. Vitamin D deficiency and risk for cardiovascular disease. Am J Med Sci 2009;338(1):40–4.
44. Beveridge LA, Struthers AD, Khan F, et al. Effect of Vitamin D Supplementation on Blood PressureA Systematic Review and Meta-analysis Incorporating Individual Patient Data. JAMA Intern Med 2015;175(5):745–54.
45. Vaidya A, Forman JP. Vitamin D and hypertension: current evidence and future directions. Hypertension 2010;56(5):774–9.
46. Beierwaltes WH. The role of calcium in the regulation of renin secretion. Am J Physiol Ren Physiol 2010;298(1):F1–11.
47. Resnick L. The role of dietary calcium in hypertension: a hierarchal overview. Am J Hypertens 1999;12(1):99–112.
48. Bohr DF. Vascular smooth muscle: dual effect of calcium. Science 1963;139(3555):597–9.
49. Mccarron DA, Reusser ME. Finding consensus in the dietary calcium-blood pressure debate. J Am Coll Nutr 1999;18(5 Suppl):398S–405S.
50. Anderson JJ, Kruszka B, Delaney JA, et al. Calcium intake from diet and supplements and the risk of coronary artery calcification and its progression among older adults: 10-year follow-up of the multi-ethnic study of atherosclerosis (MESA). J Am Heart Assoc 2016;5(10) [pii:e003815].
51. Miller PE, Van Elswyk M, Alexander DD. Long-chain omega-3 fatty acids eicosapentaenoic acid and docosahexaenoic acid and blood pressure: a meta-analysis of randomized controlled trials. Am J Hypertens 2014;27(7):885–96.
52. Sun Q, Wang B, Li Y, et al. Taurine supplementation lowers blood pressure and improves vascular function in prehypertension. Hypertension 2016;67(3):541–9.
53. Walker AF, Marakis G, Simpson E, et al. Hypotensive effects of hawthorn for patients with diabetes taking prescription drugs: a randomized controlled trial. Br J Gen Pract 2006;56(527):437–43.
54. Aviram M, Dornfeld L. Pomegranate juice consumption inhibits serum angiotensin converting enzyme activity and reduces systolic blood pressure. Atherosclerosis 2001;158:195–8.
55. Mathew AS, Capel-Williams GM, Berry SE, et al. Acute effects of pomegranate extract on postprandial lipaemia, vascular function and blood pressure. Plant Foods Hum Nutr 2012;67:351–7.
56. Corti R, Flammer AJ, Hollenberg NK, et al. Cocoa and cardiovascular health. Circulation 2009;119(10):1433–41.
57. Cornelissen VA, Smart NA. Exercise training for blood pressure: a systematic review and meta-analysis. J Am Heart Assoc 2013;2(1):e004473.
58. Available at: www.heart.org. Accessed April 25, 2017.
59. Hudnut F. Comment on "beyond medications and diet: alternative approaches to lowering blood pressure: a scientific statement from the American Heart Association". Hypertension 2014;63(1):e3.
60. Lackland DT, Townsend RR, Brook RD. Response to comment on "beyond medications and diet: alternative approaches to lowering blood pressure: a scientific statement from the American Heart Association". Hypertension 2014;63(1):e4.
61. World Health Organization. Available at: www.who.int. Accessed April 25, 2017.
62. Aadahl M, Kjaer M, Jørgensen T. Associations between overall physical activity level and cardiovascular risk factors in an adult population. Eur J Epidemiol 2007;22(6):369–78.
63. Tang WH, Wang Z, Levison BS, et al. Intestinal microbial metabolism of phosphatidylcholine and cardiovascular risk. N Engl J Med 2013;368:1575–84.

64. Cho CE, Taesuwan S, Malysheva OV, et al. Trimethylamine-N-oxide (TMAO) response to animal source foods varies among healthy young men and is influenced by their gut microbiota composition: a randomized controlled trial. Mol Nutr Food Res 2017;61(1).
65. Kleinbongard P, Dejam A, Lauer T, et al. Plasma nitrite concentrations reflect the degree of endothelial dysfunction in humans. Free Radic Biol Med 2006;40(2): 295–302.
66. Pereira EC, Ferderbar S, Bertolami MC, et al. Biomarkers of oxidative stress and endothelial dysfunction in glucose intolerance and diabetes mellitus. Clin Biochem 2008;41(18):1454–60.
67. Vogel R, Corretti M, Plotnick GD. Effect of a single high-fat meal on endothelial function in healthy subjects. Am J Cardiol 1997;79(3):350–4.
68. Ornish D, Scherwitz LW, Billings JH, et al. Intensive lifestyle changes for reversal of coronary heart disease. JAMA 1998;280(23):2001–7.
69. Hampton T. Ongoing research points to key role of gut microbes in cardiovascular health. Circulation 2016;134:1687–8.
70. Jacobs DR Jr, Meyer KA, Kushi LH, et al. Whole-grain intake may reduce the risk of ischemic heart disease death in postmenopausal women: the Iowa women's health study. Am J Clin Nutr 1998;68:248–57.
71. Liu S, Stampfer MJ, Hu FB, et al. Whole-grain consumption and risk of coronary heart disease: results from the Nurses' Health Study. Am J Clin Nutr 1999;70:412–9.
72. Hu FB, Williett WC. Optimal diets for prevention of coronary heart disease. JAMA 2002;288(20):2569–78.
73. Mensink RP, Katan MB. Effect of dietary trans fatty acids on high-density and low-density lipoprotein cholesterols levels in healthy subjects. N Engl J Med 1990;323:439–45.
74. Nestel P, Noakes M, Belling B, et al. Plasma lipoprotein lipid and Lp [a] changes with substitution of elaidic acid for oleic acid in the diet. J Lipid Res 1992;33(7): 1029–36.
75. Katan MB, Zock PL, Mensink RP. Trans fatty acids and their effects on lipoproteins in humans. Annu Rev Nutr 1995;15:473–93.
76. Salmeron J, Hu FB, Manson JE, et al. Dietary fat intake and risk of type 2 diabetes in women. Am J Clin Nutr 2001;73(6):1019–26.
77. Kushi LH, Lew RA, Stare FJ, et al. Diet and 20-year mortality from coronary heart disease: the Ireland–Boston Diet–Heart Study. N Engl J Med 1985;312(13): 811–8.
78. Hu FB, Stampfer MJ, Manson JE, et al. Dietary fat intake and the risk of coronary heart disease in women. N Engl J Med 1997;337(21):1491–9.
79. Kris-Etherton PM. AHA Science Advisory. Monounsaturated fatty acids and risk of cardiovascular disease. American Heart Association. Nutrition Committee. Circulation 1999;100:1253–8.
80. Kang JX, Leaf A. Antiarrhythmic effects of polyunsaturated fatty acids: recent studies. Circulation 1996;94:1774–80.
81. Connor SL, Connor WE. Are fish oils beneficial in the prevention and treatment of coronary artery disease? Am J Clin Nutr 1997;66(4 Suppl):1020S–31S.
82. Kromhout D, Bosschieter EB, de Lezenne Coulander C. The inverse relation between fish consumption and 20-year mortality from coronary heart disease. N Engl J Med 1985;312:1205–9.
83. Albert CM, Hennekens CH, O'Donnell CJ, et al. Fish consumption and risk of sudden cardiac death. JAMA 1998;279:23–8.

84. Dietary supplementation with N-3 polyunsaturated fatty acids and vitamin E after myocardial infarction: results of the GISSI-prevenzione trial. Lancet 1999; 354(9177):447–55.

85. Available at: www.mayoclinic.org. Accessed April 25, 2017.

86. Steinberg D, Parthasarathy S, Carew TE, et al. Beyond cholesterol: modifications of low-density lipoprotein that increase its atherogenicity. N Engl J Med 1989;320:915–24.

87. Harris WS, Mozaffarian D, Rimm E, et al. Omega-6 fatty acids and risk for cardiovascular disease: a science advisory from the American Heart Association Nutrition Subcommittee of the Council on Nutrition, Physical Activity, and Metabolism; Council on Cardiovascular Nursing; and Council on Epidemiology and Prevention. Circulation 2009;119(6):902–7.

88. Omega-6 fatty acids, University of Maryland Medical Center. Available at: http://www.umm.edu/altmed/articles/omega-6-000317.htm. Accessed April 25, 2017.

89. Estruch R, Ros E, Salas-Salvadó J, et al. Primary prevention of cardiovascular disease with a Mediterranean diet. N Engl J Med 2013;368(14):1279–90.

90. Lorgeril M, De P, Salen JL, et al. Mediterranean diet, traditional risk factors, and the rate of cardiovascular complications after myocardial infarction: final report of the Lyon Diet Heart Study. Circulation 1999;99(6):779–85.

91. Guasch-Ferré M, Hu FB, Martínez-González MA, et al. Olive oil intake and risk of cardiovascular disease and mortality in the PREDIMED Study. BMC Med 2014; 12:78.

92. Heber D, Lembertas A, Lu QY, et al. An analysis of nine proprietary Chinese red yeast rice dietary supplements: implications of variability in chemical profile and contents. J Altern Complement Med 2001;7(2):133–9.

93. Gordon RY, Cooperman T, Obermeyer W, et al. Marked variability of monacolin levels in commercial red yeast rice products: buyer beware! Arch Intern Med 2010;170(19):1722–7.

94. Lees AM, Mok HY, Lees RS, et al. Plant sterols as cholesterol-lowering agents: clinical trials in patients with hypercholesterolemia and studies of sterol balance. Atherosclerosis 1977;28:325–38.

95. Yoo EG. Sitosterolemia: a review and update of pathophysiology, clinical spectrum, diagnosis, and management. Ann Pediatr Endocrinol Metab 2016;21(1): 7–14.

96. Genser B, Silbernagel G, De Backer G, et al. Plant sterols and cardiovascular disease: a systematic review and meta-analysis. Eur Heart J 2012;33(4):444–51.

97. Cater NB. Plant stanol ester: review of cholesterol-lowering efficacy and implications for coronary heart disease risk reduction. Prev Cardiol 2000;3(3):121–30.

98. Lloyd-Jones DM, Morris PB, Ballantyne CM, et al. 2016 ACC expert consensus decision pathway on the role of non-statin therapies for LDL-cholesterol lowering in the management of atherosclerotic cardiovascular disease risk: a report of the American College of Cardiology Task Force on Clinical Expert Consensus Documents. J Am Coll Cardiol 2016;68(1):92–125.

99. Van Horn L, McCoin M, Kris-Etherton PM, et al. The evidence for dietary prevention and treatment of cardiovascular disease. J Am Diet Assoc 2008;108: 287–331.

100. James SL, Muir JG, Curtis SL, et al. Dietary fibre: a roughage guide. Intern Med J 2003;33:291–6.

101. Slavin JL, Martini MC, Jacobs DR Jr, et al. Plausible mechanisms for the protectiveness of whole grains. Am J Clin Nutr 1999;70(3 Suppl):459S–63S.

102. Threapleton DE, Greenwood DC, Evans CE, et al. Dietary fibre intake and risk of cardiovascular disease: systematic review and meta-analysis. BMJ 2013;347: f6879.

103. Ivey KL, Hodgson JM, Croft KD, et al. Flavonoid intake and all-cause mortality. Am J Clin Nutr 2015;101(5):1012–20.

104. Tresserra-Rimbau A, Rimm EB, Medina-Remón A, et al. Polyphenol intake and mortality risk: a re-analysis of the PREDIMED trial. BMC Med 2014;12:77.

105. Wallerath T, Deckert G, Ternes T. Resveratrol, a polyphenolic phytoalexin present in red wine, enhances expression and activity of endothelial nitric oxide synthase. Circulation 2002;106(13):1652–8.

106. Delmas D, Jannin B, Latruffe N. Resveratrol: preventing properties against vascular alterations and ageing. Mol Nutr Food Res 2005;49(5):377–95.

107. Mukamal KJ, Conigrave KM, Mittleman MA, et al. Roles of drinking pattern and type of alcohol consumed in coronary heart disease in men. N Engl J Med 2003; 348(2):109–18.

108. Hu FB, Willett WC. Prevention of coronary heart disease: findings from the Nurses' Health Study and health professionals' follow-up study. Coron Heart Dis Epidemiol 2005;654–68.

109. American Heart Association. Alcohol, wine and cardiovascular disease. Available at: http://www.americanheart.org/presenter.jhtml?identifier=4422. Accessed December 7, 2004.

110. Peterson J, Dwyer J, Adlercreutz H, et al. Dietary lignans: physiology and potential for cardiovascular disease risk reduction. Nutr Rev 2010;68(10):571–603.

111. Milder IE, Feskens EJ, Arts IC, et al. Intakes of 4 dietary lignans and cause-specific and all-cause mortality in the Zutphen Elderly Study. Am J Clin Nutr 2006;84(2):400–5.

112. Zhang Z, Hu G, Caballero B, et al. Habitual coffee consumption and risk of hypertension: a systematic review and meta-analysis of prospective observational studies. Am J Clin Nutr 2011;93:1212–9.

113. van Dam RM, Hu FB. Coffee consumption and risk of type 2 diabetes: a systematic review. JAMA 2005;294:97–104.

114. Ding M, Bhupathiraju SN, Satija A. Long-term coffee consumption and risk of cardiovascular disease: a systematic review and a dose-response meta-analysis of prospective cohort studies. J Vasc Surg 2014;59(5):1471.

115. Arab L, Khan F, Lam H. Tea consumption and cardiovascular disease risk. Am J Clin Nutr 2013;98(6 Suppl):1651S–9S.

116. Khalesi S, Sun J, Buys N, et al. Green tea catechins and blood pressure: a systematic review and meta-analysis of randomised controlled trials. Eur J Nutr 2014;53:1299–311.

117. Sacks FM, Lichtenstein A, Van Horn L, et al. Soy protein, isoflavones, and cardiovascular health. Circulation 2006;113:1034–44.

118. Shu XO, Zheng Y, Cai H, et al. Soy food intake and breast cancer survival. JAMA 2009;302(22):2437–43.

119. Sumner MD, Elliott-Eller M, Weidner G, et al. Effects of pomegranate juice consumption on myocardial perfusion in patients with coronary heart disease. Am J Cardiol 2005;96:810–4.

120. Aviram M, Dornfeld L, Rosenblat M, et al. Pomegranate juice consumption reduces oxidative stress, atherogenic modifications to LDL, and platelet aggregation: studies in humans and in atherosclerotic apolipoprotein E-deficient mice. Am J Clin Nutr 2000;71:1062–76.

121. Rosenblat M, Hayek T, Aviram M. Anti-oxidative effects of pomegranate juice (PJ) consumption by diabetic patients on serum and on macrophages. Atherosclerosis 2006;187:368–76.
122. Alpha-Tocopherol, Beta-Carotene Cancer Prevention Study Group. The effect of vitamin E and beta-carotene on the incidence of lung cancer and other cancers in male smokers. N Engl J Med 1994;330:1029–35.
123. Omenn GS, Goodman GE, Thornquist MD, et al. Effects of a combination of beta carotene and vitamin A on lung cancer and cardiovascular disease. N Engl J Med 1996;334:1150–5.
124. Stephens NG, Parsons A, Schofield PM, et al. Randomised controlled trial of vitamin E in patients with coronary disease: Cambridge Heart Antioxidant Study. Lancet 1996;347:781–6.
125. Rapola JM, Virtamo J, Ripatti S, et al. Randomised trial of α-tocopherol and β-carotene supplements on incidence of major coronary events in men with previous myocardial infarction. Lancet 1997;349:1715–20.
126. Kendrick J, Targher G, Smits G, et al. 25-hydroxyvitamin D deficiency is independently associated with cardiovascular disease in the third national health and nutrition examination survey. Atherosclerosis 2009;205(1):255–60.
127. Melamed ML, Michos ED, Post W, et al. 25-hydroxyvitamin D levels and the risk of mortality in the general population. Arch Intern Med 2008;168(15):1629–37.
128. Wang H, Xia N, Yang Y, et al. Influence of vitamin D supplementation on plasma lipid profiles: a meta-analysis of randomized controlled trials. Lipids Health Dis 2012;11(1):42.
129. Clinicaltrials.gov identified: NCT01169259.
130. Lamas GA, Goertz C, Boineau R, et al. Effect of disodium EDTA chelation regimen on cardiovascular events in patients with previous MI: the TACT randomized trial. JAMA 2013;309:1241–50.
131. Escolar E, Lamas GA, Mark DB, et al. The effect of an EDTA-based chelation regimen on patients with diabetes mellitus and prior myocardial infarction in the trial to assess chelation therapy (TACT). Circ Cardiovasc Qual Outcomes 2014;7:15–24.
132. Available at: https://clinicaltrials.gov/ct2/show/NCT02733185. Accessed April 25, 2017.
133. Schneider RH, Grim CE, Rainforth MV, et al. Stress reduction in the secondary prevention of cardiovascular disease randomized, controlled trial of transcendental meditation and health education in Blacks. Circ Cardiovasc Qual Outcomes 2012;5(6):750–8.
134. Writing Group Members, Mozaffarian D, Benjamin EJ, et al. Heart disease and stroke statistics-2016 update: a report from the American Heart Association. Circulation 2016;133(4):e38–360.
135. Krumholz HM, Parent EM, Tu N, et al. Readmission after hospitalization for congestive heart failure among medicare beneficiaries. Arch Intern Med 1997; 157:99–104.
136. Juenger J, Schellberg D, Kraemer S, et al. Health related quality of life in patients with congestive heart failure: comparison with other chronic diseases and relation to functional variables. Heart 2002;87(3):235–41.
137. Horowitz JD. Home-based intervention: the next step in treatment of chronic heart failure? Eur Heart J 2000;21(22):1807Y1809.
138. van der Wal MH, van Veldhuisen DJ, Veeger NJ, et al. Compliance with non-pharmacological recommendations and outcome in heart failure patients. Eur Heart J 2010;31(12):1486–93.

139. Tsuyuki RT, McKelvie RS, Arnold JM, et al. Acute precipitants of congestive heart failure exacerbations. Arch Intern Med 2001;161(19):2337–42.

140. Son YJ, Lee Y, Song EK. Adherence to a sodium-restricted diet is associated with lower symptom burden and longer cardiac event-free survival in patients with heart failure. J Clin Nurs 2011;20(21–22):3029–38.

141. Philipson H, Ekman I, Forslund HB, et al. Salt and fluid restriction is effective in patients with chronic heart failure. Eur J Heart Fail 2013;15(11):1304–10.

142. Paterna S, Parrinello G, Cannizzaro S, et al. Medium term effects of different dosage of diuretic, sodium, and fluid administration on neurohormonal and clinical outcome in patients with recently compensated heart failure. Am J Cardiol 2009;103(1):93–102.

143. Paterna S, Gaspare P, Fasullo S, et al. Normal-sodium diet compared with low-sodium diet in compensated congestive heart failure: is sodium an old enemy or a new friend? Clin Sci (Lond) 2008;114:221–30.

144. Parrinello G, Di Pasquale P, Licata G, et al. Long-term effects of dietary sodium intake on cytokines and neurohormonal activation in patients with recently compensated congestive heart failure. J Card Fail 2009;15:864–73.

145. Jessup M, Abraham WT, Casey DE, et al. 2009 Focused Update: ACCF/AHA guidelines for the diagnosis and management of heart failure in adults: a report of the American College of Cardiology Foundation/American Heart Association Task Force on practice guidelines developed in collaboration with the International Society for Heart and Lung Transplantation. J Am Coll Cardiol 2009;53: 1343–82.

146. Nieuwenhuis MM, van der Wal MH, Jaarsma T. The body of knowledge on compliance in heart failure patients: we are not there yet. J Cardiovasc Nurs 2011;26(1):21–8.

147. Molloy GJ, O'Carroll RE, Witham MD, et al. Interventions to enhance adherence to medications in patients with heart failure: a systematic review. Circ Heart Fail 2012;5(1):126–33.

148. Georgiopoulou VV, Kalogeropoulos AP, Chowdhury R, et al. Exercise capacity, heart failure risk, and mortality in older adults: the health ABC study. Am J Prev Med 2017;52(2):144–53.

149. Belardinelli R, Georgiou D, Cianci G, et al. 10-year exercise training in chronic heart failure: a randomized controlled trial. J Am Coll Cardiol 2012;60(16):1521–8.

150. Mant J, Al-Mohammad A, Swain S, et al. Guideline Development Group. Management of chronic heart failure in adults: synopsis of the National Institute for Health and Clinical Excellence guideline. Ann Intern Med 2011;155(4):252–9.

151. Giuliano C, Karahalios A, Neil C, et al. The effects of resistance training on muscle strength, quality of life and aerobic capacity in patients with chronic heart failure—a meta-analysis. Int J Cardiol 2017;227:413–23.

152. Yeh GY, McCarthy EP, Wayne PM, et al. Tai chi exercise in patients with chronic heart failure: a randomized clinical trial. Arch Intern Med 2011;171(8):750–7.

153. Sullivan MJ, Wood L, Terry J, et al. The support, education, and research in chronic heart failure study (SEARCH): a mindfulness-based psychoeducational intervention improves depression and clinical symptoms in patients with chronic heart failure. Am Heart J 2009;157(1):84–90.

154. Kemper KJ, Carmin C, Mehta B, et al. Integrative medical care plus mindfulness training for patients with congestive heart failure: proof of concept. J Evid Based Complement Altern Med 2016;21(4):282–90.

155. Curiati JA, Bocchi E, Freire JO, et al. Meditation reduces sympathetic activation and improves the quality of life in elderly patients with optimally treated heart

failure: a prospective randomized study. J Altern Complement Med 2005;11(3): 465–72.

156. Bin YS, Kiat H. Prevalence of dietary supplement use in patients with proven or suspected cardiovascular disease. Evid Based Complement Alternat Med 2011;2011:632829.

157. Chagan L, Bernstein D, Cheng JW, et al. Use of biological based therapy in patients with cardiovascular diseases in a university-hospital in New York city. BMC Complement Altern Med 2005;5:4.

158. Grant SJ, Bin YS, Kiat H, et al. The use of complementary and alternative medicine by people with cardiovascular disease: a systematic review. BMC Public Health 2012;12(1):1.

159. Madmani ME, Yusuf Solaiman A, Tamr Agha K, et al. Coenzyme Q10 for heart failure. Cochrane Database Syst Rev 2014;(6):CD008684.

160. DiNicolantonio JJ, Lavie CJ, Fares H, et al. L-carnitine in the secondary prevention of cardiovascular disease: systematic review and meta-analysis. Mayo Clin Proc 2013;88(6):544–51.

161. Institute of Medicine, Food and Nutrition Board. Dietary reference intakes: vitamin C, vitamin E, selenium, and carotenoids. Washington, DC: National Academy Press; 2000.

162. Pittler MH, Schmidt K, Ernst E. Hawthorn extract for treating chronic heart failure: meta-analysis of randomized trials. Am J Med 2003;114(8):665–74.

163. Holubarsch CJ, Colucci WS, Meinertz T, et al. The efficacy and safety of Crataegus extract WS® 1442 in patients with heart failure: the SPICE trial. Eur J Heart Fail 2008;10(12):1255–63.

164. Dasgupta A, Kidd L, Poindexter BJ, et al. Interference of hawthorn on serum digoxin measurements by immunoassays and pharmacodynamic interaction with digoxin. Arch Pathol Lab Med 2010;134(8):1188–92.

165. Kong MH, Fonarow GC, Peterson ED, et al. Systematic review of the incidence of sudden cardiac death in the United States. J Am Coll Cardiol 2011;57(7): 794–801.

166. Meissner MD, Akhtar M, Lehmann MH. Nonischemic sudden tachyarrhythmic death in atherosclerotic heart disease. Circulation 1991;84:905–12.

167. Podrid PJ, Lampert S, Graboys TB, et al. Aggravation of arrhythmia by antiarrhythmic drugs–incidence and predictors. Am J Cardiol 1987;59:38E–44E.

168. Brenyo A, Aktas MK. Review of complementary and alternative medical treatment of arrhythmias. Am J Cardiol 2014;113(5):897–903.

169. Jahangiri A, Leifert WR, Patten GS, et al. Termination of asynchronous contractile activity in rat atrial myocytes by n-3 poliun-saturated fatty acids. Mol Cell Biochem 2000;206:33–41.

170. Costanzo S, di Niro V, Di Castelnuovo A, et al. Prevention of postoperative atrial fibrillation in open heart surgery patients by preoperative supplementation of n-3 polyunsaturated fatty acids: an updated meta-analysis [review]. J Thorac Cardiovasc Surg 2013;146(4):906–11.

171. Khoueiry G, Abi Rafeh N, Sullivan E, et al. Do omega-3 polyunsaturated fatty acids reduce risk of sudden cardiac death and ventricular arrhythmias? A meta-analysis of randomized trials. Heart Lung 2013;42(4):251–6.

172. Maciejewski P, Bednarz B, Chamiec T, et al. Acute coronary syndrome: potassium, magnesium and cardiac arrhythmia. Kardiol Pol 2003;59(11):402–7.

173. Shiga T, Wajima Z, Inoue T, et al. Magnesium prophylaxis for arrhythmias after cardiac surgery: a meta-analysis of randomized controlled trials. Am J Med 2004;117(5):325–33.

174. Zehender M, Meinertz T, Faber T, et al. Antiarrhythmic effects of increasing the daily intake of magnesium and potassium in patients with frequent ventricular arrhythmias. Magnesium in cardiac arrhythmias (MAGICA) investigators. J Am Coll Cardiol 1997;29(5):1028–34.
175. Khattab K, Khattab AA, Ortak J, et al. Iyengar yoga increases cardiac parasympathetic nervous modulation among healthy yoga practitioners. Evid Based Complement Alternat Med 2007;4(4):511–7.
176. Lakkireddy D, Atkins D, Pillarisetti J, et al. Effect of yoga on arrhythmia burden, anxiety, depression, and quality of life in paroxysmal atrial fibrillation: the YOGA my heart study. J Am Coll Cardiol 2013;61(11):1177–82.
177. VanWormer AM, Lindquist R, Sendelbach SE. The effects of acupuncture on cardiac arrhythmias: a literature review. Heart Lung 2008;37(6):425–31.
178. Lomuscio A, Belletti S, Battezzati PM, et al. Efficacy of acupuncture in preventing atrial fibrillation recurrences after electrical cardioversion. J Cardiovasc Electrophysiol 2011;22(3):241–7.

Integrative Medicine for Respiratory Conditions

Asthma and Chronic Obstructive Pulmonary Disease

Gloria Y. Yeh, MD, MPH[a],*, Randy Horwitz, MD, PhD[b]

KEYWORDS

- Asthma • COPD • Respiratory disease • Integrative medicine

KEY POINTS

- An integrative approach for asthma and chronic obstructive pulmonary disease (COPD) considers a multidimensional, biopsychosocial model.
- Integrative medicine in the management of asthma and COPD includes appropriate conventional care, medications, lifestyle and self-care strategies (smoking cessation, allergen avoidance, physical activity, and nutrition), attention to mental and emotional health, and consideration of select evidence-based complementary modalities.
- Mind-body therapies may help to address psychosocial aspects of chronic disease, improve quality of life and symptoms.
- Select supplements or herbal compounds may be promising to improve symptoms and decrease exacerbations.

INTRODUCTION
Asthma and Chronic Obstructive Pulmonary Disease

Asthma and chronic obstructive pulmonary disease (COPD) are both common chronic respiratory disorders in primary care that cause considerable morbidity and mortality. Although typically classified as distinct entities, they both involve obstructive airflow limitation and inflammation, and have been described as existing along the same spectrum. In the United States, asthma affects 7.7% of the population (more than 24 million people), a prevalence that has been rising for the past several decades.[1] Although asthma can occur at any age, more than a quarter of asthma sufferers in

[a] Division of General Medicine and Primary Care, Beth Israel Deaconess Medical Center, Harvard Medical School, 1309 Beacon Street, Brookline, MA 02446, USA; [b] Arizona Center for Integrative Medicine, Department of Medicine, University of Arizona College of Medicine, PO Box 245153, Tucson, AZ 85724-5153, USA
* Corresponding author.
E-mail address: gyeh@hms.harvard.edu

Med Clin N Am 101 (2017) 925–941
http://dx.doi.org/10.1016/j.mcna.2017.04.008
0025-7125/17/© 2017 Elsevier Inc. All rights reserved.

medical.theclinics.com

the United States are children. COPD tends to have an older demographic. It has an estimated prevalence of 6.5% (14 million people) in the United States, but the condition is thought to be greatly underdiagnosed.[2–4] COPD is the third most common cause of death in the United States, behind heart disease and cancer.[5]

Although evidence-based complementary approaches to asthma and COPD can be very helpful, they are just one component of a comprehensive care plan that should include conventional therapies and regular follow-up, and should never be used in place of appropriate medical care.

ASTHMA
Pathophysiology

Early in the 1990s, asthma was categorized as either allergic or nonallergic. Since then, advanced diagnostic techniques have allowed for a marked expansion of these categories, resulting in the identification of dozens of asthma phenotypes.[6] Most of these have defined, discrete triggers, rather than unique pathophysiologic mechanisms. At its root, in people with asthma, the responses of the asthmatic airway to provocative stimuli remain constant: bronchoconstriction, bronchial hyperresponsiveness, and inflammation. Of these, airway inflammation has proven to be the most amenable to integrative modalities.

Allergic triggers are among the most predominant initiators of the asthma exacerbation and much of the pathophysiology of asthma has been delineated within the allergic model. In an atopic individual, with characteristic airway hyperresponsiveness, the introduction of an allergen into the airway triggers a well-defined series of reactions, beginning with mast cell degranulation and the release of vasoactive amines, enzymes, and leukotrienes, that trigger smooth muscle bronchoconstriction. Allergic T helper 2 cells then secrete cytokines and chemokines that further recruit other cells to the airway. The cellular influx results in mucus production that further contributes to the inflammatory cascade. In the 1970s, the recognition of an inflammatory component of asthma allowed for successful therapies using broad-spectrum anti-inflammatory drugs, such as oral corticosteroids, albeit with severe and long-term adverse effects. The recent discovery of the discrete constituents of the inflammatory pathway has allowed for targeted biological therapies using monoclonal antibodies that reduce adverse events but may have long-term sequelae that have not been observed yet.

Evaluation

The diagnosis and continuing care of the patient with asthma are standard elements of medical education and training; however, some aspects are often forgotten. Initial evaluation should characterize the frequency and severity of symptoms, the degree of airway compromise and reversibility (using spirometry with or without a bronchodilator), and any identifiable triggers. Asthma triggers are typically individualized; however, it is worth exploring the more common triggers, which include upper respiratory infections, exercise, allergen exposure, cold weather, laughing or crying, or other emotional stress. In addition, an environmental history and food diary may be helpful in discerning dietary triggers or location-specific allergen exposures (ie, dust mites in the home or office). Allergy testing is also important, especially with seasonal symptoms because the effectiveness of immunotherapy in atopic individuals has been demonstrated.[7]

Asthma diagnosis and classification relies on the presence of a set of discrete symptoms, including recurrent and reversible cough, wheezing, dyspnea, or chest tightness. Objective evidence includes spirometry that demonstrates reversal of airway obstruction following administration of a bronchodilator medication (eg, albuterol). Asthma classification is based on frequency of symptoms (including nocturnal symptoms), need and weekly use of rescue medication, interference with daily activities, lung function, and frequency of severe exacerbations. Therapeutic decisions are based on this classification. Details on assessment and classification can be found in the National Heart, Lung, and Blood Institute's expert panel review.[8]

Follow-up care in asthma is critical because it can uncover new triggers and identify the need for more or less intensive therapy. It is always prudent to use the lowest dose of drug needed to achieve and sustain control, especially when a patient is chronically using oral corticosteroids. Finally, the use of objective lung function data (spirometry) along with a standard, validated measure of asthma control is encouraged at each appointment. Two such accepted tools are the Asthma Control Test and the Asthma Control Questionnaire.[9,10] These brief forms are filled out by the patient; provide objective, quantifiable indicators of asthma symptoms; and take only minutes to administer and interpret.

Prevention

Prevention of the development of asthma is not yet possible. Studies examining genetic and epigenetic contributors, both prenatal and postnatal, have proven difficult. Much evidence points to upper respiratory viral infections early in childhood as potent catalysts to the development of asthma.[11] No dietary or environmental interventions have been shown to effectively eliminate the risk of developing asthma in susceptible or at-risk individuals. There are, however, interventions that may be useful in preventing or reducing asthma exacerbations. Avoidance of airborne triggers is difficult, given the ubiquitous nature of windblown pollens, but some commonsense recommendations may be of use, including avoidance of raking leaves (*Alternaria* exposure), vacuuming (dust mite exposure), pet ownership, or at least pet access to the bedroom (cat, dog allergens). High-efficiency particulate air (HEPA) filters can be useful for individuals with allergic rhinitis.

Treatment

Pharmaceuticals

The conventional management of asthma focuses on both immediate relief of symptoms and long-term control. Step therapy is based on asthma disease classification, and degree of symptom control.[8] The most common medications for immediate relief are the bronchodilators, mainly short-acting metered dose inhalers, including the short-acting beta agonists and anticholinergics. The medications for long-term control include inhaled corticosteroid preparations, long-acting bronchodilators, leukotriene antagonists and modifiers, and newer biological modifiers (monoclonal antibodies given intravenously).[8] Inhaled corticosteroids have become a mainstay of conventional therapy; newer formulations greatly reduce systemic corticosteroid absorption and adverse effects. Long-acting beta agonists (LABAs) have a high beta-2 receptor affinity and bronchodilate for 12 hours or more with a single administration. However, multiple studies have raised concerns about using a LABA as monotherapy, with higher numbers of asthma-related deaths observed. Studies using concomitant LABA and inhaled corticosteroid did not result in increased asthma-related deaths. Leukotriene modifiers have demonstrated efficacy in the treatment of both asthma and allergic rhinitis but only in those patients with high levels of leukotrienes.[8] The newest medications are biologically engineered antibodies designed to interfere with discrete steps in the allergic inflammatory cascade.

Cromolyn is a prime example of a drug whose active ingredient was extracted from a botanic source with a historical record of effectiveness. Isolated from an extract of the khella plant (*Ammi visnaga*), cromolyn demonstrates potent mast cell–stabilizing activity in vitro. When used prophylactically, in advance of allergenic exposure, cromolyn can markedly reduce the rate and degree of mast cell degranulation and thus allergic symptoms. Cromolyn is available by prescription in a nebulized form, as a liquid for oral use in gastrointestinal allergic conditions, and without a prescription as a nasal preparation for allergic rhinitis. This drug is regarded as a steroid-sparing anti-inflammatory, as opposed to a rescue inhaler.

Diet and nutritional supplements

The avoidance of specific foods or food additives for gastrointestinal or anaphylactic allergic reactions is an obvious and effective intervention. For asthma, however, the use of specific or elimination diets has been controversial. Although elimination diets are specific to an individual, some common classes of foods, including dairy products, wheat, and even certain animal proteins, have been popularly linked to allergic exacerbations, although published clinical data in this area are scant.

The association between milk intake and mucus production in people with allergies and asthma is a very popular belief among patients but is refuted by a small number of studies.[12] However, several biologically plausible hypotheses may support such an association. For example, patients with asthma have higher levels of a specific mucin (MUC5AC) in their airways relative to nonasthma patients.[13] Certain types of milk (from specific breeds of cow) contain a protein called β-CM-7, which has been shown to stimulate MUC5AC production. It has been hypothesized that milk ingestion may lead to stimulation of respiratory mucin production in the airway and thus increase phlegm production.[14] A brief trial (4–6 weeks) of dairy avoidance may be helpful to discern such an association in selected individuals.

An important initial step in most inflammatory conditions, including asthma, is the catabolism of cell membrane–derived fats for entry into the arachidonic acid pathway. The cell uses these fatty acids to synthesize many significant inflammatory mediators in an asthma exacerbation, including the leukotrienes. Alterations in the dietary intake of fats are known to affect the fatty acid composition of cell membranes.[15,16] Omega-3 supplementation decreases the ratio of omega-6 to omega-3 fatty acids in the inflammatory cell lipid membrane, thus creating less substrate for inflammatory mediator production. This process, in turn, decreases the production of many potent bioactive compounds (eg, leukotrienes) that are intimately involved in allergic inflammation.[17] Clinical trials of omega-3 acid supplementation from fish and plant sources in the treatment of asthma and allergic diseases have been inconsistent.[18] In one small clinical trial, subjects with asthma who consumed a diet with an elevated omega-3 to omega-6 content showed marked improvement in airway hyperresponsiveness.[19] These responders to dietary interventions could be readily identified through analysis of the leukotriene composition in the urine, a measure that predicted which patients were likely to improve with dietary intervention.[19] Unfortunately, such testing is not currently feasible for routine practice. Thus increased dietary omega-3 intake (or a trial of omega-3 supplementation) in some patients may be a useful clinical intervention.

Vitamin D deficiency has been associated with increased symptoms, exacerbations, medication use, and reduced lung function in both adults and children. Although studies have been mixed regarding the value of supplementation, a recent Cochrane meta-analysis reported that vitamin D is likely to reduce both risk of severe asthma exacerbation and health care use. It remains unclear whether this effect is limited to those with baseline vitamin deficiencies.[20] The role of antioxidants and other vitamins such as vitamin C has also received considerable attention, although the clinical value of supplementation is still largely unknown.

Magnesium is a standard of care in the emergency treatment of acute asthma exacerbations and is administered intravenously or in nebulized form.[21] Magnesium has been shown to improve forced expiratory volume in 1 second (FEV_1) and reduce intensive care unit admissions in a hospital setting.[22] In chronic asthma, inverse associations are also reported between intracellular (red blood cell) magnesium levels and asthma severity.[23] Despite this, little convincing literature supports a role for long-term magnesium supplementation in mild-to-moderate asthma. Some reports note an improvement in asthma symptoms for those subjects with a higher magnesium intake,[24] whereas others link dietary magnesium intake with an increased risk of asthma and wheezing in children.[25] A 6-month study of magnesium supplementation (340 mg of magnesium citrate daily) in adults with mild-to-moderate asthma produced improvements in bronchial hyperreactivity, peak flow, and quality of life, without significant effects on other markers of asthma control nor inflammatory markers.[26]

Other supplements The most promising of the many other supplements purported for use in asthma are the bioflavonoids. Benefits of these compounds have been demonstrated in both in vitro and animal studies; however, human studies are just beginning. It is very difficult to absorb orally administered flavonoids owing to their unique chemistry, so several compounds are routinely added to bioflavonoid formulations (eg, bromelain, vitamin C) to increase systemic absorption. Some flavonoids, such as cromolyn, have already been successfully marketed by the pharmaceutical industry and are available as prescription medications. Others are available over the counter, including Pycnogenol, quercetin, and fisetin. Because these compounds have shown remarkable in vitro activity against allergic inflammation, they are worth discussing in some detail.

Pycnogenol is a proprietary antioxidant-bioflavonoid mixed extract isolated from the bark of the maritime pine (*Pinus pinaster*). It has a variety of biological activities, ranging from blood pressure reduction to mitigation of elevated blood glucose. In terms of asthma, it has been shown to be efficacious in a murine model of airway inflammation,[27] as well as in a clinical trial of children with asthma.[28] In this study, Pycnogenol improved asthma symptoms and pulmonary function, and decreased rescue inhaler use. In addition, there was a significant reduction of urinary leukotriene production in the treated group.[28] Pycnogenol can be considered for use in adolescents and adults with persistent, mild-to-moderate asthma.

Quercetin is a bioflavonoid found in diverse foods, including apples, buckwheat, onions, and citrus fruits. In vitro, quercetin stabilizes the membranes of mast cells and reduces the release of preformed histamine.[29,30] In animal models, quercetin suppresses anaphylactic responses in sensitized rats,[31] and it inhibits asthmatic inflammation in guinea pigs and rats.[32] Quercetin also inhibits the production of enzymes responsible for synthesizing the leukotrienes.[33] Due to its ubiquity in nature, and potential benefit, quercetin can be considered for patients with allergies or allergic asthma.

Fisetin is found primarily in strawberries but also in apples, persimmons, and onions. Bioavailability is the biggest issue with fisetin, as with other flavonoids. Most studies of fisetin involving asthma animal models were done using intravenous or intraperitoneal formulations, although some used oral preparations.[34] This compound potently inhibits the transcription factor, nuclear factor-kappaB (NF-κB), is responsible for the expression of many inflammatory genes (eg, interleukin [IL]-1, IL-2, IL-6, IL-8, tumor necrosis factor, adhesins),[35] and may produce broad anti-inflammatory effects that transcend allergic disease. In animal models, the compound inhibited asthma flares with an anti-inflammatory effect that rivaled corticosteroids.[35] Human studies of fisetin are lacking to date, thus no formal clinical recommendations can be made; however, it is commonly used for asthma patients by integrative medicine practitioners.

An exciting area of future innovation worth noting is the ongoing work in the domain of Chinese herbal formulations. One herbal preparation, tested in animal models of asthma, was shown to be as effective an anti-inflammatory agent as corticosteroids but via a novel mechanism and with potentially fewer adverse effects.[36] Using a series of carefully designed experiments, the group tested the antiasthma herbal medicine intervention (ASHMI) compound in adults with mild-to-moderate asthma, compared with daily prednisone, over a 4-week period. Both ASHMI and prednisone resulted in improved peak flow, FEV_1, symptoms, and reduced need for rescue bronchodilators. However, subjects taking ASHMI did not experience prednisone-related weight gain and increased serum cortisol.[37] The provided table (**Table 1**) includes a brief summary of a few selected oral supplements used in asthma and chronic obstructive pulmonary disease (described later).

Mind-body therapy
Numerous studies document the value of mind-body approaches in the treatment of asthma. This is not unexpected considering the association of anxiety and stress with asthma exacerbations. Recall of anxious and stressful experiences adversely affect expiratory flow rates in children with chronic asthma with no pre-existing psychopathology.[38] These emotionally induced decreases in expiratory flow rates were reversed with relaxation and self-hypnosis. In addition, poor asthma control is highly associated with greater symptoms of anxiety and depression.[39] Individuals with high chronic stress exhibit a greater cortisol response to an acute stressor, as well as increases in blood and sputum eosinophils, whereas these relationships are opposite in those with low chronic stress.[39] Thus, a true psychoneuroimmunological association has been established between asthma and stress or anxiety. Although external stress can trigger or worsen chronic asthma, research has shown that intrinsic stress can have the same effect.

Interestingly, classic studies from the late 1960s demonstrated the power of the mind-body connection in asthma, Patients with moderate-to-severe asthma exhibited severe symptoms when they were exposed to saline mists that they believed were potent allergens. Even more remarkable was their prompt recovery with use of a saline inhaler that they believed to be a beta agonist.[40,41] Even standard skin test reactions that produce classic wheal-and-flare reactions to subcutaneously introduced allergens can be modulated by mind-body techniques. In one study, subjects with dust mite sensitivity who were skin tested after viewing a humorous video demonstrated lower wheal-and-flare reactivity to dust mite allergen than did subjects viewing a control video (weather documentary).[42]

Some mind-body therapies that have been studied in both adults and children with asthma include breathing exercises, relaxation, guided imagery, biofeedback, journaling, tai chi or qigong, and yoga.[43,44] Clinical hypnosis also has a long history of successful use in asthma. Another popular mind-body therapy is mindfulness meditation. One randomized controlled trial (RCT) of an 8-week Mindfulness-Based Stress Reduction (MBSR) program versus an educational program in adults with asthma showed clinically significant improvements in quality of life and perceived stress but without demonstrable improvements in lung function.[45]

CHRONIC OBSTRUCTIVE PULMONARY DISEASE
Pathophysiology

COPD is a syndrome of progressive airflow limitation which, in contrast to asthma, is not fully reversible. It is characterized by abnormal inflammatory responses

Table 1
Selected oral supplements in asthma and chronic obstructive pulmonary disease

Supplement	Asthma (A) COPD (C)	Possible Mechanism of Action	Dosing[a]	Comments
Omega-3 fatty acids (fish or plant-derived)	A, C	Decreases inflammatory mediator production	1500–2000 mg EPA daily in divided doses	Fishy breath and gastrointestinal side effects most common Lower doses being studied in COPD
Quercetin	A	Mast cell stabilizer; anti-inflammatory	400–600 mg up to tid	No human clinical study data available
Pycnogenol	A	Anti-inflammatory; decreased leukotriene production	100–200 mg bid daily in divided doses	Proprietary antioxidant-bioflavonoid mixed extract
Fisetin	A	Anti-inflammatory Nuclear factor-kappaB (NF-κB) inhibition	100–200 mg daily	No human clinical study data available
Magnesium	A	Airway smooth muscle relaxation Potentiation of beta agonist activity	300–500 mg daily	Use limited by diarrhea Magnesium glycinate may have less laxative effect Caution in kidney disease
Vitamin D-3 cholecalciferol	A, C	Immunomodulation Anti-inflammatory	800–2000 IU daily	May enhance effectiveness of corticosteroid treatment
N-acetyl cysteine	C	Mucoactive Anti-inflammatory Antioxidant	600–1200 mg daily in divided doses	Avoid nebulized form due to potential acute bronchospasm Caution with anticoagulants, such as warfarin

[a] Used in studies and/or commonly used in practice.[20,26,65,85–87]
Abbreviation: EPA, eicosapentaenoic acid.

of the lung to noxious particles or gases, leading to structural changes and narrowing of the small airways. This pathophysiology results in hyperinflation of the lungs (ie, an increase of end expiratory lung volume due to airflow limitation), weakened respiratory muscles, and inefficient gas exchange.[46] Early definitions of COPD distinguished different types (eg, chronic bronchitis, emphysema). This distinction is not in the current definition but individual patients present along a spectrum. An asthma-COPD overlap syndrome is also recently recognized.[47]

Toxic environmental exposures are central to pathogenesis, with cigarette smoking being the single most important risk factor for developing COPD. Up to 90% of all deaths from COPD are attributable to smoking.[48] Environmental exposures to occupational dusts, chemicals, and air pollution (particularly in developing worlds) also contribute to incidence. Other influences, such as infections in early life, genetic predispositions (eg, alpha-1 antitrypsin deficiency), and pre-existing asthma, may also play a role. The mechanistic basis underlying COPD is complex and involves inflammation, oxidative stress, protease-antiprotease imbalance, environmental insult, and host genetics.[5]

In general, COPD is slowly progressive with periods of exacerbations. The cardinal symptoms are dyspnea (first present with physical activity but later also at rest) and exercise intolerance. Other major symptoms are chronic cough and increased sputum production. Exacerbations worsen these symptoms, in addition to wheezing, chest tightness, tachycardia, and fevers. Skeletal muscle dysfunction, nutritional abnormalities, and systemic inflammation are important players. Fatigue, weight loss, and anorexia are common in patients with severe disease. Associated comorbidities include cardiovascular disease, metabolic syndrome, osteoporosis, lung cancer, depression, anxiety, and sleep disorders.[5]

There is increasing appreciation that COPD is a complex, multidimensional chronic disease whereby the patient experience is a consequence of not only physical and functional problems, but it is overlaid with a myriad of emotional, behavioral, spiritual considerations and psychosocial stressors. This multidimensional framework (**Fig. 1**) can be considered in all aspects of COPD management from pathophysiology to evaluation to treatment.

A conceptual model that considers one simple aspect of this framework is the anxiety or breathlessness cycle. This model (**Fig. 2**) describes an interplay between emotions and the cardinal symptom of dyspnea, which is inherently multifaceted, including physiologic, sensory, and affective dimensions.[49,50] Although this model was initially described in COPD, it is similarly relevant in asthma.

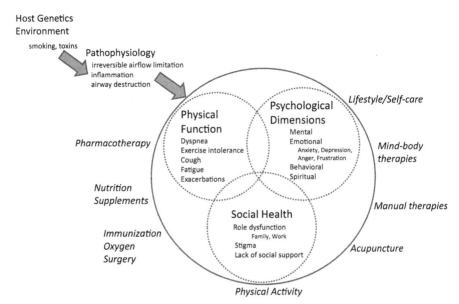

Fig. 1. Multidimensional integrative framework of COPD pathophysiology, evaluation, and management.

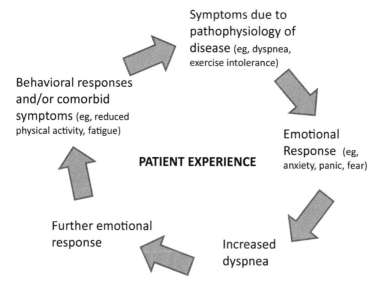

Symptoms due to pathophysiology of disease (eg, dyspnea, exercise intolerance)

Behavioral responses and/or comorbid symptoms (eg, reduced physical activity, fatigue)

PATIENT EXPERIENCE

Emotional Response (eg, anxiety, panic, fear)

Further emotional response

Increased dyspnea

Fig. 2. Anxiety-breathlessness cycle. The cycle starts with disease pathophysiology leading to dyspnea, which then exacerbates anxiety and emotional responses, which then leads to more dyspnea, further exacerbating emotional dysfunction, comorbid symptoms, or behavioral responses (eg, fatigue, reduced activity). This leads to worsening disease state, which manifests as increased dyspnea, and the cycle continues.

Evaluation

The 2016 updated Global Obstructive Lung Disease (GOLD) guidelines for the evaluation of COPD consider the following domains: severity of airflow limitation (pulmonary function testing, in particular spirometry), current level of patient's symptoms, exacerbation risk, and presence of comorbidities.[5] Degree of airflow limitation, symptoms, and impairment of quality of life are not well correlated, so independent consideration of each is needed. With spirometry, the presence of a postbronchodilator FEV_1 or forced vital capacity (FVC) less than 0.70 confirms the presence of persistent airflow limitation. GOLD severity staging is based on degree of airflow limitation ranging from stage 1 (mild, $FEV_1 \geq 80\%$ predicted) to stage 4 (very severe, $FEV_1 < 30\%$ predicted). Symptom assessment can include short questionnaires, such as the Comprehensive Assessment Test or the COPD Control Questionnaire.[51,52] Comorbidities are common at all stages of COPD and can influence mortality and hospitalizations independently. Assessment should include routine screening for comorbidities, in particular anxiety and depression.[53] In addition to physiologic and functional evaluation, a detailed assessment should explore psychosocial and behavioral issues. Important questions may probe mental, emotional, and spiritual health, including the impact of disease on daily activities, missed work, financial burdens, family routines, and social role. Assessment of lifestyle factors, for example, smoking status and motivation to quit, dietary patterns, and physical activity, is also important.

Treatment

Pharmacotherapy

Pharmacologic treatments aim to improve quality of life, control symptoms, and reduce exacerbation risk. No medications for COPD have been conclusively shown to modify long-term decline in lung function although research is ongoing with long-acting bronchodilators and/or inhaled corticosteroids.[54,55] COPD pharmacotreatment is guided by GOLD stage. As disease severity increases, treatment step-ups occur and therapies are added to provide additional symptom control and reduce the risk of exacerbations. Medications include bronchodilators (short-acting and long-acting beta 2 agonists and anticholinergics; methylxanthines are less frequently used), anti-inflammatory agents (inhaled and systemic corticosteroids and phosphodiesterase-4 inhibitors), leukotriene modifiers, and antibiotics for respiratory infections. Some of these medications also have a mucoactive effect (facilitating clearance or decreasing hypersecretion of mucus).[5]

Diet and nutritional supplements

Vitamins and antioxidants As with any other chronic condition, proper nutrition and a healthy diet are extremely important. For COPD in particular, inflammation and oxidative stress and the potential role of antioxidants have received considerable attention.[56] Most available data are observational and suggest there is a protective effect on COPD associated with antioxidant vitamins, particularly vitamin C and to a lesser extent vitamin E, beta carotenoids, and omega-3 FA.[57] There may be an association of individual vitamins with decreased symptoms, infections, and exacerbation. Possible benefits of omega-3 fatty acids for muscle oxidative metabolism as this relates to exercise performance have been suggested.[58,59] Low levels of certain minerals, including potassium, magnesium, selenium, and zinc, are also associated with risk of COPD and poor lung function. However, intervention studies for supplementation are lacking or inconclusive. Higher consumption of fruits and vegetables is associated with higher FEV_1 and reduced rate of lung function decline, and diets rich in oily fish may protect against COPD.[59,60] One recent RCT showed that a shift to a higher antioxidant diet improved lung function.[61] Thus, it may be reasonable at this point to consider antioxidant supplementation only in those with extreme oxidative stress challenges, for example, exposure to high levels of air pollution. Otherwise, for most patients with COPD, it is best to recommend a prudent diet rich in antioxidants, magnesium, other minerals, and omega-3 fatty acids (including fruits, vegetables, and fish).

Also of note, vitamin D deficiency is highly prevalent in COPD and associated with disease severity, decreased lung function, muscle dysfunction, osteoporosis, and immune dysfunction. There are hypothesized genetic subgroups of COPD patients with different responses to supplementation and COPD exacerbations. Current studies are ongoing.[62,63]

It is also important to note that anorexia and protein-calorie malnutrition is present in more than 30% of patients with severe disease and this is associated with increased mortality, impaired respiratory muscle function, and immune dysfunction.[59] Oral nutritional supplementation in malnourished patients with COPD improves nutritional status, respiratory muscle strength, and quality of life but the benefits are less clear in the average nourished patient with stable disease.[64]

Mucoactive agents Mucoactive agents facilitate clearance or decrease hypersecretion of mucus. For patients with bothersome sputum production that is refractory to smoking cessation and routine therapies for COPD, N-acetyl cysteine (NAC), an oral thiol preparation, has had some reported benefits.[65,66] NAC may also have anti-inflammatory and antioxidant properties. Although some practices use nebulized NAC, this is best avoided due to the potential for acute bronchospasm.

Hypertonic saline inhalation, oral expectorants (eg, guaifenesin), iodide preparations (eg, saturated solution of potassium iodide), inhaled cromoglycate, and DNase have also been suggested as mucoactive agents but currently lack evidence of clinical efficacy. Other agents that decrease sputum adhesiveness, viscosity, or production are currently being studied, such as surfactants, actin-severing agents, and prostaglandin inhibitors.[67]

Other potential supplements Several other supplements have purported benefits, although further clinical studies are needed before any recommendations in COPD can be made. Among these are: L-carnitine; echinacea-containing formulas; polyphenols, such as curcumin and resveratrol; and Chinese herbs, such as *Astragalus membranaceus*, *Panax ginseng*, *Cordyceps sinensis*, and combination formulas made from isolated herbal compounds.[56,64,68–70]

Immunization
Yearly influenza vaccination is recommended and reduces COPD exacerbations. The Centers for Disease Control and Prevention also recommends pneumococcal vaccination for adults with chronic lung disease, although the benefit on pneumonia rates, hospital admissions, and emergency room (ER) visits in COPD is unclear.[5]

Lifestyle and self-care
Environmental exposures and toxins Smoking cessation should be targeted as one of the most important self-care interventions, with counseling, nicotine replacement, and other medications recommended as appropriate for individual patients.[5] The American Academy of Family Physicians' Ask and Act Tobacco Cessation Program provides excellent online resources for physicians and patients.[71] Acupuncture, hypnosis, meditation and mind-body practices may be considered as helpful adjunctive therapies to aid in smoking cessation.[72,73]

Physical activity Physical inactivity has been demonstrated to be the strongest predictor of all-cause mortality in COPD.[74] This finding underscores the importance of exercise in the management of COPD.[5,75] Conventional exercise programs, both high-intensity and low-intensity, improve endurance, dyspnea, and quality of life, even in patients with severe disease and poor exercise tolerance. Optimal regimens are not known; however, a combination of endurance and strength training has been proposed to best treat peripheral muscle dysfunction. Current guidelines recommend formal pulmonary rehabilitation for all patients. These programs are heterogeneous; however, they typically include both lower extremity (eg, stationary cycle ergometer, treadmill, walking) as well as upper extremity exercise (eg, arm cycle ergometer, free weights, elastic bands), breathing exercises (eg, pursed lip technique, diaphragmatic breathing, spirometry), and education. Guidelines also recognize the importance of psychosocial stressors and include stress reduction as a recommended component of pulmonary rehabilitation. Symptoms of depression and anxiety can limit the benefits of exercise training due to poor motivation or fear of symptoms such as exertional dyspnea and should, therefore, be addressed concomitantly.[76] Mind-body exercise, such as tai chi and yoga, may be helpful to engage deconditioned patients in physical activity either as a bridge, adjunct, and/or alternative to conventional choices.[77,78]

Mind-body therapy Because COPD is a chronic disease that affects not only physical and functional but also behavioral, emotional, and spiritual domains in a patient's life, addressing the whole person in the course and management of the disease is crucial. Mind-body therapies may play a role in multiple levels of impairment in COPD. Inherent in these therapies is often an attention to the breath, which may be particularly salient to a population whose main symptom is breathlessness. There is some overlap between controlled breathing exercises and respiratory muscle training used conventionally with techniques of diaphragmatic breathing or yogic breathing. Mind-body approaches may also play a role in addressing a myriad of psychosocial aspects of living with the disease, including complex emotions surrounding loss of independence and self-efficacy, anger, depression, frustration, guilt, and family and social role dysfunction.[77]

Mindfulness has been shown to be effective for anxiety in many populations through promoting self-awareness and body awareness. Interestingly, in COPD, some have suggested that mindfulness may trigger anxiety and that perhaps other meditation styles may be better suited.[78] In practice, however, elements of mindfulness are common to many styles and it is unclear why patients with COPD would be different from other chronic disease populations, including asthma. In fact, studies have shown that mindfulness programs in other chronic disease populations can promote self-care, improve sleep and well-being, and increase adherence to medical recommendations. Mind-body exercise, such as tai chi and yoga, may theoretically provide both gentle exercise as well as the benefits of mindfulness, meditative breathing, and stress reduction. There are limited data to suggest benefit of tai chi for exercise capacity, quality of life, symptoms of dyspnea, and pulmonary function.[79,80] Data in other chronic diseases suggest mind-body exercise may promote self-efficacy and empowerment.[81]

Cognitive behavioral therapy (CBT) includes cognitive restructuring, behavioral activation, competency enhancement through skill-building exercises, and psychoeducation. Some studies suggest CBT may reduce symptoms of depression or anxiety and lower dyspnea, as well as improve walking distance, quality of life, and hospital admissions in patients with COPD.[77]

Other small studies in COPD have suggested benefits of progressive muscle relaxation (improved fatigue and sleep quality) and various physiologic biofeedback techniques.[77]

Other integrative modalities

Acupuncture Data on the use of acupuncture in COPD suggest benefit but is still limited, thus recommendations for use are premature. Several RCTs have reported safety.[82] One promising relatively small RCT investigated acupuncture versus placebo needling in stage 2 to 4 COPD and reported improved dyspnea, 6-minute walk distance, oxygenation, quality of life, nutritional status, spirometry, and chest wall biomechanics.[83]

Manual therapies Although there is a proposed theoretic rationale for manual therapies such as spinal manipulation and soft tissue therapies to reduce chest wall rigidity and thereby improve breathing mechanics, the data on the use of manual therapies in COPD are sparse. One systematic review of spinal manipulation and osteopathic manipulation suggested improved symptoms, lung function, and exercise.[84]

Other considerations

Oxygen Supplemental oxygen improves endurance and exercise capacity in patients with moderate-to-severe COPD. Long-term therapy is recommended for patients with severe hypoxemia (oxygen saturation less than 88% or partial arterial oxygen pressure <55 mm Hg). Prescriptions are tailored based on need (eg, differential flow delivery and timing of use [continuous, nocturnal, with exercise]).[5]

Surgery Lung volume reduction surgery may be helpful in select patients with severe COPD and heterogeneous distribution of emphysema with upper lobe predominance.

Criteria for referral include a score greater than 5 on the Body mass index, Obstruction, Dyspnea, Exercise (BODE) Index.[5]

SUMMARY

For both asthma and COPD, an integrative approach may emphasize a more holistic strategy of patient management and recognizes the multidimensional aspects of disease. Undoubtedly, there are well-studied and effective conventional medications and treatments. However, integrative medicine may offer beneficial adjuncts or address areas that are more often overlooked. An integrative approach may help to bring commonsense self-care to the fore, including healthy lifestyle modifications, allergen avoidance, smoking cessation, physical activity, and a prudent diet. Mind-body therapies may help to address psychosocial aspects; however, benefits in physical and functional dimensions are closely intertwined. Several supplements or herbal compounds may have benefit to consider further as research grows. Open communication between patients and providers is strongly emphasized. It is important to stress that the foundational tenet of integrative medicine is that it promotes a treatment plan together with, and not as a replacement for, appropriate conventional care.

REFERENCES

1. CDC. Most Recent Asthma Data Website. 2016. Available at: http://www.cdc.gov/asthma/most_recent_data.htm. Accessed October 29, 2016.
2. Ford ES, Croft JB, Mannino DM, et al. COPD surveillance—United States, 1999-2011. Chest 2013;144(1):284–305.
3. Halbert RJ, Natoli JL, Gano A, et al. Global burden of COPD: systematic review and meta-analysis. Eur Respir J 2006;28:523–32.
4. Vestbo J, Hurd SS, Agustí AG, et al. Global strategy for the diagnosis, management, and prevention of chronic obstructive pulmonary disease: GOLD executive summary. Am J Respir Crit Care Med 2013;187(4):347–65.
5. From the Global Strategy for the diagnosis, management and prevention of COPD, Global Initiative for Chronic Obstructive Lung Disease (GOLD) 2016. Available at: http://goldcopd.org/. Accessed November 6, 2016.
6. Hekking PW, Bel EH. Developing and emerging clinical asthma phenotypes. J Allergy Clin Immunol Pract 2014;2:671–80.
7. Ross RN, Nelson HS, Finegold I. Effectiveness of specific immunotherapy in the treatment of asthma: a meta-analysis of prospective, randomized, double-blind, placebo-controlled studies. Clin Ther 2000;22:329–41.
8. National Heart, Lung, and Blood Institute. National Asthma Education and Prevention Program. Expert Panel Report 3: Guidelines for the Diagnosis and Management of Asthma. 2007. http://www.nhlbi.nih.gov/guidelines/asthma/asthgdln.pdf. Accessed October 29, 2016.
9. Nathan RA, Sorkness CA, Kosinski M, et al. Development of the asthma control test: a survey for assessing asthma control. J Allergy Clin Immunol 2004;113:59–65.
10. Juniper EF, Svensson K, Mork AC, et al. Measurement properties and interpretation of three shortened versions of the asthma control questionnaire. Respir Med 2005;99:553–8.
11. Sly PD, Kusel M, Holt PG. Do early-life viral infections cause asthma? J Allergy Clin Immunol 2010;125(6):1202–5.
12. Wüthrich B, Schmid A, Walther B, et al. Milk consumption does not lead to mucus production or occurrence of asthma. J Am Coll Nutr 2005;24(suppl):547S–55S.

13. Kirkham S, Sheehan JK, Knight D, et al. Heterogeneity of airways mucus: variations in the amounts and glycoforms of the major oligomeric mucins MUC5AC and MUC5B. Biochem J 2002;361(Pt 3):537–46.
14. Bartley J, McGlashan SR. Does milk increase mucus production? Med Hypotheses 2010;74:732–4.
15. Lee TH, Hoover RL, Williams JD, et al. Effect of dietary enrichment with eicosapentaenoic and docosahexaenoic acids on in vitro neutrophil and monocyte leukotriene generation and neutrophil function. N Engl J Med 1985;312:1217–23.
16. Arm JP, Horton CE, Mencia-Huerta JM, et al. Effect of dietary supplementation with fish oil lipids on mild asthma. Thorax 1988;43:84–92.
17. Horwitz R. Controlling asthma: the role of nutrition. Explore (NY) 2005;1:393–5.
18. Miyata J, Arita M. Role of omega-3 fatty acids and their metabolites in asthma and allergic diseases. Allergol Int 2015;64(1):27–34.
19. Broughton KS, Johnson CS, Pace BK, et al. Reduced asthma symptoms with w-3 fatty acid ingestion are related to 5-series leukotriene production. Am J Clin Nutr 1997;65:1011–7.
20. Martineau AR, Cates CJ, Urashima M, et al. Vitamin D for the management of asthma. Cochrane Database Syst Rev 2016;(9):CD011511.
21. Powell CV. The role of magnesium sulfate in acute asthma: does route of administration make a difference? Curr Opin Pulm Med 2014;20(1):103–8.
22. Powell CV, Kolamunnage-Dona R, Lowe J, the MAGNETIC study group. MAGNEsium Trial In Children (MAGNETIC): a randomised, placebo-controlled trial and economic evaluation of nebulised magnesium sulphate in acute severe asthma in children. Health Technol Assess 2013;17:v–vi, 1–216.
23. Dominguez LJ, Barbagallo M, Di Lorenzo M, et al. Bronchial reactivity and intracellular magnesium: a possible mechanism for the bronchodilating effects of magnesium in asthma. Clin Sci 1998;95:137–42.
24. Britton J, Pavord I, Richards K, et al. Dietary magnesium, lung function, wheezing, and airway hyperreactivity in a random adult population sample. Lancet 1994;344:357–62.
25. Emmanouil E, Manios Y, Grammatikaki E, et al. Association of nutrient intake and wheeze or asthma in a Greek pre-school population. Pediatr Allergy Immunol 2010;21:90–5.
26. Kazaks AG, Uriu-Adams JY, Albertson TE, et al. Effect of oral magnesium supplementation on measures of airway resistance and subjective assessment of asthma control and quality of life in men and women with mild to moderate asthma: a randomized placebo controlled trial. J Asthma 2010;47(1):83–92.
27. Shin I, Shin N, Jeon C, et al. Inhibitory effects of Pycnogenol (French maritime pine bark extract) on airway inflammation in ovalbumin-induced allergic asthma. Food Chem Toxicol 2013;62:681–6.
28. Lau B, Riesen SK, Truong KP, et al. Pycnogenol® as an adjunct in the management of childhood asthma. J Asthma 2004;41(8):825–32.
29. Otsuka H, Inaba M, Fujikura T, et al. Histochemical and functional characteristics of metachromic cells in the nasal epithelium in allergic rhinitis: studies of nasal scrapings and their dispersed cells. J Allergy Clin Immunol 1995;96:528–36.
30. Haggag EG, Abou-Moustafa MA, Boucher W, et al. The effect of a herbal water-extract on histamine release from mast cells and on allergic asthma. J Herb Pharmacother 2003;3:41–54.
31. Shishehbor F, Behroo L, Broujerdnia G, et al. Quercetin effectively quells peanut-induced anaphylactic reactions in the peanut sensitized rats. Iran J Allergy Asthma Immunol 2010;9:27–34.

32. Moon H, Choi HH, Lee JY, et al. Quercetin inhalation inhibits the asthmatic responses by exposure to aerosolized-ovalbumin in conscious guinea-pigs. Arch Pharm Res 2008;31:771–8.
33. Yoshimoto T, Furukawa M, Yamamoto S, et al. Flavonoids: potent inhibitors of arachidonate 5-lipoxygenase. Biochem Biophys Res Commun 1983;116:612–8.
34. Maher P, Akaishi T, Abe K. Flavonoid fisetin promotes ERK-dependent long-term potentiation and enhances memory. Proc Natl Acad Sci U S A 2006;103(44):16568–73.
35. Goh FY, Upton N, Guan S, et al. Fisetin, a bioactive flavonol, attenuates allergic airway inflammation through negative regulation of NF-κB. Eur J Pharmacol 2012;679:109–16.
36. Srivastava K, Teper AA, Zhang T, et al. Immunomodulatory effect of the anti-asthma Chinese herbal formula MSSM-002 on TH2 cells. J Allergy Clin Immunol 2004;113:268–76.
37. Kelly-Pieper K, Patil SP, Busse P, et al. Safety and Tolerability of an Antiasthma Herbal Formula (ASHMI™) in adult subjects with asthma: a randomized, double-blinded, placebo-controlled, dose-escalation phase I study. J Altern Complement Med 2009;15(7):735–43.
38. Tal A, Miklich DR. Emotionally induced decreases in pulmonary flow rates in asthmatic children. Psychosom Med 1976;38:190–200.
39. Rosenkranz MA, Esnault S, Christian BT, et al. Mind-body interactions in the regulation of airway inflammation in asthma: a PET study of acute and chronic stress. Brain Behav Immun 2016;58:18–30.
40. Radulovic S, Calderon MA, Wilson D, et al. Sublingual immunotherapy for allergic rhinitis. Cochrane Database Syst Rev 2010;(12):CD002893. [update of Cochrane Database Syst Rev 2003;(2):CD002893].
41. McFadden ER, Luparello T, Lons HA, et al. The mechanism of suggestion in the induction of acute asthma attacks. Psychosom Med 1969;31:134–43.
42. Luparello TJ, Lyons HA, Bleeker ER, et al. Influence of suggestion on airways reactivity in asthmatic subjects. Psychosom Med 1968;30:819.
43. Smyth JM, Stone AA, Hurewitz A, et al. Effects of writing about stressful experiences on stressful experiences on symptom reduction in patients with asthma or rheumatoid arthritis: a randomized trial. JAMA 1999;281(14):1304–9.
44. McClafferty H. An overview of integrative therapies in asthma treatment. Curr Allergy Asthma Rep 2014;14:464.
45. Pbert L, Madison JM, Druker S, et al. Effect of mindfulness training on asthma quality of life and lung function: a randomised controlled trial. Thorax 2012;67:769–76.
46. Sutherland ER, Cherniack RM. Management of chronic obstructive pulmonary disease. N Engl J Med 2004;350(26):2689–97.
47. Postma DS, Rabe KF. The asthma-COPD overlap syndrome. N Engl J Med 2015;373:1241.
48. Chen JC, Mannino DM. Worldwide epidemiology of chronic obstructive pulmonary disease. Curr Opin Pulm Med 1999;5:93–9.
49. Bailey PH. The Dyspnea-Anxiety-Dyspnea Cycle – COPD patients' stories of breathlessness: "It's scary /when you can't breathe". Qual Health Res 2005;14(6):760–78.
50. Smoller JW, Pollack MH, Otto MW, et al. Panic anxiety, dyspnea, and respiratory disease. Theoretical and clinical considerations. Am J Respir Crit Care Med 1996;154(1):6–17.

51. Jones PW, Harding G, Berry P, et al. Development and first validation of the COPD Assessment Test. Eur Respir J 2009;34:648–54.

52. Reda AA, Kotz D, Kocks JW, et al. Reliability and validity of the clinical COPD questionniare and chronic respiratory questionnaire. Respir Med 2010;104(11):1675–82.

53. Pumar MI, Gray CR, Walsh JR, et al. Anxiety and depression-Important psychological comorbidities of COPD. J Thorac Dis 2014;6(11):1615–31.

54. Decramer M, Celli B, Kesten S, et al. Effect of tiotropium on outcomes in patients with moderate chronic obstructive pulmonary disease (UPLIFT): a prespecified subgroup analysis of a randomised controlled trial. Lancet 2009;374:1171–8.

55. Celli BR, Thomas NE, Anderson JA, et al. Effect of pharmacotherapy on rate of decline of lung function in chronic obstructive pulmonary disease: results from the TORCH study. Am J Respir Crit Care Med 2008;178:332–8.

56. Fischer BM, Voynow JA, Ghio AJ. COPD: balancing oxidants and antioxidants. Int J Chron Obstruct Pulmon Dis 2015;10:261–76.

57. Tsigliani IG, van der Molen T. A systematic review of the role of vitamin insufficiencies and supplementation in COPD. Respir Res 2010;11:171.

58. Broekhuizen R, Wouters EF, Creutzberg EC, et al. Polyunsaturated fatty acids improve exercise capacity in chronic obstructive pulmonary disease. Thorax 2005;60:376–82.

59. Schols AM. Nutrition as a metabolic modulator in COPD. Chest 2013;144:1340–5.

60. Romieu I, Trenga C. Diet and obstructive lung diseases. Epidemiol Rev 2001;23(2):268–87.

61. Keranis E, Makris D, Rodopoulou P, et al. Impact of dietary shift to hgher antioxidant foods in COPD: a randomized trial. Eur Respir J 2010;36:774–80.

62. de Tena JG, El Hachem Debek A, Hernandez Guttierez C, et al. The role of vitamin D in chronic obstructive pulmonary disease, asthma, and other respiratory diseases. Arch Bronconeumol 2014;50:179–84.

63. Janssens W, Bouillon R, Claes B, et al. Vitamin D deficiency is highly prevalent in COPD and correlates with variants in the vitamin D-binding gene. Thorax 2010;65(3):215–20.

64. Ferreira IM, Brooks D, White J, et al. Nutritional supplementation for stable chronic obstructive pulmonary disease. Cochrane Database Syst Rev 2012;12:CD000998.

65. Cazzola M, Calzetta L, Page C, et al. Influence of N-acetylcysteine on chronic bronchitis or COPD exacerbations: a meta-analysis. Eur Respir Rev 2015;24(137):451–61.

66. Tse HN, Tseng CZ. Update on the pathological processes, molecular biology, and clinical utility of N-acetylcysteine in chronic obstructive pulmonary disease. Int J Chron Obstruct Pulmon Dis 2014;9:825–36.

67. Rogers DF. Mucoactive agents for airway mucus hypersecretory diseases. Chemotherapy 2002;48:259–66.

68. Hauke W, Köhler G, Henneicke-Von Zepelin HH, et al. Esberitox N as supportive therapy when providing standard antibiotic treatment in subjects with a severe bacterial infection (acute exacerbation of chronic bronchitis). A multicentric, prospective, double-blind, placebo-controlled study. Respir Care 2007;52:1176–93 [discussion: 1193–7].

69. Chen HY, Ma CH, Cao KJ, et al. A systematic review and meta-analysis of herbal medicine on chronic obstructive pulmonary diseases. Evid Based Complement Alternat Med 2014;2014:925069.

70. Li J, Zhao P, Li Y, et al. Systems pharmacology-based dissection of mechanisms of Chinese medicinal formula Bufei Yishen as an effective treatment for chronic obstructive pulmonary disease. Sci Rep 2015;5:15290.

71. The American Academy of Family Physicians' Ask and Act Tobacco Cessation Program. http://www.aafp.org/patient-care/public-health/tobacco-nicotine/ask-act.html. Accessed October 31, 2016.

72. Tahiri M, Mottillo S, Joseph L, et al. Alternative smoking cessation aids: a meta-analysis of randomized controlled trials. Am J Med 2012;125:576–84.

73. Carim-Todd L, Mitchell SH, Oken BS. Mind-body practices: an alternative, drug-free treatment for smoking cessation? A systematic review of the literature. Drug Alcohol Depend 2013;132:399–410.

74. Waschki B, Kirsten A, Holz O, et al. Physical activity is the strongest predictor of all-cause mortality in patients with COPD: a prospective cohort study. Chest 2011;140:331–42.

75. Garvey C, Bayles MP, Hamm LF, et al. Pulmonary rehabilitation exercise prescription in chronic obstructive pulmonary disease: review of selected guidelines: an official statement from the American Association of Cardiovascular and Pulmonary Rehabilitation. J Cardiopulm Rehabil Prev 2016;36:75–83.

76. von Leupoldt A, Taube K, Lehmann K, et al. The impact of anxiety and depression on outcomes of pulmonary rehabilitation in patients with COPD. Chest 2011;140:730–6.

77. von Leupoldt A, Fritzsche A, Trueba AF, et al. Behavioral medicine approaches to chronic obstructive pulmonary disease. Ann Behav Med 2012;44:52–65.

78. Chan RR, Giardino N, Larson JL. A pilot study: mindfulness meditation intervention in COPD. Int J Chron Obstruct Pulmon Dis 2015;10:445–54.

79. Ngai SP, Jones AY, Tam WW. Tai Chi for chronic obstructive pulmonary disease (COPD). Cochrane Database Syst Rev 2016;(6):CD009953.

80. Liu XC, Pan L, Hu Q, et al. Effects of yoga training in patients with chronic obstructive pulmonary disease: a systematic review and meta-analysis. J Thorac Dis 2014;6:795–802.

81. Farver-Vestergaard I, Jacobsen D, Zachariae R. Efficacy of psychosocial interventions on psychological and physical health outcomes in chronic obstructive pulmonary disease: a systematic review and meta-analysis. Psychother Psychosom 2015;84:37–50.

82. Coyle ME, Shergis JL, Huang ET, et al. Acupuncture therapies for chronic obstructive pulmonary disease: a systematic review of randomized, controlled trials. Altern Ther Health Med 2014;20:10–23.

83. Suzuki M, Muro S, Ando Y, et al. A randomized, placebo-controlled trial of acupuncture in patients with chronic obstructive pulmonary disease (COPD): the COPD-acupuncture trial (CAT). Arch Intern Med 2012;172:878–86.

84. Wearing J, Beaumont S, Forbes D, et al. The use of spinal manipulative therapy in the management of chronic obstructive pulmonary disease: a systematic review. J Altern Complement Med 2016;22:108–14.

85. Sarah-Egert S, Wolffram S, Bosy-Westphal A, et al. Daily quercetin supplementation dose-dependently increases plasma quercetin concentrations in healthy humans. J Nutr 2008;138:1615–21.

86. Hosseini S, Pishnamazi S, Sadrzadeh SM, et al. Pycnogenol((R)) in the management of asthma. J Med Food 2001;4:201–9.

87. Mickleborough TD, Lindley MR, Ionescu AA, et al. Protective effect of fish oil supplementation on exercise-induced bronchoconstriction in asthma. Chest 2006;129:39–49.

Complementary and Integrative Gastroenterology

Joshua Korzenik, MD[a],*, Anna K. Koch, MSc(Psych)[b,c],
Jost Langhorst, MD[b,c]

KEYWORDS

- Gastroenterology • Complementary and alternative medicine
- Inflammatory bowel disease • Crohn disease • Ulcerative colitis • Yoga

KEY POINTS

- Polyphenols, including curcumin, resveratrol, and epigallocatechin-3-gallate (EGCG), have supportive data for the treatment of ulcerative colitis (UC) flares.
- Quality of life for patients with inflammatory bowel disease (IBD) and irritable bowel syndrome (IBS) benefit from lifestyle interventions and stress management techniques, although without a clear benefit for reduction of disease flares.
- Yoga has beneficial effects on symptoms, anxiety, physical functioning, and quality of life for patients with IBS.
- A large randomized trial demonstrated superiority of melatonin and nutritional supplements compared with omeprazole for reduction of gastroesophageal reflux disease (GERD) symptoms.

INTRODUCTION

The use of complementary and alternative medicine (CAM) has grown tremendously within gastroenterology. Use is particularly high for chronic conditions, such as IBD, IBS, and reflux esophagitis, where a considerable unmet need to treat the underlying

Disclosure Statement: Disclosure of any relationship with a commercial company that has a direct financial interest in subject matter or materials discussed in article or with a company making a competing product.
[a] Division of Gastroenterology, Hepatology, and Endoscopy, Department of Medicine, Brigham and Women's Hospital, Harvard Medical School, Boston, MA, USA; [b] Department of Integrative Gastroenterology, Kliniken Essen-Mitte, Faculty of Medicine, University of Duisburg-Essen, Am Deimelsberg 34 a, 45276 Essen, Germany; [c] Department of Internal and Integrative Medicine, Kliniken Essen-Mitte, Faculty of Medicine, University of Duisburg-Essen, Am Deimelsberg 34 a, 45276 Essen, Germany
* Corresponding author. Crohn's and Colitis Center, 2nd Floor, 850 Boylston Street, Chestnut Hill, MA.
E-mail address: jkorzenik@bwh.harvard.edu

Med Clin N Am 101 (2017) 943–954
http://dx.doi.org/10.1016/j.mcna.2017.04.009
0025-7125/17/© 2017 Elsevier Inc. All rights reserved.

process or control symptoms persists.[1–5] People with IBD are more motivated by ongoing symptoms and concerns over adverse events from medications that suppress the immune system. The remarkable diversity of CAM compounds and approaches used in gastrointestinal (GI) disorders makes a comprehensive review not feasible in this article. In addition, the line between CAM approaches and mainstream therapies sometimes moves as growing evidence moves an alternative therapy to the mainstream. Herbal therapies, such as curcumin for UC, is one such example where larger trials have been performed. Another example is the ascendency of mainstream interest in the intestinal microbiome. The popular appeal of probiotics, the expanding interest in the microbiome in medical research, and the dramatic results in fecal transplant have fueled a renewed focus on probiotics and prebiotics as potential medical therapies. This thrust has been embraced by mainstream medicine with research and by pharma with investments. This likely will lead to multiple microbial-based therapies in the near future not only for GI disorders but also for areas seemingly further outside the GI tract, such as hypertension and depression.[6–8] Thus, a review of probiotics or the more extreme version with fecal microbial transplant is beyond the scope of this review and is not discussed in this article. This review surveys CAM treatment modalities for IBD and IBS following the proposed categorization system by Wieland and colleagues[9] for the Cochrane Collaboration: mind-body medicine, whole medical systems, natural product–based therapies, manipulative and body-based practices, and energy medicine. Many of these trials of CAM in GI, however, tend to be single-center studies and small without the thoroughness of costly, multicentered, sponsored conventional studies. With those acknowledged limitations, the range of options studied with some supportive data opens up a new set of approaches for many patients.

INFLAMMATORY BOWEL DISEASES
Mind-body Medicine

Although the contribution of stress in provoking IBD flares has been difficult to quantify, studies have suggested stress, anxiety, and depression influence the likelihood of flares in UC and Crohn disease (CD).[10] These data are reinforced by patients' impressions that stressful events are implicated in initiating disease activity. Because GI diseases may be modified by stress, treatments like mind-body interventions, which aim to strengthen patients' resources and resiliency, have been studied and used. Mind-body treatments include, for example, lifestyle modification, mindfulness interventions, relaxation techniques, and hypnotherapy. In addition, anxiety and depression are increased in patients with IBD, particularly in those with more active disease. Nonpharmacologic approaches to counter this issues have been also examined in IBD.

Clinical trials of mind-body interventions show promising results: a lifestyle-modification program with 60 patients with UC led to improvements in psychological quality of life and reduction of anxiety.[11] The program consisted of a structured 60-hour training program over a period of 10 weeks, which included stress management training, psychoeducational elements, and self-care strategies. Regarding inactive UC, mindfulness-based stress reduction was found to positively influence facets of quality of life compared with attention control.[12] Those findings, however, could not be confirmed within a study that included both UC and CD patients.[13] Both studies did not find significant group differences regarding disease activity, relapse, or psychological variables in the main analysis. Subset analyses revealed that significant effects on quality of life were found in patients with IBS-type symptoms. Furthermore, mindfulness-based stress reduction decreased perceived stress and C-reactive protein during flare.

Stress management techniques are another promising treatment modality for decreasing symptoms.[14] A further study in which patients attended 3 relaxation-training sessions and received an audio disc for home practice found that relaxation training can lead to significant improvements in pain, anxiety, depression, mood, stress, and quality of life, including bowel symptoms.[15] To test the effects of hypnotherapy, 26 patients received 7 sessions of gut-directed hypnotherapy (a special form of hypnotherapy for IBS) and were compared with 29 patients within an attention control group. Findings suggest that gut-directed hypnotherapy has the potential to prolong clinical remission. It did not, however, improve quality of life or other psychological measures.[16] Another study enrolled patients with IBD and IBS and used a specific mind-body program to address stress management through mindfulness and other relaxation response techniques. Benefits were demonstrated after the 9-week program with improvements in disease-specific measures, trait anxiety, and pain catastrophizing. In addition, altered gene expression of inflammatory markers, such as nuclear factor κB was observed.[17]

Yoga is a special form of physical exercise, often described as a meditative movement therapy. It consists of body postures, breathing techniques, and meditation and has been shown to have beneficial effects on quality of life and mental health for patients with UC.[18,19] Regarding patients with CD, yoga had no effects.[18] Also, physical exercise in general seems to improve quality of life of patients with IBD. Ten weeks of moderate physical activity improved quality of life of patients with IBD.[20]

Whole Medical Systems

Clinical trials for patients with active UC[21] show that acupuncture and moxibustion induced significant decreases in disease activity compared with the control group. An increase in well-being and quality of life compared with baseline was also observed, but there was no significant difference in these measures compared with sham acupuncture.[21] Regarding active CD, significant decreases in disease activity and increases in well-being with acupuncture and moxibustion compared with control patients were found. Compared with baseline, serum markers of inflammation were also reduced.[22] A meta-analysis examined the effects of acupuncture and moxibustion for IBD included a total of 43 randomized controlled trials (RCTs) (42 regarding UC and 1 regarding CD) with a total of 4021 patients with IBD. The investigators concluded that although acupuncture and moxibustion were superior compared with oral sulfasalazine, definitive conclusions could not be drawn due to a lack of high-quality trials.[23]

Natural Product–based Therapies

Numerous natural product–based therapies have been evaluated regarding the treatment effects on IBD. Regarding active UC, HMPL-004, which contains *Andrographis paniculata* extract, was compared with mesalamine. The compound is thought to suppress inflammation through several pathways, including tumor necrosis factor (TNF)-α, interleukin (IL)-1β, and IL-6. Both treatment groups showed significant improvements on all outcomes. Side effects were more frequent, however, in the mesalamine group compared with HMPL-004 group (27% vs 13%, respectively).[24] Another study compared mesalamine and HMPL-004 to mesalamine and placebo. Patients receiving mesalamine and HMPL-004 (1800 mg daily) showed significantly higher clinical response rates.[25] Phase 3 trials are now under way (clinical trials.gov).

Boswellia serrata (Indian frankincense) has evidence for beneficial effects in the treatment of patients suffering from CD[26,27] and from UC.[28,29] Wormwood (*Artemisia absinthium*) and a steroid taper were compared with a placebo and steroid taper in patients with CD. At weeks 6, 8, and 20, the intervention group reported significantly lower severity of symptoms. At weeks 8, 10 and 12, the intervention group reported increased well-being. Therefore, wormwood might have the potential to decrease symptoms and increase well-being of patients with CD.[30] A further study found that in active CD, wormwood added to their usual CD therapy was more effective than usual therapy alone. There was a significant decrease in disease activity, depression, and TNF-α and an increase in quality of life after 6 weeks. No such differences were found for standard therapy alone.[31]

A great deal of use of cannabis in CD and UC has been documented with patient-reported benefit, particularly for abdominal pain associated with CD. Whether there is an anti-inflammatory effect is uncertain. In active CD, Cannabis sativa cigarettes might have a positive influence on CD activity index and quality of life.[32] The study was small (21 patients) but a benefit was suggested with remission in 45% (5/11) and 10% (1/10) in the cannabis and placebo groups, respectively. No difference was seen in C-reactive protein.

Several polyphenols have been studied in UC with promising results. Best studied is curcumin, also known as turmeric, which has been investigated for both maintenance of remission of UC and more recently induction of remission. Numerous potential mechanisms of action have been identified with regard to anti-inflammatory actions. Curcumin has been demonstrated to reduce p38 mitogen-activated protein kinase activity and inhibit Il-1β, Il-6, and TNF-α. Widely studied for numerous indications in addition to IBD, doses as high as 8 g are rapidly metabolized and found to be safe. Regarding maintenance of remission in UC, 89 patients were randomized to treatment with curcumin at a dose of 1 g twice daily in addition to sulfasalazine or mesalamine or with placebo plus sulfasalazine or mesalamine. The curcumin-containing group showed significantly less disease activity and lower recurrence rate at 6 months (4.4% vs 15% for the curcumin and placebo-containing arms, respectively).[33] The benefit was not statistically significant, however, at 12 months. A larger, multicenter study was recently performed using a slightly higher dose of curcumin (1.5 g twice daily) for 4 weeks in an RCT while both groups continued on mesalamine. Clinical remission was seen in 53.8% (14/26) of the curcumin group versus none in the placebo group (0/24). Endoscopic remission was seen in 38% of the curcumin group and none in the placebo arm.[34,35]

Polyphenols other than curcumin, such as EGCG, resveratrol, and bilberry, have also been studied in UC. Resveratrol is a polyphenol in the class of stilbenes that are derived from grapes and other berries. Bilberry, also studied in UC, has been investigated in cardiovascular disease and is thought to be rich with sirtuins—stress protective enzymes—and considered for longevity as well. Resveratrol was studied in a single-center RCT in active UC.[36] The trial enrolled 56 people randomized to 500 mg of resveratrol or placebo for 6 weeks. The resveratrol group showed a significant although modest improvement in disease activity and quality of life with decreases in inflammatory cytokines.[37] EGCG, derived from green tea, has considerable preclinical data in animal models showing a benefit as well as a small pilot study in UC suggesting effectiveness. Another dietary phenol found in bilberries—anthocyanins—has some promising open-label pilot data as well.[37] Wheatgrass juice is another promising and safe treatment option that has been studied in a small RCT and may help patients with active UC. A mechanism is unclear and suggested to act as an antioxidant. Patients who drank wheatgrass juice showed significantly less disease activity, less rectal bleeding, and less abdominal pain.[38] Germinated barley compared with standard therapy might add additional benefit compared with a treatment with standard therapy alone: after 3 months, 6 months, and 12 months, the severity of clinical symptoms and the recurrence of UC in patients achieving remission were significantly lower in patients treated with additional germinated barley.[39]

An assortment of other herbal compounds has been studied in small human trials as well. A treatment with *Plantago ovata* showed no significant differences from a treatment with mesalamine or a combination of both for patients with UC in remission.[40] Super evening primrose oil showed no significant benefits in treatment of active UC compared with placebo and with a high-dose omega-3 oil. Only stool consistency after 6 months and 9 months was superior in the super evening primrose oil group.[41] A combination of myrrh, chamomile extract, and coffee charcoal (Myrrhinil-Intest) might be a promising and safe treatment alternative for treating UC because it shows potential to be noninferior to the gold standard therapy.[42] Within the study, a total of 96 patients with inactive UC received either Myrrhinil-Intest or mesalamine. Results showed that the herbal preparation is well tolerated and shows a good safety profile and potential to be noninferior to mesalamine. In active UC, treatment with aloe vera gel, at a dose of 100 mL twice daily, as a mucosal protectant compared with placebo led to significant improvements in clinical signs and quality of life after 4 weeks and a reduction in histologic score but not in sigmoidoscopic scores and laboratory variables.[43] The treatment with sophora (Japanese pagoda tree) might be a promising and safe treatment option because it did not reveal any differences regarding disease activity or laboratory measurements compared with mesalamine in patients with UC diagnosed as internal dampness–heat syndrome type according to traditional Chinese medicine.[44] Silymarin shows promising effects on hemoglobin levels, erythrocyte sedimentation rate, and disease activity in patients with inactive UC.[45] Phosphatidylcholine as a treatment option for patients with UC has been shown to significantly improve disease activity in comparison with placebo and was found safe.[46] Additional trials are ongoing.

Even though there are a variety of promising herbal products for treating IBD, most herbal products are only evaluated within 1 or a few clinical studies. More than 50 herbal compounds have been studied and a benefit suggested in animal models but human studies are lacking.[47] Further research needs to be conducted to confirm the results.

IRRITABLE BOWEL SYNDROME

IBS and other functional GI disorders are not well understood with regard to pathophysiology. Few therapies are effective and the benefit of approved therapies over placebo is modest. A great unmet need continues to exist for these patients, with many people turning to CAM for relief of symptoms.

Mind-body Medicine

Mindfulness-based therapies—which often include stress management techniques—have a positive effect on quality of life, stress, disease symptoms and physiologic markers.[48,49] To determine the effects of relaxation techniques on IBS, 90-minute sessions of relaxation training in small groups in addition to standard medical care were applied to 52 patients. The effects were compared with 46 patients who received standard medical care. In the relaxation training group, IBS symptom severity was reduced and quality of life increased compared with the standard care group at 3 months, 6 months, and 12 months after treatment. Relaxation techniques like progressive muscle relaxation, therefore, have potential for positive short-term and long-term effects on quality of life and symptom severity of patients with IBS.[50] Furthermore, a recent review reports hypnotherapy is beneficial for overall GI symptoms in IBS.[51] According to a recent systematic review of 6 RCTs (n = 273 patients), yoga has beneficial effects on symptoms, anxiety, physical functioning, and quality of life of patients with IBS.[52] Also, physical exercise in general yields potential in treating IBS. A slight increase of physical activity, for example, aerobic exercise, walking, or biking—adapted to a patient's individual constitution—had positive short-term and long-term effects on symptom severity, quality of life, and fatigue.[53,54]

Whole Medical Systems

A Cochrane review of 17 RCTs with a total of 1806 patients concluded that acupuncture in comparison to pharmacologic interventions led to decreased IBS symptoms. Acupuncture showed no difference in comparison to probiotics and psychotherapy. Acupuncture as an adjunct to psychotherapy and traditional Chinese medicine was effective in the treatment of IBS. Acupuncture showed no superiority, however, compared with sham acupuncture.[55] The exact modes of actions regarding acupuncture in the treatment of IBS need to be evaluated.

There is sparse evidence for the efficacy of homeopathy in the treatment of IBS. According to a recent Cochrane review that included 3 RCTs with a total of 213 patients, the homeopathic remedy asafoetida might be beneficial for patients suffering from IBS. But findings should be interpreted with caution due to the low study quality and few RCTs concerning this matter.[56]

Regarding functional GI disorders, the traditional Japanese Kampo preparation keishi-ka-shakuyaku-to, with *Paeoniae radix*, *Cinnamomi cortex*, *Zizyphi fructus*, *Glycyrrhizae radix*, and *Zingiberis rhizoma* as main ingredients, shows initial promising effects on abdominal pain, bloating, and general IBS symptoms.[57] Other Kampo preparations lack high-quality trials to determine their effects on IBS.

Natural Product–based Therapies

Like yoga, Ayurvedic therapy has its roots in traditional Indian medicine and philosophy. Data concerning IBS are mixed. Ayurvedic therapy consisting of *Aegle marmelos correa* plus *Bacopa monniere Linn* was particularly beneficial in diarrhea predominant form of IBS.[58] No beneficial effects were found for Ayurvedic herbs consisting of *Murraya koenigii*, *Punica granatum*, and *Curcuma longa*.[59] Hot caraway oil poultices applied to the abdomen have been shown effective and safe and, therefore, serve as a good self-management treatment. Their effects may be a result, however, mainly of the heat application.[60] Compared with placebo, red pepper, psyllium husks, a 9-plant extract (STW 5), a 6-plant extract (STW 5-II), and Dinggui oil might exert beneficial effects on patients with IBS.[61–64] Compared with conventional therapy, an herbal preparation (*Mentha longifolia*, *Cyperus rotundus*, and *Zingiber officinale*) showed beneficial effects.[65] Combined with probiotic therapy, Gwakhyangjeonggisan, an herbal preparation (*Melissa officinalis*, *Mentha spicata*, and *Coriandrum sativum*), might yield additional benefit compared with probiotic therapy alone.[66] A systematic review that included 9 RCTs with a total of 726 patients concluded that peppermint oil seems a safe and effective short-term treatment. Patients treated with peppermint oil, however, are more likely to experience mild and transient adverse events—such as heartburn, dry mouth, belching, and peppermint taste—than patients in the control groups.[67] There is no evidence for the efficacy of bitter candytuft, St. John's wort, ginger, curcuma, and furmitory.[62,68–71]

Similar to IBD, in IBS there is a variety of promising herbal products but most of them have only been evaluated within 1 or a few clinical studies. Further research needs to be conducted to confirm the results.

A subset of patients with IBS–diarrhea predominant have small intestine bacterial overgrowth (SIBO), bacterial growth in the small intestine, where excessive amounts of bacteria are not common, diagnosed with a noninvasive hydrogen breath test. Conventional therapy uses a broad-spectrum antibiotic, such as rifaximin, for treatment of SIBO. A recent RCT compared an herbal preparation with numerous components to rifaxamin in individuals with symptoms and SIBO as determined by a positive lactulose breath test. They found equivalent results between the 2 treatments, although it was underpowered for determination of true noninferiority.[72]

REFLUX ESOPHAGITIS

CAM approaches to GERD have been studied far less than in IBD and IBS. An herbal preparation with polyphenols from *Olea europaea* and *Opuntia ficus indica* (Mucosave) was compared with placebo in 118 patients, with a benefit demonstrated in 73% versus 18% of the herbal and placebo arms, respectively.[73] After resolution of GERD symptoms by omeprazole, a pectin-based medicine (Aflurax) was superior to placebo for maintaining remission at 6 months (48% vs 8%).[74] A head-to-head comparison of the proton pump inhibitor (PPI) esomeprazole and Aflurax, however, failed to show a benefit in a pragmatic RCT of on-demand use.[75] The best studied dietary supplement has been melatonin. A randomized trial of 351 patients compared melatonin (6 mg daily) and nutritional supplements (including methionine, L-tryptophan, vitamin B_6, folic acid, vitamin B_{12}, methionine, and betaine) to omeprazole (20 mg daily)[76]; 100% of patients taking the melatonin/nutrient combination experienced relief after 7 days compared with 66% of those on omeprazole ($P<.001$). Although impressive, the remarkably high response rate in the melatonin/nutrient medication and the low success rate of the PPI compared with other studies brings skepticism along with interest. Other studies suggest a physiologic role for melatonin in preventing reflux and smaller studies do suggest a potential benefit though larger trials are needed.[77,78] Although a variety of other alternative approaches have been reported to be useful for GERD, including ginger, STW 5 (Iberogast), curcumin, quercetin, and vitamin E,[79] these additional compounds have not been evaluated.

SUMMARY

Complementary therapies offer potential approaches for common gastroenterological conditions with the hope of benefit with little harm. Alternative approaches, such as melatonin for reflux or curcumin for UC, likely have better safety profiles than a PPI or an anti-TNF, but the risk-benefit ratios have not been adequately assessed. The efficacy data for these approaches are promising but sufficiently robust trials have not been conducted to be confident in the benefits. Similarly the safety has not been fully established. The most convincing evidence for UC and CD is present for treatment approaches, like lifestyle-modification programs, stress management techniques, and herbal medicine. For IBS especially, physical exercise, peppermint oil, relaxation techniques, and stress management seem fruitful. Although additional data for GERD treatment are needed, these approaches have the potential of fulfilling a substantial unmet need for these GI diseases. Where these medications firmly fit in the algorithms for treatment remains uncertain, but likely some of these compounds will cross over from being alternative therapies to being more widely considered and benefiting a larger group of patients.

REFERENCES

1. Langhorst J, Anthonisen IB, Steder-Neukamm U, et al. Patterns of complementary and alternative medicine (CAM) use in patients with inflammatory bowel

disease: perceived stress is a potential indicator for CAM use. Complement Ther Med 2007;15(1):30–7.

2. Langhorst J, Anthonisen IB, Steder-Neukamm U, et al. Amount of systemic steroid medication is a strong predictor for the use of complementary and alternative medicine in patients with inflammatory bowel disease: results from a German national survey. Inflamm Bowel Dis 2005;11(3):287–95.

3. Kong SC, Hurlstone DP, Pocock CY, et al. The Incidence of self-prescribed oral complementary and alternative medicine use by patients with gastrointestinal diseases. J Clin Gastroenterol 2005;39(2):138–41.

4. Hung A, Kang N, Bollom A, et al. Complementary and alternative medicine use is prevalent among patients with gastrointestinal diseases. Dig Dis Sci 2015;60(7): 1883–8.

5. Hilsden RJ, Verhoef MJ, Rasmussen H, et al. Use of complementary and alternative medicine by patients with inflammatory bowel disease. Inflamm Bowel Dis 2011;17(2):655–62.

6. Eales J, Gibson P, Whorwell P, et al. Systematic review and meta-analysis: The effects of fermented milk with Bifidobacterium lactis CNCM I-2494 and lactic acid bacteria on gastrointestinal discomfort in the general adult population. Therap Adv Gastroenterol 2017;10(1):74–88.

7. Robles-Vera I, Toral M, Romero M, et al. Antihypertensive effects of probiotics. Curr Hypertens Rep 2017;19(4):26.

8. Wallace CJ, Milev R. The effets of probiotics on depressive symptoms in humans: a systematic review. Ann Gen Psychiatry 2017;16:14.

9. Wieland LS, Manheimer E, Berman BM. Development and classification of an operational definition of complementary and alternative medicine for the Cochrane collaboration. Altern Ther Health Med 2011;17(2):50–9.

10. Mittermaier C, Dejaco C, Waldhoer T, et al. Impact of depressive mood on relapse in patients with inflammatory bowel disease: a prospective 18-month follow-up study. Psychosom Med 2004;66(1):79–84.

11. Langhorst J, Mueller T, Luedtke R, et al. Effects of a comprehensive lifestyle modification program on quality-of-life in patients with ulcerative colitis: a twelve-month follow-up. Scand J Gastroenterol 2007;42(6):734–45.

12. Jedel S, Hoffman A, Merriman P, et al. A randomized controlled trial of mindfulness-based stress reduction to prevent flare-up in patients with inactive ulcerative colitis. Digestion 2014;89(2):142–55.

13. Berrill JW, Sadlier M, Hood K, et al. Mindfulness-based therapy for inflammatory bowel disease patients with functional abdominal symptoms or high perceived stress levels. J Crohns colitis 2014;8(9):945–55. Available at: http://onlinelibrary. wiley.com/o/cochrane/clcentral/articles/744/CN-01041744/frame.html.

14. Milne B, Joachim G, Niedhardt J. A stress management programme for inflammatory bowel disease patients. J Adv Nurs 1986;11(5):561–7.

15. Mizrahi MC, Reicher-Atir R, Levy S, et al. Effects of guided imagery with relaxation training on anxiety and quality of life among patients with inflammatory bowel disease. Psychol Health 2012;27(12):1463–79.

16. Keefer L, Taft TH, Kiebles JL, et al. Gut-directed hypnotherapy significantly augments clinical remission in quiescent ulcerative colitis. Aliment Pharmacol Ther 2013;38(7):761–71.

17. Kuo B, Bhasin M, Jacquart J, et al. Genomic and clinical effects associated with a relaxation response mind-body intervention in patients with irritable bowel syndrome and inflammatory bowel disease. PLoS One 2015;10(4):e0123861.

18. Sharma P, Poojary G, Velez DM, et al. Effect of yoga-based intervention in patients with inflammatory bowel disease. Int J Yoga Therap 2015;25(1):101–12.
19. Langhorst J, Schaefer M, Schoels M, et al. A randomized controlled trial of yoga for ulcerative colitis. United Eur Gastroenterol J 2016;146(5, Suppl 1 P0317): A267.
20. Klare P, Nigg J, Nold J, et al. The impact of a ten-week physical exercise program on health-related quality of life in patients with inflammatory bowel disease: A prospective randomized controlled trial. Digestion 2015;91(3):239–47.
21. Joos S, Wildau N, Kohnen R, et al. Acupuncture and moxibustion in the treatment of ulcerative colitis: a randomized controlled study. Scand J Gastroenterol 2006; 41(9):1056–63.
22. Joos S, Brinkhaus B, Maluche C, et al. Acupuncture and moxibustion in the treatment of active Crohn's disease: a randomized controlled study. Digestion 2004; 69(3):131–9.
23. Ji J, Lu Y, Liu H, et al. Acupuncture and moxibustion for inflammatory bowel diseases: a systematic review and meta-analysis of randomized controlled trials. Evid Based Complement Alternat Med 2013;2013:158352.
24. Tang T, Targan SR, Li ZS, et al. Randomised clinical trial: herbal extract HMPL-004 in active ulcerative colitis - a double-blind comparison with sustained release mesalazine. Aliment Pharmacol Ther 2011;33(2):194–202.
25. Sandborn WJ, Targan SR, Byers VS, et al. Andrographis paniculata extract (HMPL-004) for active ulcerative colitis. Am J Gastroenterol 2013;108(1):90–8.
26. Holtmeier W, Zeuzem S, Preiss J, et al. Randomized, placebo-controlled, double-blind trial of Boswellia serrata in maintaining remission of Crohn's disease: good safety profile but lack of efficacy. Inflamm Bowel Dis 2011;17(2):573–82.
27. Gerhardt H, Seifert F, Buvari P, et al. Therapy of active Crohn disease with Boswellia serrata extract H 15. Z Gastroenterol 2001;39(1):11–7 [in German].
28. Gupta I, Parihar A, Malhotra P, et al. Effects of Boswellia serrata gum resin in patients with ulcerative colitis. Eur J Med Res 1997;2(1):37–43.
29. Gupta I, Parihar A, Malhotra P, et al. Effects of gum resin of Boswellia serrata in patients with chronic colitis. Planta Med 2001;67(5):391–5.
30. Omer B, Krebs S, Omer H, et al. Steroid-sparing effect of wormwood (Artemisia absinthium) in Crohn's disease: a double-blind placebo-controlled study. Phytomedicine 2007;14(2–3):87–95.
31. Krebs S, Omer TN, Omer B. Wormwood (Artemisia absinthium) suppresses tumour necrosis factor alpha and accelerates healing in patients with Crohn's disease - A controlled clinical trial. Phytomedicine 2010;17(5):305–9. Available at: http://onlinelibrary.wiley.com/o/cochrane/clcentral/articles/449/CN-00753449/frame.html.
32. Naftali T, Bar-Lev Schleider L, Dotan I, et al. Cannabis induces a clinical response in patients with Crohn's disease: a prospective placebo-controlled study. Clin Gastroenterol Hepatol 2013;11(10):1276–80.e1.
33. Hanai H, Sugimoto K. Curcumin has bright prospects for the treatment of inflammatory bowel disease. Curr Pharm Des 2009;15(18):2087–94.
34. Lang A, Salomon N, Wu JCY, et al. Curcumin in Combination With Mesalamine Induces Remission in Patients With Mild-to-Moderate Ulcerative Colitis in a Randomized Controlled Trial. Clin Gastroenterol Hepatol 2015;13(8):1444–9.e1.
35. Singla V, Pratap Mouli V, Garg SK, et al. Induction with NCB-02 (curcumin) enema for mild-to-moderate distal ulcerative colitis - a randomized, placebo-controlled, pilot study. J Crohns Colitis 2014;8(3):208–14.

36. Samsamikor M, Daryani NE, Asl PR, et al. Resveratrol supplementation and oxidative/anti-oxidative status in patients with ulcerative colitis: a randomized, double-blind, placebo-controlled pilot study. Arch Med Res 2016;47(4):304–9.

37. Dryden GW, Lam A, Beatty K, et al. A pilot study to evaluate the safety and efficacy of an oral dose of (-)-epigallocatechin-3-gallate-rich polyphenon E in patients with mild to moderate ulcerative colitis. Inflamm Bowel Dis 2013;19(9): 1904–12.

38. Ben-Arye E, Goldin E, Wengrower D, et al. Wheat grass juice in the treatment of active distal ulcerative colitis: a randomized double-blind placebo-controlled trial. Scand J Gastroenterol 2002;37(4):444–9.

39. Hanai H, Kanauchi O, Mitsuyama K, et al. Germinated barley foodstuff prolongs remission in patients with ulcerative colitis. Int J Mol Med 2004;13(5):643–7.

40. Fernandez-Banares F, Hinojosa J, Sanchez-Lombrana JL, et al. Randomized clinical trial of Plantago ovata seeds (dietary fiber) as compared with mesalamine in maintaining remission in ulcerative colitis. Spanish Group for the Study of Crohn's Disease and Ulcerative Colitis (GETECCU). Am J Gastroenterol 1999;94(2): 427–33.

41. Greenfield SM, Green AT, Teare JP, et al. A randomized controlled study of evening primrose oil and fish oil in ulcerative colitis. Aliment Pharmacol Ther 1993; 7(2):159–66.

42. Langhorst J, Varnhagen I, Schneider SB, et al. Randomised clinical trial: a herbal preparation of myrrh, chamomile and coffee charcoal compared with mesalazine in maintaining remission in ulcerative colitis–a double-blind, double-dummy study. Aliment Pharmacol Ther 2013;38(5):490–500.

43. Langmead L, Feakins RM, Goldthorpe S, et al. Randomized, double-blind, placebo-controlled trial of oral aloe vera gel for active ulcerative colitis. Aliment Pharmacol Ther 2004;19(7):739–47.

44. Tong ZQ, Yang B, Tong XY. A multi-center randomized double-blinded, placebo-controlled clinical study on efficacy of composite sophora colon-soluble capsules in treating ulcerative colitis of internal dampness-heat accumulation syndrome type. Zhongguo Zhong Xi Yi Jie He Za Zhi 2011;31(2):172–6 [in Chinese].

45. Rastegarpanah M, Malekzadeh R, Vahedi H, et al. A randomized, double blinded, placebo-controlled clinical trial of silymarin in ulcerative colitis. Chin J Integr Med 2015;21(12):902–6.

46. Karner M, Kocjan A, Stein J, et al. First multicenter study of modified release phosphatidylcholine "LT-02" in ulcerative colitis: a randomized, placebo-controlled trial in mesalazine-refractory courses. Am J Gastroenterol 2014; 109(7):1041–51.

47. Martin DA, Bolling BW. A review of the efficacy of dietary polyphenols in experimental models of inflammatory bowel diseases. Food Funct 2015;6(6):1773–86.

48. Lakhan SE, Schofield KL. Mindfulness-based therapies in the treatment of somatization disorders: a systematic review and meta-analysis. PLoS One 2013;8(8): e71834.

49. Aucoin M, Lalonde-Parsi MJ, Cooley K. Mindfulness-based therapies in the treatment of functional gastrointestinal disorders: a meta-analysis. Evid Based Complement Alternat Med 2014;2014:140724.

50. van der Veek PP, van Rood YR, Masclee AA. Clinical trial: short- and long-term benefit of relaxation training for irritable bowel syndrome. Aliment Pharmacol Ther 2007;26(6):943–52.

51. Lee HH, Choi YY, Choi MG. The efficacy of hypnotherapy in the treatment of irritable bowel syndrome: a systematic review and meta-analysis. J Neurogastroenterology Motil 2014;20(2):152–62.
52. Schumann D, Anheyer D, Lauche R, et al. Effect of yoga in the therapy of irritable bowel syndrome: a systematic review. Clin Gastroenterol Hepatol 2016;14(12):1720–31.
53. Johannesson E, Simren M, Strid H, et al. Physical activity improves symptoms in irritable bowel syndrome: a randomized controlled trial. Am J Gastroenterol 2011;106(5):915–22.
54. Johannesson E, Ringström G, Abrahamsson H, et al. Intervention to increase physical activity in irritable bowel syndrome shows long-term positive effects. World J Gastroenterol 2015;21(2):600–8. Available at: http://onlinelibrary.wiley.com/o/cochrane/clcentral/articles/322/CN-01101322/frame.html.
55. Manheimer E, Cheng K, Wieland LS, et al. Acupuncture for treatment of irritable bowel syndrome. Cochrane Database Syst Rev 2012;(5):CD005111.
56. Peckham EJ, Nelson EA, Greenhalgh J, et al. Homeopathy for treatment of irritable bowel syndrome. Cochrane Database Syst Rev 2013;(11):CD009710.
57. Oka T, Okumi H, Nishida S, et al. Effects of Kampo on functional gastrointestinal disorders. Biopsychosoc Med 2014;8(1):5.
58. Yadav SK, Jain AK, Tripathi SN, et al. Irritable bowel syndrome: therapeutic evaluation of indigenous drugs. Indian J Med Res 1989;90:496–503.
59. Lauche R, Kumar S, Hallmann J, et al. Efficacy and safety of Ayurvedic herbs in diarrhoea-predominant irritable bowel syndrome: a randomised controlled crossover trial. Complement Ther Med 2016;26:171–7.
60. Lauche R, Janzen A, Ludtke R, et al. Efficacy of caraway oil poultices in treating irritable bowel syndrome–a randomized controlled cross-over trial. Digestion 2015;92(1):22–31.
61. Zhang RM, Wang L, Yang XN, et al. Dinggui Oil Capsule in treating irritable bowel syndrome with stagnation of qi and cold: a prospective, multi-center, randomized, placebo-controlled, double-blind trial. Zhong Xi Yi Jie He Xue Bao 2007;5(4):392–7 [in Chinese].
62. Madisch A, Holtmann G, Plein K, et al. Treatment of irritable bowel syndrome with herbal preparations: results of a double-blind, randomized, placebo-controlled, multi-centre trial. Aliment Pharmacol Ther 2004;19(3):271–9.
63. Jalihal A, Kurian G. Ispaghula therapy in irritable bowel syndrome: Improvement in overall well-being is related to reduction in bowel dissatisfaction. J Gastroenterol Hepatol 1990;5(5):507–13.
64. Bortolotti M, Porta S. Effect of red pepper on symptoms of irritable bowel syndrome: preliminary study. Dig Dis Sci 2011;56(11):3288–95.
65. Sahib AS. Treatment of irritable bowel syndrome using a selected herbal combination of Iraqi folk medicines. J Ethnopharmacol 2013;148(3):1008–12.
66. Jae-Woo P, Seok-Jae K, Gajin H, et al. A randomised, double-blind, placebo-controlled study of effect of probiotics combined with a herbal mixture on irritable bowel syndrome with diarrhoea. Eur J Integr Med 2012;4:179. Available at: http://onlinelibrary.wiley.com/o/cochrane/clcentral/articles/842/CN-01029842/frame.html.
67. Khanna R, MacDonald JK, Levesque BG. Peppermint oil for the treatment of irritable bowel syndrome: a systematic review and meta-analysis. J Clin Gastroenterol 2014;48(6):505–12.
68. Van Tilburg MAL, Palsson OS, Ringel Y, et al. Is ginger effective for the treatment of irritable bowel syndrome? A double blind randomized controlled pilot trial. Complement Therap Med 2014;22(1):17–20.

69. Saito YA, Rey E, Almazar-Elder AE, et al. A randomized, double-blind, placebo-controlled trial of St John's wort for treating irritable bowel syndrome. Am J Gastroenterol 2010;105(1):170–7.

70. Davis K, Philpott S, Kumar D, et al. Randomised double-blind placebo-controlled trial of aloe vera for irritable bowel syndrome. Int J Clin Pract 2006;60(9):1080–6.

71. Brinkhaus B, Hentschel C, Von Keudell C, et al. Herbal medicine with curcuma and fumitory in the treatment of irritable bowel syndrome: a randomized, placebo-controlled, double-blind clinical trial. Scand J Gastroenterol 2005; 40(8):936–43.

72. Chedid V, Dhalla S, Clarke JO, et al. Herbal therapy is equivalent to rifaximin for the treatment of small intestinal bacterial overgrowth. Glob Adv Health Med 2014; 3(3):16–24.

73. Alecci U, Bonina F, Bonina A, et al. Efficacy and safety of a natural remedy for the treatment of gastroesophageal reflux: a double-blinded randomized-controlled study. evidence-based complementary and alternative medicine. Evid Based Complement Alternat Med 2016;2016:2581461.

74. Havelund T, Aalykke C, Rasmussen L. Efficacy of a pectin-based anti-reflux agent on acid reflux and recurrence of symptoms and oesophagitis in gastro-oesophageal reflux disease. Eur J Gastroenterol Hepatol 1997;9(5):509–14.

75. Farup PG, Heibert M, Hoeg V. Alternative vs. conventional treatment given on-demand for gastroesophageal reflux disease: a randomised controlled trial. BMC Complement Altern Med 2009;9:3.

76. Pereira Rde S. Regression of gastroesophageal reflux disease symptoms using dietary supplementation with melatonin, vitamins and aminoacids: comparison with omeprazole. J pineal Res 2006;41(3):195–200.

77. Brzozowska I, Strzalka M, Drozdowicz D, et al. Mechanisms of esophageal protection, gastroprotection and ulcer healing by melatonin: implications for the therapeutic use of melatonin in gastroesophageal reflux disease (GERD) and peptic ulcer disease. Curr Pharm Des 2014;20(3):4807–15.

78. Kandil T, Mousa A, El-Gendy A. The potential therapeutic effect of melatonin in gastroesophageal reflux disease. BMC Gastroenterol 2010;10:7.

79. Patrick L. Gastroesophageal reflux disease (GERD): a review of conventional and alternative treatments. Altern Med Rev 2011;16(2):116–33.

Integrative Women's Health

Delia Chiaramonte, MD[a,b,*], Melinda Ring, MD[c], Amy B. Locke, MD[d]

KEYWORDS

- Integrative women's health • Menopause • Premenstrual syndrome
- Premenstrual dysphoric disorder • Chronic pelvic pain • Vulvodynia
- Interstitial cystitis • Central sensitization

KEY POINTS

- More than 50% of women seek integrative approaches to help manage menopause-related symptoms.
- Although menopause hormone therapy is the gold standard for alleviating vasomotor symptoms, there is evidence of benefit for other approaches, including mind-body therapies, acupuncture, and phytoestrogens.
- Premenstrual syndrome (PMS) is a common, heterogeneous disorder with symptoms limited to the luteal phase of the menstrual cycle, which can be improved with lifestyle and mind-body interventions.
- Calcium, magnesium, vitamin B_6, and chaste tree berry are dietary supplements that have the best evidence for treatment of PMS.
- Chronic pelvic pain is multifactorial, can be associated with central sensitization, and negatively impacts quality of life.
- An integrative approach that addresses both physical and psychological contributors to pain may be most effective at improving chronic pelvic pain symptoms and restoring function.

The authors have nothing to disclose.
[a] Department of Family and Community Medicine, Center for Integrative Medicine, University of Maryland School of Medicine, 520 West Lombard Street, East Hall, Baltimore, MD 21201, USA; [b] Department of Epidemiology and Public Health, Center for Integrative Medicine, University of Maryland School of Medicine, 520 West Lombard Street, East Hall, Baltimore, MD 21201, USA; [c] Osher Center for Integrative Medicine at Northwestern University, Northwestern University Feinberg School of Medicine, 150 East Huron Avenue, Suite 1100, Chicago, IL 60611, USA; [d] Co-Director Resiliency Center, Office of Wellness and Integrative Health, Department of Family and Preventive Medicine, University of Utah, 555 Foothill Boulevard, Salt Lake City, UT 84112, USA
* Corresponding author. Departments of Family and Community Medicine and Epidemiology and Public Health, Center for Integrative Medicine, University of Maryland School of Medicine, 520 West Lombard Street, East Hall, Baltimore, MD 21201.
E-mail address: dchiaramonte@som.umaryland.edu

http://dx.doi.org/10.1016/j.mcna.2017.04.010
medical.theclinics.com

INTRODUCTION

As many as 75% of women use complementary therapies[1,2]; the most commonly used interventions are dietary supplements and mind-body modalities,[1] often by self-referral.[2] Complementary medicine use is particularly common in women with menopausal symptoms.[3] Women are frequently influenced by nonprofessional sources when choosing complementary therapies, relying on information provided by friends, family, and the media.[4] Physicians, therefore, should educate themselves about the integrative approach to women's health to effectively counsel their patients.

MENOPAUSE

An estimated 6000 US women reach menopause every day; by 2020, the number of US women older than 51 is expected to exceed 50 million.[5] Just more than 50% of menopausal women in a 2013 systematic review reported the use of integrative medicine therapies specifically for menopausal symptoms.[6] Any primary care provider who cares for adult women is thus certain to be confronted with women seeking options for symptom relief and support as a partner in the aging process.

Pathophysiology

The natural process of menopause results from the progressive loss of ovarian follicle function. Natural menopause, defined as 1 year after cessation of menstruation, occurs on average at age 51, with most women falling between age 45 to 55. Certain factors are associated with an earlier age of menopause, including smoking, high-fiber or vegetarian diet, low body mass index, type 1 diabetes mellitus, and nulligravida. Menopause also may be induced from surgery or medications, such as chemotherapy.

The perimenopause transition time may begin when a woman is in her late 30s to early 40s, with episodic symptoms, such as night sweats and changes in cycle length. The Stages of Reproductive Aging Workshop (STRAW) classification (**Fig. 1**) is a useful construct for explaining to women the progression from reproductive years through late postmenopause, and helping her understand that her symptoms are normal and expected.[7]

Evaluation

In general, laboratory testing is not required to establish menopause, although some measurements may be beneficial in staging during the perimenopausal years. A primary care provider instead can focus on taking a thorough history to elucidate any symptoms related to hormone changes, review preventive strategies to maintain health, and partner with the patient to help her define and achieve her goals. Laboratory markers of menopause, when used, include an increase in serum follicle stimulating hormone (FSH) and decreases in estradiol. In perimenopause, the progesterone decline often precedes changes in estrogen, leading to a relative estrogen dominance, with associated increasing premenstrual syndrome and breast tenderness. When hormones such as testosterone are being considered for use alongside estrogens and progestogen for hyposexual sexual disorder, levels of androgens and baseline chemistries and blood counts should be obtained. The measurement of hormones during perimenopause and postmenopause in blood, urine, or saliva is an area of controversy.

Treatment/Management

Up to 80% of perimenopausal and postmenopausal women report having vasomotor symptoms (VMS), including hot flashes and night sweats, with up to half reporting

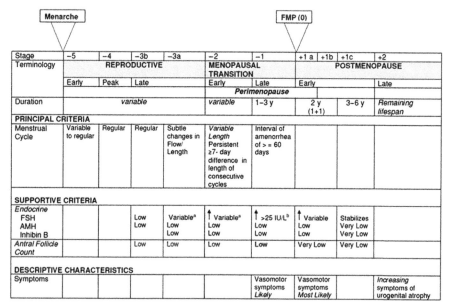

Fig. 1. Stages of reproductive aging workshop (STRAW) classification. [a] Blood draw on cycle days 2–5 ↑ = elevated. [b] Approximate expected level based on assays using current international pituitary standard. (*From* Harlow SD, Gass M, Hall JE, et al. Executive summary of the Stages of Reproductive Aging Workshop þ 10: addressing the unfinished agenda of staging reproductive aging. J Clin Endocrinol Metab 2012;97(4):1159–68; with permission.)

moderate or severe symptoms.[8] Vasomotor symptoms peak during the menopausal transition, but up to 25% of women in their 60s and 70s report VMS.[9] Given the broad spectrum of symptoms a woman may experience during the menopausal transition, the following summary focuses on integrative therapies for vasomotor symptoms.

Lifestyle

Dietary factors commonly reported by women as triggers for vasomotor symptoms include caffeine, alcohol, and spicy and hot foods and beverages. Studies on specific dietary factors are limited, with the primary interventions studied being weight loss and phytoestrogens.

Weight In one trial of women not using hormones, those who lost weight via reduced fat and increased fruit, vegetable, and fiber intake reported a reduction or elimination of VMS over 1 year.[10] The diet appeared to impact symptoms over and above the effect of weight change. A 2015 pilot study in 40 overweight or obese women found that weight loss was significantly associated with a greater reduction in the number of hot flashes, although not on reported VMS severity.[11]

Dietary phytoestrogens Many plants produce chemicals that mimic or interact with hormone signals. Soy isoflavones genistein and daidzein can bind estrogen receptors, resulting in both estrogen agonist and antagonist actions. Prior meta-analyses and systematic reviews have shown mixed results of soy isoflavones on VMS.[12,13] However, a 2016 *JAMA* meta-analysis of 21 randomized controlled trials concludes that both composite phytoestrogen supplementation and individual phytoestrogen interventions, such as dietary and supplemental soy isoflavones, are associated with modest reductions in the frequency of hot flashes and vaginal dryness but not night sweats.[14] Soy protein is generally safe when used in moderation, although some patients note gastrointestinal side effects, such as bloating and loose stool. Lignans in ground flaxseed are polyphenolic sterols that produce weakly estrogenic sterols when acted on by gut microbiota. A review of 5 controlled studies of ground flaxseed for VMS reported no significant change in VMS compared with placebo.[15]

Mind-body practices

Acupuncture A 2015 meta-analysis of 12 studies (n = 869) examined the effect of acupuncture once to twice weekly over 5 to 12 weeks.[16] Acupuncture significantly reduced the frequency and severity of hot flashes, with effects lasting up to 3 months. Additional benefits were noted in psychological, somatic, and urogenital subscale scores. Acupuncture is increasingly available within hospitals and health systems and in the community setting. Referral to a provider trained in acupuncture, with appropriate licensure and credentials, should be considered for menopausal women seeking a holistic strategy.

Movement and meditation-based practices A 2010 systematic review explored interventions such as yoga, meditation, tai chi, muscle relaxation, breath-based techniques, and relaxation response training.[17] The conclusion, despite variable study quality, was that mind-body practices should play a prominent role in a menopause management strategy. Eight of the 9 studies of yoga, tai chi, and meditation-based programs reported improvement in overall menopausal and vasomotor symptoms. A 2014 review examined how mind-body therapies could impact not just isolated symptoms, but clusters of symptoms, such as hot flashes co-occurring with impaired sleep, cognitive dysfunction, dysphoric mood, or pain.[18] In this report, mindfulness-based stress reduction, in particular, was found to improve sleep, mood symptoms, and hot flashes.

Natural products

Although good-quality data are lacking in general for dietary supplements, the following show the greatest promise in menopause.

Sage Sage *(Salvia officinalis)* has been used in traditional herbal medicine for excessive sweating and hot flashes, and may have some estrogenic and neuromodulatory activity. In 71 women with at least 5 hot flashes daily, a 280-mg extract led to a significant decrease in intensity-rated hot flashes by 50% within 4 weeks and by 64% within 8 weeks.[19] Additional studies are warranted to explore the potential role of sage in treatment of VMS.

Black cohosh Black cohosh *(Cimicifuga racemosa)* is frequently used for menopause in the United States and Europe. The mechanism for its effect is unclear. Black cohosh does not directly bind estrogen receptors or stimulate the growth of estrogen-dependent tumors.[20,21] The most consistent evidence is for a specific extract called Remifemin, shown in multiple studies to significantly reduce menopausal symptom indices and hot flash frequency compared with placebo.[22,23] However, other studies and systematic reviews on black cohosh have been inconclusive.[24,25] Some issues of safety, in particular with regard to hepatotoxicity, have been raised, although in general, long-term use has been shown to be very safe.[26,27] Black cohosh may be considered at a dosage of 20 mg twice daily, standardized to contain 1 mg of 27-deoxyactein.

Other herbals Chaste berry, kudzu, alfalfa, hops, licorice, evening primrose oil, *Panax ginseng*, maca, wild yam, and vitamin E have all been promoted for menopausal symptom relief, but studies are limited.

Pharmacologic

Pharmaceuticals Selective serotonin reuptake inhibitors (SSRIs) and serotonin-norepinephrine reuptake inhibitors, as well as gabapentin and pregabalin, are the most common medications prescribed for VMS based on studies showing mild-moderate improvements. These medications have the potential for significant side effects, and the antidepressants carry black box warnings regarding the risk of suicidal thoughts and behaviors. Although of benefit for some women, nonpharmacologic approaches may be preferable as initial treatment.

Menopausal hormone therapy A full guide to prescribing menopausal hormone therapy (MHT) is beyond the scope of this article. Primary care providers caring for menopausal women must stay up-to-date on MHT recommendations. Current guidelines support MHT in women without contraindications within 10 years of menopause and before age 60, especially when significant VMSs are present.[28,29] Chronic VMSs can negatively impact quality of life and reanalysis of data on MHT suggest a potential cardioprotective effect. This, along with reanalysis of data on MHT-related cancer risk, has led to a call for a more individualized risk-benefit assessment. Decisions about whether or not to initiate MHT should consider a woman's preference, the severity of vasomotor symptoms, impact of symptoms on quality of life, and family or personal history of hormone-dependent cancer, venous thrombosis, or cardiovascular disease.[30] Understanding terminology related to MHT formulations is important in integrative care:

Natural: implies that hormones are derived from a naturally occurring source but tells nothing about the actual content. This term should be avoided.

Synthetic: hormone formulations with a chemical structure not produced by the human body.

Bioidentical: the molecular structure of the hormones is identical to endogenous hormones. Bioidentical hormones are available both through compounding pharmacies and in pharmaceutical versions. Proponents of bioidentical hormones point to differential effects of bioidentical versus synthetic hormones on lipids, glucose regulation, sleep, mood, breast tenderness, and breast cancer risk.[31–34] Given the widespread availability of bioidentical hormones, efficacy in addressing the symptoms of menopause, and possible preferential risk and side-effect profile, the use of bioidentical versions is reasonable and appropriate for any woman seeking MHT.

Summary

The menopausal transition is a time when women may be experiencing significant life issues, such as aging parents, growing children, employment issues, and marital stress. The physical symptoms and changes in their bodies can add an additional burden. The support of a primary care provider who uses a team-based approach and encourages a whole-person, integrative wellness plan can make all the difference to a woman, and help her see this period as a transition that is a meaningful part of her growth and life work.

PREMENSTRUAL SYNDROME

Premenstrual syndrome (PMS) is defined as "recurrent moderate psychological and physical symptoms that occur during the luteal phase of menses and resolve with menstruation."[35] Although 80% of women have some luteal symptoms, 20% to 32% have mild to moderate symptoms that are significant enough to be considered PMS.[36] A further 3% to 8% of women have severe debilitating symptoms; these fall into the category of premenstrual dysphoric disorder (PMDD).

Pathophysiology

The classically identified peak in luteinizing hormone and FSH before ovulation and their effect on estrogen and progesterone are well known. The peak of estrogen just before ovulation and the smaller rise in the mid-luteal phase along with the peak of progesterone are important, but they are only a portion of the cyclical changes that occur. Prolactin peaks near the time of ovulation and remains high in the luteal phase. There is blunting of cortisol and melatonin rhythms in the luteal phase.[37] Aldosterone levels rise at ovulation and remain elevated during the luteal phase. Calcium, parathyroid hormone, and vitamin D levels fluctuate across the cycle.[38] Alterations in any of these can affect symptomatology. Classic symptoms of PMS are numerous and are included in **Box 1**. Symptoms must be isolated in the luteal phase, otherwise, they likely represent a different cause.

There are many theories as to the cause of PMS, and it is likely multifactorial. Some hypothesize hormone imbalance, such as low luteal progesterone, high prolactin, increased aldosterone, or renin activity, but differences between those with and without symptoms are not clear.[39] Neurotransmitter deregulation, vitamin deficiency, hypoglycemia, prostaglandins, and psychosocial stressors also have been linked to PMS. Aldosterone fluctuation might lead to edema, bloating, weight gain, and headache. Prostaglandin shifts could be associated with breast pain, fluid retention, headache, cramping, irritability, and depression. A response to nonsteroidal anti-inflammatory drugs might support this link.

For some individuals, it may be increased sensitivity to normal phenomena. For others, the complex changes that occur in the luteal phase may unmask underlying weaknesses or deficiencies. For example, high stress, poor sleep, or a marginal diet

---

Box 1
Common symptoms of premenstrual syndrome

- Mood
  - Irritability
  - Depressive symptoms
  - Anxiety
- Libido change
- Appetite change
- Poor sleep
- Fatigue
- Physical symptoms
  - Myalgia
  - Bloating
  - Mastalgia
  - Weight gain
  - Edema
  - Nausea
  - Abdominal cramping
  - Headache

may be less well tolerated during the luteal phase. The luteal phase may be more susceptible to underlying disorders as well, such as menstrual migraines. Additionally, one set of symptoms can lead to behavioral changes that then cause other symptoms (eg, mood symptoms may drive changes in diet that then can lead to changes in bowel habits).

During adolescence and perimenopause, there are unique concerns. Adolescence is a time of frequent mood shifts and psychosocial change. This overlay of issues can complicate diagnosis. In addition, there are issues particular to perimenopause. During this time, frequently defined as the 10 years before menopause, hormone fluctuations are common, resulting in cycle irregularity. Poor lifestyle effects can be amplified and can unmask chronic stress-related fatigue. Mood issues and migraines often flare.

Diagnosis and Evaluation

To diagnosis PMS or PMDD, the symptoms must be isolated to the luteal phase. Many women have difficulty clearly determining this correlation. The Daily Record of Severity of Problems (DRSP) is a measure used for prospective charting of symptoms. It is administered for 2 months and is sensitive and reliable, particularly for PMDD.[40] Administration of the DRSP at the beginning of a cycle can help rule out PMS.[41] A short retrospective questionnaire is similarly sensitive and can hasten diagnosis.[42] The DRSP is most useful with a confusing diagnostic picture.

Treatment/Management

Lifestyle

The most consistently demonstrated association of worsened PMS symptoms has been secondary to alcohol and tobacco.[43] Alcohol is associated with increased headache and mood symptoms.[43] Cravings for nicotine increase during the luteal phase.[44]

There is no clear evidence that specific dietary interventions treat PMS, but good dietary advice can help with underlying problems. A Mediterranean diet is a reasonable recommendation. Women with diets higher in thiamine and riboflavin have lower symptoms of PMS.[45] Women with PMS are more likely to change their diet for the worse during the luteal phase, with increased refined carbohydrates, sugars, and fat.[46] Recognizing this may allow for dietary modification. The most common foods identified by women as exacerbating PMS symptoms include caffeine, salt, simple sugars/starches, and alcohol. Although there is a dose-dependent relationship between caffeine and symptoms in some studies,[47] newer studies suggest there may not be a relationship.[48] Caffeine may be associated with irritability and salty foods with bloating. Some advocate for a diet low in exogenous estrogens, consisting of high fiber, plant-based, and low saturated fat. Phytoestrogens are not thought to be problematic. Based on the level of data to support specific dietary interventions, advice will need to be individualized to the experiences of the individual.

Physical activity has not been extensively studied in PMS; however, studies suggest benefit,[49] and it is recommended by the American College of Obstetrics and Gynecology. Aerobic activity affects progesterone, estrogen, and prolactin levels.[50] Moderate-level activity decreases fatigue and improves concentration among other benefits.[50] One small study found an effect on skin blemishes in addition to mood, pain, loneliness, and crying.[51] Those with underlying conditions, such as depression and anxiety, may have additional benefit. Recommendations mirror those for the larger population: 30 minutes of moderate activity daily along with some vigorous strengthening and stretching activities.

Sleep is commonly disrupted in those with PMS. Sleep changes in the luteal phase regardless of PMS. Rapid eye movement sleep decreases in the luteal phase along with an increase in stage 2 sleep.[52] This change can be accentuated in those with PMS.[53] Additionally, patients with PMDD exhibit decreased melatonin, slow-wave sleep,[52] and reduced parasympathetic activity during the luteal phase.[54] Examination of shift workers shows further disruption in menstrual cycles with increased cycle length and irregularity.[37] Strategies to reduce PMS-related insomnia are similar to those used for other causes.

Mind-body therapies

Significant emotional distress can accompany the presence of PMS. Several studies examine the role of mind-body therapies for treatment. Meditation has strong effects on PMS.[55] Herbert Benson's Relaxation Response method, combining progressive muscle relaxation, breathing exercises, and meditation using word (ie, mantra) repetition, decreases symptoms when practiced 15 to 20 minutes twice daily.[56] Guided imagery has positive preliminary data.[57] Cognitive behavioral therapy (CBT) is effective, particularly for acceptance-based CBT and mindfulness.[58] CBT is as effective as fluoxetine in PMDD.[59] Yoga can be considered, as small studies in healthy women show reduction in weight, anger, anxiety, and depression during the premenstrual portion of the cycle when practiced for 35 to 40 minutes 6 days a week.[60]

Acupuncture has been examined in several small trials. A 2014 systematic review found a 50% improvement of physical symptoms for those with PMS and PMDD but no significant improvement in psychological symptoms compared with controls.[61] Different acupuncture techniques, including traditional acupuncture, hand acupuncture with moxibustion, and auricular acupuncture were used.

Natural products

The popularity of natural products often precedes medical evidence of efficacy. There are biological reasons to suspect that certain vitamins may have an effect on PMS. Several B vitamins and magnesium are required for synthesis of the neurotransmitters that play a role in PMS. Vitamin B6 (pyridoxine) has positive effects on serotonin, norepinephrine, and dopamine. A systematic review of B_6 found small sample sizes but improved PMS symptoms overall, including depressive symptoms.[62] Other studies have suggested only dietary B vitamins have an effect.[45] Common dosage: B-complex 50 to 100 mg daily.

Low intake of calcium and vitamin D are associated with PMS.[63] Calcium is modulated by estrogen.[64] Some have drawn comparisons between the symptoms of PMS and hypocalcemia, suggesting that estrogen levels in the luteal phase unmask calcium deficiency, contributing to symptoms.[64] Calcium at a dosage of 1200 mg daily showed a 48% reduction in symptoms.[65] Magnesium may be helpful for overall symptoms, especially mood.[66] It is particularly beneficial for cramps and the prevention of menstrual migraine. It appears to have additive benefit when combined with B6. Common dosage: Calcium 1200 mg daily. Magnesium chelate, glycinate, or malate 400 mg daily.

Chaste tree berry (*Vitex agnus-castus*) decreases estrogen and prolactin while increasing progesterone.[67] In randomized placebo-controlled studies, it has been shown to impact women's assessment of irritability, mood, anger, headache, breast fullness, and bloating.[67] A systematic review found *Vitex* extracts to be superior to placebo (5 of 6 studies), pyridoxine (1 study), and magnesium oxide (1 study). In PMDD, *Vitex* was equivalent to fluoxetine in 1 study, and was outperformed by fluoxetine in another.[68] Common dose: 20 to 40 mL standardized extract or 250 to 500 mg crude herb.

Evening primrose oil may be helpful for cyclic mastalgia at a dosage of 1.5 g twice daily. However, there are several negative trials of evening primrose oil for more general PMS symptoms[69] Gingko (*Gingko biloba*) and black cohosh are often used for PMS symptoms, but do not have strong evidence supporting their use.

In addition to treatments for general PMS symptoms, targeting specific symptoms for therapy should be considered. For menstrual migraine, treatment may include a focus on magnesium or chaste tree.[66] For depression and anxiety, vitamin B_6 or chaste tree may be a better choice.[62,67] For mastalgia, evening primrose oil or chaste tree may have more of an effect.[69] Interventions should be tailored to symptomatology.

Pharmacologic

Hormonal therapies include oral contraceptives (OCPs), progesterone, and estrogen. OCPs are the mainstay of conventional treatment due to their efficacy in reducing symptoms. Although some prefer the progesterone drospirenone, it is not clearly superior.[70] There is a high placebo effect of OCPs. Aggression, irritability, and fatigue are consistently associated with lower luteal progesterone.[71] Progesterone alone dosed in the luteal phase either orally or topically is a popular treatment.[72–74] However, a Cochrane review was unable to evaluate its effect due to heterogeneity in studies and study quality.[75] Common dosage: 100 mg progesterone (Prometrium) or 5 to 20 mg topical compounded formulation on days 14 to 25. Estrogen is sometimes added in perimenopause.

SSRIs are also an effective treatment for PMS. Luteal dosing and continuous dosing are equally efficacious.[76]

Summary

PMS and PMDD are common conditions frequently treated by conventional therapies without complete resolution of symptoms, making them good targets for an integrative approach to care. Identification and treatment of underlying conditions can help make progress toward resolution of symptoms. Understanding the complex hormonal changes of the menstrual cycle can help in understanding correlations. Treatment modalities should target the level of intervention to symptoms and the interest of the patient.

CHRONIC PELVIC PAIN

Chronic pelvic pain (CPP) is defined as pain in the lower abdomen or pelvis lasting 6 months or more.[77] It is a common yet frustrating pain condition, which can adversely affect physical functioning, psychological well-being, sexual functioning, sleep, and quality of life.[78–81] Impairment in functioning may be related to the severity of coexisting anxiety or depression[78] or to a history of adolescent or adult sexual abuse.[82] Approximately 74% of women with CPP experience pain with sexual activity.[83] Studies have suggested prevalence rates of 5.7% to 26.6%.[84]

Pelvic pain can be cyclic or noncyclic. This article focuses on noncyclic CPP. CPP is well-suited to be addressed with an integrative approach; 51% of women with CPP have used at least 1 complementary health approach in the past year, often improving their health-related quality of life.[85] Common etiologies of noncyclic CPP include vulvodynia, interstitial cystitis (IC), irritable bowel syndrome, and myofascial pain.

Pathophysiology

Vulvodynia

Vulvodynia can be defined as vulvar pain, burning, or discomfort without a clear etiology. Underlying contributors may include inflammation, peripheral and central sensitization, candida infection, alterations in vaginal flora, and pudendal neuralgia. Vulvodynia can be associated with painful intercourse and subsequent sexual dysfunction. Women with vulvodynia often have coexisting undifferentiated CPP symptoms and irritable bowel syndrome.[86] Anxiety, fear of pain, catastrophizing, and depression are all more common in this population.[87]

Interstitial cystitis

Women with IC, sometimes called painful bladder syndrome, experience urinary urgency, frequency, and bladder and/or pelvic pain in the absence of urinary tract infection. These symptoms often coexist with undifferentiated pelvic pain. In one study, 89% of women undergoing laparoscopy for CPP had concomitant IC confirmed by cystoscopy.[88] Symptoms can be continuous or intermittent.

Gastrointestinal etiologies

Irritable bowel syndrome is a functional gastrointestinal condition that causes pelvic and abdominal pain, cramping, and changes in stool frequency and consistency. Celiac disease also may cause CPP.[89]

Myofascial pain

CPP can result from pelvic floor dysfunction, myofascial pain, and trigger points in the low back, pelvis, and abdominal wall.

Undifferentiated chronic pelvic pain

CPP is often multifactorial and in many cases a direct cause cannot be found.[90] Even if pathology is found, pain is frequently out of proportion to the extent of disease identified.

Central sensitization

Central sensitization is a condition of the nervous system brought about by chronic pain that results in a heightened sensitivity to pain and touch. Increased signal transmission and reduced inhibition create a state in which the pain is no longer coupled to the presence or intensity of tissue damage. Instead, central sensitization creates pain hypersensitivity by changing the sensory response elicited by non-noxious inputs.[91] The nervous system becomes regulated in a persistently reactive state, which can maintain pain even after the inciting condition has healed. Central sensitization has been shown in multiple pain conditions, including CPP.[92] A heightened sense of "threat" supports the development of central sensitization. Physicians and other health care providers may inadvertently enhance this effect by eliciting the nocebo response during discussions of test results or prognosis. Patients may catastrophize and practice fear-based avoidance of activities.

Endometriosis

Although endometriosis is a common cause of cyclic CPP, and discussion of standard endometriosis management is beyond the scope of this article, women with a diagnosis of endometriosis may have other coexisting etiologies of CPP. In a recent study, central sensitization was present in more than 80% of women with CPP, and was approximately equally common in women with and without endometriosis. More than 90% of these women, both with and without endometriosis, also had myofascial trigger points.[93] Thus, sensitization and myofascial trigger points are common in women with CPP, regardless of whether or not they have endometriosis. Endometriosis-associated pain may be multifactorial and responsive to an integrative approach.

Evaluation

Evaluation of CPP should be 2-pronged. Underlying contributing conditions should be identified *and* CPP should be considered a diagnosis in and of itself. These 2 approaches are not mutually exclusive and may work best if addressed simultaneously.[94] Anxiety and depression commonly co-occur with chronic pain and active treatment is important for the management of CPP. When considering underlying contributors, it can be helpful to organize potential etiologies into 3 categories: visceral causes (eg, reproductive organs, bowel, or bladder), musculoskeletal and neuropathic causes (eg, pelvic floor muscle spasm), and psychosocial contributors (eg, depression, anxiety).[95]

History should include assessment of the urinary, gastrointestinal, reproductive, and musculoskeletal systems, as well as screening for depression, anxiety, sexual dysfunction, adverse childhood events, and current and prior abuse history. Consider prescribing a pain diary (**Fig. 2**) to assess pain triggers, treatment effectiveness, impact of mood, and other pain modifiers. Online pain diaries are available.[96]

Physical Examination

In addition to a standard gynecologic examination, consider assessment of the gastrointestinal system, back, lower extremities, pelvic floor, and abdominal musculature, looking for spasm, tenderness, or trigger points, and assess the vulva for tenderness using a cotton swab. A 12-point manual examination of the vagina can

Pain Scale

| 0 | 1 | 2 | 3 | 4 | 5 | 6 | 7 | 8 | 9 | 10 |

No Pain   Mild Pain   Moderate Pain   Severe Pain   Worst Pain

Date	Pain Level 0–10	Pain description & how long did it last?	What made it worse?	What helped?	Stress/ Negative Mood 0–10

Fig. 2. Pain diary.

be used to help identify the etiology of CPP symptoms.[95] This involves an examination of the 4 vaginal walls at varying depths of the vagina and includes assessment of the introitus, urethra, rectum, bladder, and pelvic floor musculature.

Treatment/Management

Vulvodynia

Conventional treatment options include both topical treatments, such as anesthetic gels and estrogen cream, as well as oral treatments, such as tricyclic antidepressants and antifungals. DeAndres and colleagues[97] recently published a comprehensive review of conventional vulvodynia management.

Gabapentin, used both topically[98] and orally,[99] has been shown to decrease pain. Nitroglycerin cream (0.2%) can decrease intercourse-related pain when used immediately before sexual activity.[100] Surgical interventions are reserved for the most severe and intractable cases.

Physical therapy is an important component of vulvodynia management. Treatments may include pelvic floor exercises, myofascial release, trigger point therapy, massage, joint mobilization, and soft tissue mobilization, with the goal of rehabilitating and desensitizing the pelvic musculature. Both CBT and physical therapy have been shown to decrease vulvodynia pain and pain catastrophizing, but CBT more effectively improved sexual function.[101] In addition, acupuncture may improve pain and sexual function in vulvodynia.[97]

Interstitial cystitis

As with all other contributors to CPP, IC is best handled with a multifactorial approach. Pelvic floor manual therapy, dietary modifications, medications, behavioral strategies, and stress management all can be helpful. Physical therapy interventions are similar to those for vulvodynia and have been shown to be effective in IC.[102] Dietary modifications focus on decreasing bladder irritants by elimination of foods such as "the 4 Cs": carbonated beverages, caffeine, citrus foods, and those with high vitamin C content. It also may be helpful to eliminate tomatoes, alcohol, spicy foods, and artificial sweeteners.[103] Medication options include tricyclic antidepressants, antihistamines, and pentosan polysulfate sodium, which may improve symptoms by protecting the bladder wall. Timed voiding, in which elimination is tied to the clock rather than the urge to urinate, is used to decrease symptoms of urgency and frequency. Other interventions include transcutaneous electrical nerve stimulation, sacral nerve stimulation, intravesicular dimethyl sulfoxide, and bladder distension. Stress management is an important component of IC treatment. Despite the varied treatment options, treatment for IC is challenging. This may explain why, in one study, more than 80% of patients with IC reported using complementary medicine approaches.[104] Therapies reported by patients to be most effective include dietary modifications, physical therapy, relaxation strategies, acupuncture, stress management, exercise, and sleep hygiene.[104]

Pelvic floor dysfunction/myofascial pain

Women suspected of having pelvic floor dysfunction or myofascial pain, such as those with a history of physical trauma or back pain, or in whom a urogenital diagnosis cannot be found, should be referred to a physical therapist or other practitioner with specialized training in pelvic soft tissue manipulation and rehabilitation. Therapeutic interventions may include myofascial release, trigger point compression or injection, biofeedback, and strengthening and stretching of the pelvic floor muscles. Physical therapy showed significant improvement in myofascial CPP, with improvements proportional to the number of physical therapy visits.[105] Botulinum toxin type A injected into the pelvic floor muscles may be helpful for CPP associated with pelvic floor muscle spasm.[106,107]

Undifferentiated chronic pelvic pain

Many cases of CPP have no clear etiology. CBT, which teaches self-management skills that support self-efficacy and resourcefulness, is a useful adjunct in the treatment of chronic pain, and may be more effective than supportive psychotherapy.[108] Somatocognitive therapy, a hybrid of physical therapy principles and CBT, improved psychological distress, pain experience, and function in women with CPP better than gynecologic treatment alone.[109] Group visits have been used successfully in the treatment of CPP[110] and positive psychology interventions have been successful in decreasing chronic pain of varied etiologies.[111] Patients should be screened for post-traumatic stress disorder and adverse childhood experiences and referred for psychotherapy and eye movement desensitization and reprocessing (EMDR) as appropriate. EMDR uses rhythmic eye movements or alternating bilateral stimuli to modulate, and facilitate processing of, emotionally charged memories.[112,113] Even those without a trauma history can benefit from referral for psychological care. Dietary modifications that focus on increasing antioxidant-containing foods may also help some patients with CPP.[114]

Mind-Body Practices

Mindfulness-based interventions can benefit patients with chronic pain[115–117] and have been shown to improve coexisting anxiety and depression.[118] Such interventions have resulted in enhanced vitality, psychological well-being, pain acceptance, and feelings of control over one's pain.[119] A small study of mindfulness meditation in patients with CPP showed significant improvement in pain scores and physical functioning.[120] Mindfulness meditation appears to control pain through a neural mechanism distinct from the placebo response.[121] It has been shown to increase gray matter in areas of the brain involved in emotion regulation and perspective taking,[122] which may explain its effectiveness in mood and pain regulation.

Because central sensitization contributes to chronic pain states, decreasing the patient's sense of "threat" is an important component of pain management. Active stress management, pain education, and treatment of anxiety and depression are key. Medications such as gabapentin, duloxetine, and pregabalin may be useful, in addition to mind-body interventions, such as meditation, guided imagery, diaphragmatic breathing, tai chi, qi gong, and yoga.[123,124] Catastrophizing is associated with increased central sensitization,[125] and mind-body interventions can modulate catastrophizing.[126]

Although acupuncture has shown benefit in CPP in men,[127] studies on noncyclic pelvic pain in women are lacking. A randomized controlled trial comparing electroacupuncture, Chinese medicine, and standard care in women with CPP[128] is in progress.

Summary

CPP is a complex, multidimensional condition resulting in significant physical, psychological, and sexual dysfunction. Diagnosis and treatment of CPP have evolved from targeting a specific organ to adopting a multifactorial and interdisciplinary approach.[129] Effective management integrates information from diverse fields, including gynecology, gastroenterology, urology, neurology, physical therapy, psychology, and psychiatry. Focus is on pain reduction to facilitate improved function and quality of life rather than on complete elimination of pain.

ARTICLE SUMMARY

Many common women's health conditions are best managed with an integrative approach. Combining conventional interventions with complementary modalities and lifestyle counseling can decrease women's suffering and increase physical and psychological functioning. It is important for physicians to be aware of the integrative approach to common women's health conditions to effectively care for and advise their patients.

REFERENCES

1. Murthy V, Sibbritt D, Adams J, et al. Self-prescribed complementary and alternative medicine use for back pain amongst a range of care options: results from a nationally representative sample of 1310 women aged 60-65 years. Complement Ther Med 2014;22(1):133–40.
2. Bowe S, Adams J, Lui CW, et al. A longitudinal analysis of self-prescribed complementary and alternative medicine use by a nationally representative sample of 19,783 Australian women, 2006-2010. Complement Ther Med 2015;23(5): 699–704.
3. Peng W, Adams J, Hickman L, et al. Longitudinal analysis of associations between women's consultations with complementary and alternative medicine practitioners/use of self-prescribed complementary and alternative medicine and menopause-related symptoms, 2007-2010. Menopause 2016;23(1):74–80.
4. Frawley J, Adams J, Broom A, et al. Majority of women are influenced by nonprofessional information sources when deciding to consult a complementary and alternative medicine practitioner during pregnancy. J Altern Complement Med 2014;20(7):571–7.
5. Manson JE, Kaunitz AM. Menopause management–getting clinical care back on track. N Engl J Med 2016;374:803.
6. Posadzki P, Lee MS, Moon TW, et al. Prevalence of complementary and alternative medicine (CAM) use by menopausal women: a systematic review of surveys. Maturitas 2013;75(1):34–43.
7. Harlow SD, Gass M, Hall JE, et al. Executive summary of the Stages of Reproductive Aging Workshop þ 10: addressing the unfinished agenda of staging reproductive aging. J Clin Endocrinol Metab 2012;97(4):1159–68.
8. Brown WJ, Mishra GD, Dobson A. Changes in physical symptoms during the menopause transition. Int J Behav Med 2002;9:53–67.
9. Col NF, Guthrie JR, Politi M, et al. Duration of vasomotor symptoms in middle-aged women: a longitudinal study. Menopause 2009;16:453–7.
10. Kroenke CH, Caan B, Stefanick M, et al. Effects of a dietary intervention and weight change on vasomotor symptoms in the women's health initiative. Menopause 2012;19.9:980–8.
11. Thurston RC, Ewing LJ, Low CA, et al. Behavioral weight loss for the management of menopausal hot flashes: a pilot study. Menopause 2015;22:59–65.
12. Chen MN, Lin CC, Liu CF. Efficacy of phytoestrogens for menopausal symptoms: a meta-analysis and systematic review. Climacteric 2015;18:260–9.
13. Lethaby A, Marjoribanks J, Kronenberg F, et al. Phytoestrogens for menopausal VMS. Cochrane Database Syst Rev 2013;(12):CD001395.
14. Franco OH, Chowdhury R, Troup J, et al. Use of plant-based therapies and menopausal symptoms: a systematic review and meta-analysis. JAMA 2016; 315(23):2554–63.

15. Dew TP, Williamson G. Controlled flax interventions for the improvement of menopausal symptoms and postmenopausal bone health: a systematic review. Menopause 2013;20:1207–15.

16. Chiu HY, Pan CH, Shyu YK, et al. Effects of acupuncture on menopause-related symptoms and quality of life in women in natural menopause: a meta-analysis of randomized controlled trials. Menopause 2015;22(2):234–44.

17. Innes KE, Selfe TK, Vishnu A. Mind-body therapies for menopausal symptoms: a systematic review. Maturitas 2010;66(2):135–49.

18. Woods NF, Pan CH, Shyu YK, et al. Effects of mind–body therapies on symptom clusters during the menopausal transition. Climacteric 2014;17(1):10–22.

19. Bommer S, Klein P, Suter A. First time proof of sage's tolerability and efficacy in menopausal women with hot flushes. Adv Ther 2011;28(6):490–500.

20. Liske E, Hänggi W, Henneicke-von Zepelin HH, et al. Physiological investigation of a unique extract of black cohosh (*Cimicifugae racemosae rhizoma*): a 6-month clinical study demonstrates no systemic estrogenic effect. J Womens Health Gend Based Med 2002;11(2):163–74.

21. Jacobson JS, Troxel AB, Evans J, et al. Randomized trial of black cohosh for the treatment of hot flashes among women with a history of breast cancer. J Clin Oncol 2001;19(10):2739–45.

22. Vermes G, Bánhidy F, Ács N. The effects of Remifemin® on subjective symptoms of menopause. Adv Ther 2005;22(2):148–54.

23. Ross SM. Menopause: a standardized isopropanolic black cohosh extract (remifemin) is found to be safe and effective for menopausal symptoms. Holist Nurs Pract 2012;26(1):58–61.

24. Newton KM, Reed SD, LaCroix AZ, et al. Treatment of vasomotor symptoms of menopause with black cohosh, multibotanicals, soy, hormone therapy, or placebo: a randomized trial. Ann Intern Med 2006;145.12:869–79.

25. Borrelli F, Ernst E. Black cohosh (*Cimicifuga racemosa*) for menopausal symptoms: a systematic review of its efficacy. Pharmacol Res 2008;58(1):8–14.

26. Huntley A, Ernst E. A systematic review of the safety of black cohosh. Menopause 2003;10(1):58–64.

27. Low Dog T, Powell KL, Weisman SM. Critical evaluation of the safety of *Cimicifuga racemosa* in menopause symptom relief. Menopause 2003;10(4):299–313.

28. North American Menopause Society. The 2012 hormone therapy position statement of: The North American Menopause Society. Menopause 2012;19:257–71.

29. Stuenkel CA, Davis SR, Gompel A, et al. Treatment of symptoms of the menopause: an endocrine society clinical practice guideline. J Clin Endocrinol Metab 2015;100(11):3975–4011.

30. Lipold LD, Batur P, Kagan R. Is there a time limit for systemic menopausal hormone therapy? Cleveland Clinic J Med 2016;83(8):605.

31. Bakken K, Fournier A, Lund E, et al. Menopausal hormone therapy and breast cancer risk: impact of different treatments. The European Prospective Investigation into Cancer and Nutrition. Int J Cancer 2011;128(1):144–56.

32. Cummings JA, Brizendine L. Comparison of physical and emotional side effects of progesterone or medroxyprogesterone in early postmenopausal women. Menopause 2002;9(4):253–63.

33. de Lignières B. Oral micronized progesterone. Clin Ther 1999;21(1):41–60.

34. Fournier A, Fabre A, Mesrine S, et al. Use of different postmenopausal hormone therapies and risk of histology-and hormone receptor–defined invasive breast cancer. J Clin Oncol 2008;26(8):1260–8.

35. Biggs WS, Demuth RH. Premenstrual syndrome and premenstrual dysphoric disorder. Am Fam Physician 2011;84(8):918–24.
36. Yonkers KA, O'Brien PM, Eriksson E. Premenstrual syndrome. Lancet 2008; 371(9619):1200–10.
37. Baker FC, Driver HS. Circadian rhythms, sleep, and the menstrual cycle. Sleep Med 2007;8(6):613–22.
38. Thys-Jacobs S, McMahon D, Bilezikian JP. Cyclical changes in calcium metabolism across the menstrual cycle in women with premenstrual dysphoric disorder. J Clin Endocrinol Metab 2007;92(8):2952–9.
39. Rubinow DR, Hoban MC, Grover GN, et al. Changes in plasma hormones across the menstrual cycle in patients with menstrually related mood disorder and in control subjects. Am J Obstet Gynecol 1988;158:5–11.
40. Endicott J, Nee J, Harrison W. Daily Record of Severity of Problems (DRSP): reliability and validity. Arch Womens Ment Health 2006;9(1):41–9.
41. Borenstein JE, Dean BB, Yonkers KA, et al. Using the daily record of severity of problems as a screening instrument for premenstrual syndrome. Obstet Gynecol 2007;109(5):1068–75.
42. Bertone-Johnson ER, Hankinson SE, Johnson SR, et al. A simple method of assessing premenstrual syndrome in large prospective studies. J Reprod Med 2007;52(9):779–86.
43. Gold EB, Bair Y, Block G, et al. Diet and lifestyle factors associated with premenstrual symptoms in a racially diverse community sample: Study of Women's Health Across the Nation (SWAN). J Womens Health (Larchmt) 2007;16(5): 641–56.
44. Carpenter MJ, Upadhyaya HP, LaRowe SD, et al. Menstrual cycle phase effects on nicotine withdrawal and cigarette craving: a review. Nicotine Tob Res 2006; 8(5):627–38.
45. Chocano-Bedoya PO, Manson JE, Hankinson SE, et al. Dietary B vitamin intake and incident premenstrual syndrome. Am J Clin Nutr 2011;93(5):1080–6.
46. Cross GB, Marley J, Miles H, et al. Changes in nutrient intake during the menstrual cycle of overweight women with premenstrual syndrome. Br J Nutr 2001;85(4):475–82.
47. Rossignol AM, Bonnlander H. Caffeine-containing beverages, total fluid consumption, and premenstrual syndrome. Am J Public Health 1990;80(9): 1106–10.
48. Purdue-Smithe AC, Manson JE, Hankinson SE, et al. A prospective study of caffeine and coffee intake and premenstrual syndrome. Am J Clin Nutr 2016; 104(2):499–507.
49. Daley A. Exercise and premenstrual symptomatology: a comprehensive review. J Womens Health (Larchmt) 2009;18(6):895–9.
50. El-Lithy A, El-Mazny A, Sabbour A, et al. Effect of aerobic exercise on premenstrual symptoms, haematological and hormonal parameters in young women. J Obstet Gynaecol 2015;35(4):389–92.
51. Stoddard JL, Dent CW, Shames L, et al. Exercise training effects on premenstrual distress and ovarian steroid hormones. Eur J Appl Physiol 2007;99(1): 27–37.
52. Shechter A, Lespérance P, Ng Ying Kin NM, et al. Nocturnal polysomnographic sleep across the menstrual cycle in premenstrual dysphoric disorder. Sleep Med 2012;13(8):1071–8.
53. de Zambotti M, Nicholas CL, Colrain IM, et al. Autonomic regulation across phases of the menstrual cycle and sleep stages in women with premenstrual

syndrome and healthy controls. Psychoneuroendocrinology 2013;38(11): 2618–27.

54. Baker FC, Colrain IM, Trinder J. Reduced parasympathetic activity during sleep in the symptomatic phase of severe premenstrual syndrome. J Psychosom Res 2008;65(1):13–22.

55. Arias AJ, Steinberg K, Banga A, et al. Systematic review of the efficacy of meditation techniques as treatments for medical illness. J Altern Complement Med 2006;12(8):817–32.

56. Goodale IL, Domar AD, Benson H. Alleviation of premenstrual syndrome symptoms with the relaxation response. Strong effects for meditation for PMS and menopausal symptoms. Obstet Gynecol 1990;75(4):649–55.

57. Groër M, Ohnesorge C. Menstrual-cycle lengthening and reduction in premenstrual distress through guided imagery. J Holist Nurs 1993;11(3):286–94.

58. Lusky MK, Gerrish WG, Shaver S, et al. Cognitive-behavioral therapy for premenstrual syndrome and premenstrual dysphoric disorder: a systematic review. Arch Womens Ment Health 2009;12(2):85–96.

59. Hunter MS, Ussher JM, Browne SJ, et al. A randomized comparison of psychological (cognitive behavior therapy), medical (fluoxetine) and combined treatment for women with premenstrual dysphoric disorder. J Psychosom Obstet Gynaecol 2002;23(3):193–9.

60. Kanojia S, Sharma VK, Gandhi A, et al. Effect of yoga on autonomic functions and psychological status during both phases of menstrual cycle in young healthy females. J Clin Diagn Res 2013;7(10):2133–9.

61. Jang SH, Kim DI, Choi MS. Effects and treatment methods of acupuncture and herbal medicine for premenstrual syndrome/premenstrual dysphoric disorder: systematic review. BMC Complement Altern Med 2014;14:11.

62. Wyatt KM, Dimmock PW, Jones PW, et al. Efficacy of vitamin B-6 in the treatment of premenstrual syndrome: systematic review. BMJ 1999;318(7195):1375–81.

63. Bertone-Johnson ER, Hankinson SE, Bendich A, et al. Calcium and vitamin D intake and risk of incident premenstrual syndrome. Arch Intern Med 2005; 165(11):1246–52.

64. Thys-Jacobs S. Micronutrients and the premenstrual syndrome: the case for calcium. J Am Coll Nutr 2000;19(2):220–7.

65. Thys-Jacobs S, Starkey P, Bernstein D, et al. Calcium carbonate and the premenstrual syndrome: effects on premenstrual and menstrual symptoms. Premenstrual Syndrome Study Group. Am J Obstet Gynecol 1998;179(2):444–52.

66. Allais G, Castagnoli Gabellari I, Burzio C, et al. Premenstrual syndrome and migraine. Neurol Sci 2012;33(Suppl 1):S111–5.

67. Schellenberg R. Treatment for the premenstrual syndrome with agnus castus fruit extract: prospective, randomised, placebo controlled study. BMJ 2001; 322(7279):134–7.

68. van Die MD, Burger HG, Teede HJ, et al. Vitex agnus-castus extracts for female reproductive disorders: a systematic review of clinical trials. Planta Med 2013; 79(7):562–75.

69. Pruthi S, Wahner-Roedler DL, Torkelson CJ, et al. Vitamin E and evening primrose oil for management of cyclical mastalgia: a randomized pilot study. Altern Med Rev 2010;15(1):59–67.

70. Lopez LM, Kaptein AA, Helmerhorst FM. Oral contraceptives containing drospirenone for premenstrual syndrome. Cochrane Database Syst Rev 2012;(2):CD006586.

71. Ziomkiewicz A, Pawlowski B, Ellison PT, et al. Higher luteal progesterone is associated with low levels of premenstrual aggressive behavior and fatigue. Biol Psychol 2012;91(3):376–82.

72. Keye W. Medical treatment of premenstrual syndrome. Can J Psychol 1985;30: 483–7.

73. Dennerstein L, Spencer-Gardner C, Gotts G, et al. Progesterone and the premenstrual syndrome: a double blind crossover trial. Br Med J (Clin Res Ed) 1985;290(6482):1617–21.

74. Maddocks S, Hahn P, Moller F, et al. A double-blind placebo-controlled trial of progesterone vaginal suppositories in the treatment of premenstrual syndrome. Am J Obstet Gynecol 1986;154(3):573–81.

75. Ford O, Lethaby A, Roberts H, et al. Progesterone for premenstrual syndrome. Cochrane Database Syst Rev 2012;(3):CD003415.

76. Marjoribanks J, Brown J, O'Brien PM, et al. Selective serotonin reuptake inhibitors for premenstrual syndrome. Cochrane Database Syst Rev 2013;(6):CD001396.

77. Williams R, Hartmann K, Steege J. Documenting the current definitions of chronic pelvic pain: implications for research. Obstet Gynecol 2004;103: 686–91.

78. Miller-Matero LR, Saulino C, Clark S, et al. When treating the pain is not enough: a multidisciplinary approach for chronic pelvic pain. Arch Womens Ment Health 2016;19(2):349–54.

79. Cosar E, Çakır Güngör A, Gencer M, et al. Sleep disturbance among women with chronic pelvic pain. Int J Gynaecol Obstet 2014;126(3):232–4.

80. Romão AP, Gorayeb R, Romão GS, et al. High levels of anxiety and depression have a negative effect on quality of life of women with chronic pelvic pain. Int J Clin Pract 2009;63(5):707–11.

81. Tripoli TM, Sato H, Sartori MG, et al. Evaluation of quality of life and sexual satisfaction in women suffering from chronic pelvic pain with or without endometriosis. J Sex Med 2011;8(2):497–503.

82. As-Sanie S, Clevenger LA, Geisser ME, et al. History of abuse and its relationship to pain experience and depression in women with chronic pelvic pain. Am J Obstet Gynecol 2014;210(4):317.e1-8.

83. Verit F, Verit A, Yeni E. The prevalence of sexual dysfunction and associated risk factors in women with chronic pelvic pain; a cross-sectional study. Arch Gynecol Obstet 2006;274:297–302.

84. Ahangari A. Prevalence of chronic pelvic pain among women: an updated review. Pain Physician 2014;17(2):E141–7.

85. Chao MT, Abercrombie PD, Nakagawa S, et al. Prevalence and use of complementary health approaches among women with chronic pelvic pain in a prospective cohort study. Pain Med 2015;16(2):328–40.

86. Lamvu G, Nguyen RH, Burrows LJ, et al. The Evidence-based Vulvodynia Assessment Project. A National Registry for the Study of Vulvodynia. J Reprod Med 2015;60(5–6):223–35.

87. Alappattu MJ, Bishop MD. Psychological factors in chronic pelvic pain in women: relevance and application of the fear-avoidance model of pain. Phys Ther 2011;91:1542–50.

88. Chung MK, Chung RP, Gordon D. Interstitial cystitis and endometriosis in patients with chronic pelvic pain: the "evil twins" syndrome. JSLS 2005;9(1):25–9.

89. Porpora MG, Picarelli A, Prosperi Porta R, et al. Celiac disease as a cause of chronic pelvic pain, dysmenorrhea, and deep dyspareunia. Obstet Gynecol 2002;99:937–9.

90. Tirlapur SA, Daniels JP, Khan KS, MEDAL trial collaboration. Chronic pelvic pain: how does noninvasive imaging compare with diagnostic laparoscopy? Curr Opin Obstet Gynecol 2015;27(6):445–8.

91. Latremoliere A, Woolf CJ. Central sensitization: a generator of pain hypersensitivity by central neural plasticity. J Pain 2009;10(9):895–926.

92. Brawn J, Morotti M, Zondervan KT, et al. Central changes associated with chronic pelvic pain and endometriosis. Hum Reprod Update 2014;20(5):737–47.

93. Stratton P, Khachikyan I, Sinaii N, et al. Association of chronic pelvic pain and endometriosis with signs of sensitization and myofascial pain. Obstet Gynecol 2015;125(3):719–28.

94. Howard FM. Chronic pelvic pain. Obstet Gynecol 2003;101(3):594–611.

95. Abercrombie P, Learman L. Providing holistic care for women with chronic pelvic pain. J Obstet Gynecol Neonatal Nurs 2012;41:668–79.

96. Available at: http://mypaindiary.com. Accessed January 13, 2017.

97. De Andres J, Sanchis-Lopez N, Asensio-Samper JM, et al. Vulvodynia–an evidence-based literature review and proposed treatment algorithm. Pain Pract 2016;16(2):204–36.

98. Sator-Katzenschlager SM, Scharbert G, Kress HG, et al. Chronic pelvic pain treated with gabapentin and amitriptyline: a randomized controlled pilot study. Wien Klin Wochenschr 2005;117:761–8.

99. Walsh KE, Berman JR, Berman LA, et al. Safety and efficacy of topical nitroglycerin for treatment of vulvar pain in women with vulvodynia: a pilot study. J Gend Specif Med 2002;5:21–7.

100. Goldfinger C, Pukall CF, Thibault-Gagnon S, et al. Effectiveness of cognitive-behavioral therapy and physical therapy for provoked vestibulodynia: a randomized pilot study. J Sex Med 2016;13(1):88–94.

101. Schlaeger JM, Xu N, Mejta CL, et al. Acupuncture for the treatment of vulvodynia: a randomized wait-list controlled pilot study. J Sex Med 2015;12(4):1019–27.

102. Weiss JM. Pelvic floor myofascial trigger points: manual therapy for interstitial cystitis and the urgency-frequency syndrome. J Urol 2001;166(6):2226–31.

103. Bassaly R, Downes K, Hart S. Dietary consumption triggers in interstitial cystitis/bladder pain syndrome patients. Female Pelvic Med Reconstr Surg 2011;17(1):36–9.

104. O'Hare PG 3rd, Hoffmann AR, Allen P, et al. Interstitial cystitis patients' use and rating of complementary and alternative medicine therapies. Int Urogynecol J 2013;24(6):977–82.

105. Bedaiwy MA, Patterson B, Mahajan S. Prevalence of myofascial chronic pelvic pain and the effectiveness of pelvic floor physical therapy. J Reprod Med 2013;58(11–12):504–10.

106. Abbott JA, Jarvis SK, Lyons SD, et al. Botulinum toxin type A for chronic pelvic pain and pelvic floor spasm in women: a randomized controlled trial. Obstet Gynecol 2006;108(4):915–23.

107. Morrissey D, El-Khawand D, Ginzburg N, et al. Botulinum toxin A injections into pelvic floor muscles under electromyographic guidance for women with refractory high-tone pelvic floor dysfunction: a 6-month prospective pilot study. Female Pelvic Med Reconstr Surg 2015;21(5):277–82.

108. Haugstad GK, Haugstad TS, Kirste UM, et al. Continuing improvement of chronic pelvic pain in women after short-term Mensendieck somatocognitive therapy: results of a 1-year follow-up study. Am J Obstet Gynecol 2008; 199(6):615.e1-8.
109. Masheb RM, Kerns RD, Lozano C, et al. A randomized clinical trial for women with vulvodynia: cognitive-behavioral therapy vs. supportive psychotherapy. Pain 2009;141(1–2):31–40.
110. Chao MT, Abercrombie PD, Duncan LG. Centering as a model for group visits among women with chronic pelvic pain. J Obstet Gynecol Neonatal Nurs 2012;41:703–10.
111. Müller R, Gertz KJ, Molton IR, et al. Effects of a tailored positive psychology intervention on well-being and pain in individuals with chronic pain and a physical disability: a feasibility trial. Clin J Pain 2016;32(1):32–44.
112. Cvetek R. EMDR treatment of stressful experiences that fail to meet the criteria for PTSD. J EMDR Pract Res 2008;2:2–14.
113. van der Kolk B, Spinazzola J, Blaustein M, et al. A randomized clinical trial of EMDR, fluoxetine and pill placebo in the treatment of PTSD: treatment effects and long-term maintenance. J Clin Psychiatry 2007;68:37–46.
114. Sesti F, Capozzolo T, Pietropolli A, et al. Dietary therapy: a new strategy for management of chronic pelvic pain. Nutr Res Rev 2011;24(1):31–8.
115. Cherkin DC, Sherman KJ, Balderson BH, et al. Effect of mindfulness-based stress reduction vs cognitive behavioral therapy or usual care on back pain and functional limitations in adults with chronic low back pain: a randomized clinical trial. JAMA 2016;315(12):1240–9.
116. Chiesa A, Serretti A. Mindfulness-based interventions for chronic pain: a systematic review of the evidence. J Altern Complement Med 2011;17(1):83–93.
117. Bakhshani NM, Amirani A, Amirifard H, et al. The effectiveness of mindfulness-based stress reduction on perceived pain intensity and quality of life in patients with chronic headache. Glob J Health Sci 2015;8(4):142–51.
118. Rod K. Observing the effects of mindfulness-based meditation on anxiety and depression in chronic pain patients. Psychiatr Danub 2015;27(Suppl 1): S209–11.
119. la Cour P, Petersen M. Effects of mindfulness meditation on chronic pain: a randomized controlled trial. Pain Med 2015;16(4):641–52.
120. Fox SD, Flynn E, Allen RH. Mindfulness meditation for women with chronic pelvic pain: a pilot study. J Reprod Med 2011;56(3–4):158–62.
121. Zeidan F, Emerson NM, Farris SR, et al. Mindfulness meditation-based pain relief employs different neural mechanisms than placebo and sham mindfulness meditation-induced analgesia. J Neurosci 2015;35(46):15307–25.
122. Hölzel BK, Carmody J, Vangel M, et al. Mindfulness practice leads to increases in regional brain gray matter density. Psychiatry Res 2011;191(1):36–43.
123. Morone NE, Greco CM, Moore CG, et al. A mind-body program for older adults with chronic low back pain: a randomized clinical trial. JAMA Intern Med 2016; 176(3):329–37.
124. Lauche R, Stumpe C, Fehr J, et al. The effects of tai chi and neck exercises in the treatment of chronic nonspecific neck pain: a randomized controlled trial. J Pain 2016;17(9):1013–27.
125. Campbell CM, Buenaver LF, Finan P, et al. Sleep, pain catastrophizing, and central sensitization in knee osteoarthritis patients with and without insomnia. Arthritis Care Res (Hoboken) 2015;67(10):1387–96.

126. Turner JA, Anderson ML, Balderson BH, et al. Mindfulness-based stress reduction and cognitive behavioral therapy for chronic low back pain: similar effects on mindfulness, catastrophizing, self-efficacy, and acceptance in a randomized controlled trial. Pain 2016;157(11):2434–44.

127. Liu BP, Wang YT, Chen SD. Effect of acupuncture on clinical symptoms and laboratory indicators for chronic prostatitis/chronic pelvic pain syndrome: a systematic review and meta-analysis. Int Urol Nephrol 2016;48(12):1977–91.

128. Chong OT, Critchley HO, Horne AW, et al. The BMEA study: the impact of meridian balanced method electroacupuncture on women with chronic pelvic pain—a three-arm randomised controlled pilot study using a mixed-methods approach. BMJ Open 2015;5(11):1–9.

129. Morrissey D, Ginzburg N, Whitmore K. Current advancements in the diagnosis and treatment of chronic pelvic pain. Curr Opin Urol 2014;24(4):336–44.

Integrative Oncology

Gabriel Lopez, MD[a],*, Jun J. Mao, MD, MSCE[b], Lorenzo Cohen, PhD[c]

KEYWORDS

- Integrative oncology • Cancer • Symptoms • Complementary health approaches
- Lifestyle

KEY POINTS

- Integrative oncology is an emerging field that helps support the health of patients with cancer and their caregivers through an evidence-informed approach to lifestyle and behavior modification and use of complementary health therapies in the context of conventional cancer care delivery.
- A significant number of patients with cancer are seeking complementary health approaches and have a desire to engage in discussions regarding this subject area with their health care providers.
- Integrative approaches (eg, lifestyle, meditation, yoga, acupuncture, massage) can provide patients relief from cancer and cancer treatment–related symptoms and improve their physical and psychosocial health.
- An evidence-informed approach is important when recommending an integrative cancer plan, taking into account potential toxicities (eg, direct organ toxicity, bleeding, herb-drug interactions) and precautions (eg, low blood counts, fracture risk).
- Efforts at enhancing communication between patients and health care professionals, as well as between integrative practitioners and conventional health care teams, are critical to achieving optimal health and healing for patients with cancer, from diagnosis through treatment and into survivorship or end of life.

INTEGRATIVE ONCOLOGY: DEFINITION

Integrative medicine is an approach to health care delivery that balances complementary health approaches and lifestyle medicine with conventional medicine in a deliberate manner that is personalized, evidence-informed, and safe. According to the

Disclosure: The authors have nothing to disclose.
[a] Section of Integrative Medicine, Department of Palliative, Rehabilitation and Integrative Medicine, Integrative Medicine Center, University of Texas, MD Anderson Cancer Center, 1515 Holcombe Blvd, Unit 1414, Houston, TX 77030, USA; [b] Integrative Medicine Service, Memorial Sloan Kettering Cancer Center, 1429 First Avenue, New York, NY 10021, USA; [c] Integrative Medicine, Integrative Medicine Program, Department of Palliative, Rehabilitation and Integrative Medicine, University of Texas, MD Anderson Cancer Center, 1515 Holcombe Blvd, Houston, TX 77030, USA
* Corresponding author.
E-mail address: gabriel.lopez@mdanderson.org

Med Clin N Am 101 (2017) 977–985
http://dx.doi.org/10.1016/j.mcna.2017.04.011
0025-7125/17/© 2017 Elsevier Inc. All rights reserved.

National Center for Complementary and Integrative Health, complementary health approaches refer to natural products (eg, dietary supplements, herbals), mind and body practices (eg, meditation, yoga, massage, acupuncture), and other systems of care such as traditional Chinese medicine, Ayurvedic medicine, or naturopathy. In a recent survey reviewing use of complementary health approaches among adults in the United States, the most commonly used approaches include natural products (dietary supplements other than vitamins and minerals); deep breathing; and practices such as yoga, tai chi, or qigong.[1] Integrative oncology is the application of integrative medicine to the care of patients with cancer and their caregivers. According to the Academic Consortium for Integrative Medicine & Health,[2] "integrative medicine and health reaffirms the importance of the relationship between practitioner and patient, focuses on the whole person, is informed by evidence, and makes use of all appropriate therapeutic and lifestyle approaches, healthcare professionals and disciplines to achieve optimal health and healing."

CLINICAL CONSULTATION AND COMMUNICATION

Interest in and use of complementary health approaches is highest among individuals with cancer. Although up to 38% of the general US population has engaged in complementary health approaches, this number increases to 68% in surveys of patients with cancer, with even greater use in those with breast cancer or advanced/incurable illness.[3–5] Patients with cancer look to these approaches to improve wellness, enhance immune function, and find relief for pain and other symptoms. When looking for guidance regarding how to use complementary health approaches, patients may make decisions based on recommendations gathered from resources of varying reliability, including the media, Internet, other patients, family members, and health care professionals.[6,7] In addition, patient experience of unmet needs from their health care providers, a desire to engage in health-supporting behaviors, and finding meaning related to cancer have motivated patients to seek complementary therapies to augment the current approach to cancer prevention and treatment.[6,8–10]

A significant number of patients are seeking complementary health approaches and have a desire to engage in discussions regarding this subject area with their health care providers.[11] To encourage effective dialogue, it is important for health care providers to enter into an open, nonjudgmental discussion with their patients regarding their past or present use of or interest in complementary health approaches. A thoughtful approach to entering into a dialogue about integrative medicine interests can play an important role in developing an integrative care plan (**Box 1**). Not only can these open discussions strengthen the therapeutic alliance between patient and provider but there are implications for patient safety. An open, nonjudgmental inquiry into the use of complementary health approaches leads to increased disclosure and ability to guide patients safely, which is especially important for specific approaches such as natural products, which can have the potential for harm, causing organ injury, increased cancer risk, or interference with treatment efficacy.[12]

In an attempt to meet patients' needs and guide the appropriate use of complementary therapies, an increasing number of cancer centers have developed, or are in the process of developing, integrative oncology programs.[13,14] Integrative oncology programs may include clinical services such as a physician consultation, oncology massage, acupuncture, nutrition counseling, health psychology (eg, stress management, support for behavior change, and lifestyle counseling), exercise counseling,

---

Box 1
Approach to integrative oncology consultation

Baseline assessment may include interest, symptom, or quality of life survey.

Create comfortable environment encouraging open communication. Pay attention to your own as well as patient (and caregiver) verbal and nonverbal cues.

Assess patient/caregiver goals and level of understanding regarding complementary integrative medicine.

Ask about current or prior experience with and interest in complementary integrative approaches, including herb/supplement use, diet, level of physical activity, and engagement in mind-body practices.

Provide education and evidence-informed recommendations regarding topics of interest as appropriate.

Ask about resources past or present used for learning about complementary integrative medicine (eg, Internet, textbook, complementary health provider).

Check for understanding regarding education provided and topics reviewed.

Provide education materials, relevant references and resources, as well as summary of recommendations as part of an integrative care plan.

Encourage follow-up as appropriate to review progress with integrative care plan and address any new questions that may develop.

Communicate integrative care plan with multidisciplinary team of providers, including oncology care team and complementary health practitioners.

---

expressive arts (eg, music therapy, art therapy), and group classes (eg, meditation, yoga, tai chi/qigong).

COMPLEMENTARY HEALTH APPROACHES FOR SYMPTOM MANAGEMENT

Cancer and its treatments can contribute to significant morbidity through immediate and delayed effects on either physical or psychosocial health. Integrative approaches can provide patients relief from these symptoms and also help provide support for lifestyle changes across the continuum of cancer care, from diagnosis through survivorship and into advanced disease and end of life.

Mind-Body Approaches

Mind-body practices can contribute to the health of patients with cancer through their influence on physical and psychosocial health. Such practices may have beneficial effects on aspects of mental health such as stress, anxiety, and depression, as well as physical symptoms such as pain, nausea, sleep disturbances, and mobility issues. Mind-body practices may incorporate movement or be conducted in a seated, stationary position. Examples include meditation, yoga, tai chi, qigong, and expressive arts (art, music, and dance therapy). Meditation is a contemplative practice that allows individuals to focus attention on themselves, using sound, breathing, or movement.[15] Research suggests that the highest level of evidence exists for the use of relaxation techniques to help with anxiety, insomnia, and nausea caused by chemotherapy.[16] For practices such as yoga, tai chi, qigong, and meditation, benefits include improving well-being, mood, and sleep quality, as well as physical function.[17–21] Expressive arts interventions such as music therapy can have positive effects on management of symptoms such as pain, anxiety, and mood disturbance, and help improve quality of life.[22]

Acupuncture

With roots in traditional Chinese medicine, acupuncture has shown benefits for the relief of symptoms including nausea, pain, hot flashes, radiation-induced dry mouth, sleep disturbance, prolonged postoperative ileus, and fatigue.[23] Needles are placed at specific points throughout the body as part of an overall treatment plan that can include the management of 1 or more symptoms. Acupuncture has an excellent safety profile, with minimal risk of complications, most commonly fainting, bruising, and mild pain.[24] Precautions are needed in the setting of low platelet counts, low neutrophil counts, and compromised skin integrity, or with the concurrent use of anticoagulants.[24]

Massage

Oncology massage is the modification of massage techniques in the context of cancer care. Modifications can include site restrictions, changes in pressure, and additional precautions in the setting of low blood counts, recent surgery, or metastatic disease. Evidence from multiple studies points to the benefits of massage for relieving symptoms such as pain, anxiety, fatigue, and general aspects of quality of life.[25,26] Recent data also suggest that massage can be safely integrated into chemotherapy suites to provide symptom relief such as reduction of pain, nausea, and anxiety.[27] Two studies have shown that massage is effective in the treatment of constipation.[28,29] Initial evidence in the form of a case report and expert opinion suggests a role for massage in the relief of symptoms such as chemotherapy-induced peripheral neuropathy.[30] The beneficial effects of massage tend to be short lasting. Additional research is needed to better understand the symptoms that massage can help treat as well as the optimal length and frequency of treatments.

SAFETY, TOXICITY, PRECAUTIONS

Most individuals engage in the use of complementary health approaches without the guidance of their health care providers. Concerns arising from the uninformed use of these approaches include the potential for harm.[31] Harm can come in the form of toxicity from the use of natural products or injury from engaging in movement practices without proper supervision or modifications. Interventions such as oncology massage, acupuncture, and yoga can be safely incorporated into the care of patients with cancer. Health care providers can play a significant role in reducing risk from injury by helping their patients understand risks versus benefits of such interventions, as well as helping them identify complementary health practitioners with appropriate expertise and certification. In the case of a health care practitioner who is unsure of which approaches to recommend, referrals can be made to individuals with expertise in this area, such as physicians practicing integrative oncology, palliative/supportive medicine, or cancer rehabilitation.

Quality Control

Concerns surround the quality of supplements and natural products made available through retailers. The manufacture of these herbal supplements and natural products has limited oversight, with potential for inaccurate labeling, contamination, product substitution, and use of fillers.[32] Studies of supplements have revealed cases in which none of the desired product is present in the formulation assessed.[33] Other studies have revealed contamination with toxic levels of harmful substances such as arsenic, lead, and mercury.[34] Such uncertainty in product quality and content poses a potential for harm in the setting of individuals receiving cancer therapeutics.

Drug-Herb Interactions

Dietary supplements or herbal products may contribute to harm when combined with cancer therapies such as chemotherapy, targeted therapies, radiation, and surgery.[35] Herbal products and high-dose antioxidants may interfere with the efficacy of treatments such as radiation and chemotherapy.[31,36,37] There is also concern that certain natural products use similar metabolic pathways to chemotherapeutic agents and, when combined with chemotherapy, may have inadvertent effects on the therapeutic dose. Certain herbal products can increase bleeding risk, presenting risk to patients with anticipated or recent surgical procedures.[12] Agents such as mushroom extracts have immune-modulatory properties and may have unpredictable effects on the immune system, which is of particular concern in the context of immune-based therapies.[38] The potential also exists for some of these herbals and natural products to cause direct organ toxicity, with harmful effects on the liver and/or kidneys.[39]

CANCER PREVENTION AND CONTROL

There has been increasing evidence linking obesity and modifiable lifestyle behaviors such as tobacco and alcohol use, physical inactivity, and dietary factors to cancer development. For individuals with cancer, there is also evidence supporting the importance of physical activity and nutrition during and after cancer care for improving quality of life, maintaining health, decreasing the risk of recurrence of disease, and increasing survival time.[40–43] The American Institute for Cancer Research recommends that, for cancer prevention and for cancer survivors, focus in the area of diet and lifestyle should follow these basic principles: (1) maintain a normal weight; (2) be physically active for at least 30 minutes every day, and limit sedentary habits; (3) avoid sugary drinks and limit consumption of energy-dense foods; (4) eat more of a variety of vegetables, fruits, whole grains, and legumes such as beans; (5) limit consumption of red meats (such as beef, pork, and lamb) and avoid processed meats; and (6) if consumed at all, limit daily alcoholic drinks to 2 for men and 1 for women. Mounting evidence also shows that stress and depression are associated with cancer growth and progression of disease.[44–48] The National Comprehensive Cancer Network has issued guidelines mandating regular screening and referral for distress management. Conventional treatments such as cognitive behavioral therapy or individual or group psychotherapy are effective treatments for mood disorders in oncology as well as mind-body approaches such as mindfulness-based stress reduction, meditation, yoga, and tai chi.[21] Cancer survivors commonly look to complementary health approaches as a way to improve their treatment outcomes, manage residual cancer or cancer treatment–related symptoms, or help manage or prevent other illness. Communication between health care professionals such as the oncology care team and primary care physician is critical to the success of implementing an effective multidisciplinary team approach to cancer prevention for cancer survivors and other high-risk individuals.

EVIDENCE-INFORMED RESOURCES

Several reliable resources exist for finding the latest information regarding complementary health approaches (**Table 1**). Although patients and health care practitioners alike are increasingly using the Internet as a resource for health-related information, it is important to realize that not all information available is reliable and that it can be based on varying levels of evidence. Identifying trustworthy resources for patients and providers can come in the form of seeking information from academic institutions,

Table 1 Recommended Internet resources for integrative oncology	
Memorial Sloan Kettering Cancer Center	www.mskcc.org/cancer-care/treatments/symptom-management/integrative-medicine/herbs
University of Texas MD Anderson Cancer Center, Integrative Medicine Program	www.mdanderson.org/integrativemedcenter
Natural Medicines Comprehensive Database	www.naturaldatabase.com
National Center for Complementary and Integrative Health	www.nccih.nih.gov
National Cancer Institute Office of Cancer Complementary and Alternative Medicine	www.cancer.gov
American Institute for Cancer Research	www.aicr.org
Society for Integrative Oncology	www.integrativeonc.org

governmental organizations, and organizations committed to the use of peer-reviewed research and expert opinion for development of evidence-informed resources. Guidelines from organizations such as the National Cancer Institute, American Cancer Society,[49] American Institute for Cancer Research, and the Society for Integrative Oncology[50,51] can provide a starting point for making evidence-informed decisions in the area of complementary and integrative oncology.

SUMMARY

Integrative medicine as applied to the care of patients with cancer can have beneficial effects on physical and psychosocial aspects of health. Open communication with patients and health care teams regarding available complementary health approaches can help with the development of evidence-informed, personalized, and safe integrative care plans.

REFERENCES

1. Clarke TC, Black LI, Stussman BJ, et al. Trends in the use of complementary health approaches among adults: United States, 2002-2012. Natl Health Stat Rep 2015;1(79):16.
2. Academic Consortium for Integrative Medicine & Health. Available at: https://www.imconsortium.org/about/about-us.cfm. Accessed May 24, 2017.
3. Richardson MA, Sanders T, Palmer JL, et al. Complementary/alternative medicine use in a comprehensive cancer center and the implications for oncology. J Clin Ocnol 2000;18:2505–16.
4. Navo MA, Phan J, Vaughan C, et al. An assessment of the utilization of complementary and alternative medication in women with gynecologic or breast malignancies. J Clin Oncol 2004;22:671–7.
5. Barnes PM, Bloom B, Nahin RL. Complementary and alternative medicine use among adults and children: United States, 2007. Natl Health Stat Rep 2008;12:1–23.
6. Verhoef MJ, Mulkins A, Carslon LE, et al. Assessing the role of evidence in patients' evaluation of complementary therapies: a quality study. Integr Cancer Ther 2007;6(4):345–53.

7. Mao JJ, Palmer SC, Straton JB, et al. Cancer survivors with unmet needs were more likely to use complementary and alternative medicine. J Cancer Surviv 2008;2(2):116–24.

8. Bauml JM, Chokshi S, Schapira MM, et al. Do attitudes and beliefs regarding complementary and alternative medicine impact its use among patients with cancer? A cross-sectional survey. Cancer 2015;121:2431–8.

9. Garland SN, Valentine D, Desai K, et al. Complementary and alternative medicine use and benefit finding among cancer patients. J Altern Complement Med 2013; 19(11):876–81.

10. Garland SN, Stainken C, Ahluwalia K, et al. Cancer-related search for meaning increases willingness to participate in mindfulness-based stress reduction. Integr Cancer Ther 2015;14(3):231–9.

11. Verhoef MJ, White MA, Doll R. Cancer patients' expectations of the role of family physicians in communication about complementary therapies. Cancer Prev Control 1999;3:181–7.

12. Ulbricht C, Chao W, Costa D, et al. Clinical evidence of herb-drug interactions: a systematic review by the natural standard research collaboration. Curr Drug Metab 2008;9:1063–120.

13. Lopez G, McQuade J, Cohen L, et al. Integrative oncology physician consultations at a comprehensive cancer center: analysis of demographic, clinical and patient reported outcomes. J Cancer 2017;8(3):395–402.

14. Brauer JA, Sehamy AE, Metz J, et al. Complementary and alternative medicine (CAM) and supportive care at leading cancer centers: a systematic analysis of websites. J Altern Complement Med 2010;16(2):183–6.

15. Biegler KA, Chaoul MA, Cohen L. Cancer, cognitive impairment, and meditation. Acta Oncol 2009;8:18–26.

16. Ernst E, Pittler MH, Wider B, et al. Mind-body therapies: are the trial data getting stronger? Altern Ther Health Med 2007;13(5):62–4.

17. Cohen L, Warneke CL, Fouladi RT, et al. Psychological adjustment and sleep quality in a randomized trial of the effects of a Tibetan yoga intervention in patients with lymphoma. Cancer 2004;100(10):2253–60.

18. Bower JE, Woolery A, Sternlieb B, et al. Yoga for cancer patients and survivors. Cancer Control 2005;12(3):165–71.

19. Chandwani KD, Thornton B, Perkins GH, et al. Yoga improves quality of life and benefit finding in women undergoing radiotherapy for breast cancer. J Soc Integr Oncol 2010;8(2):43–55.

20. Oh B, Butow PN, Mullan BA, et al. Effect of medical qigong on cognitive function, quality of life, and a biomarker of inflammation in cancer patients: a randomized controlled trial. Support Care Cancer 2012;20(6):1235–42.

21. Chaoul A, Milbury K, Sood A, et al. Mind-body practices in cancer care. Curr Oncol Rep 2014;16(12):417.

22. Archie P, Bruera E, Cohen L. Music-based interventions in palliative cancer care: a review of quantitative studies and neurobiological literature. Support Care Cancer 2013;21(9):2609–24.

23. Garcia MK, McQuade J, Haddad R, et al. Systematic review of acupuncture in cancer care: a synthesis of the evidence. J Clin Oncol 2013;31(7):952–60.

24. Lu W, Doherty-Gilman AM, Rosenthal DS. Recent advances in oncology acupuncture and safety considerations in practice. Curr Treat Options Oncol 2010;11(3–4):141–6.

25. Cassileth BR, Vickers AJ. Massage therapy for symptom control: outcome study at a major cancer center. J Pain Symptom Manage 2004;28(3):244–9.

26. Russell NC, Sumler SS, Beinhorn CM, et al. Role of massage therapy in cancer care. J Altern Complement Med 2008;14(2):209–14.
27. Mao JJ, Wagner KE, Seluzicki CM, et al. Integrating oncology massage into chemoinfusion suites: a program evaluation. J Oncol Pract 2017;13(3):e207–16.
28. Lamas K, Lindholm L, Stenlund H, et al. Effects of abdominal massage in management of constipation—a randomized controlled trial. Int J Nurs Stud 2009; 46(6):759–67.
29. Lai TK, Cheung MC, Lo CK, et al. Effectiveness of aroma massage on advanced cancer patients with constipation: a pilot study. Complement Ther Clin Prac 2011; 17(1):37–43.
30. Cunningham JE, Kelechi T, Sterba K, et al. Case report of a patient with chemotherapy-induced peripheral neuropathy treated with manual therapy (massage). Support Care Cancer 2011;19(9):1473–6.
31. Palmer ME, Haller C, McKinney PE, et al. Adverse events associated with dietary supplements: an observational study. Lancet 2003;361:101–6.
32. Newmaster SG, Grguric M, Shanmughanandhan D, et al. DNA barcoding detects contamination and substitution in North American herbal products. BMC Med 2013;11:222.
33. Gilroy CM, Steiner JF, Byers T, et al. Echinacea and truth in labeling. Arch Intern Med 2003;163:699–704.
34. Saper RB, Philips RS, Sehgal A, et al. Lead, mercury, and arsenic in US- and Indian-manufactured ayurvedic medicines sold via the Internet. JAMA 2008; 300(8):915–23.
35. Block KI, Koch AC, Mead MN, et al. Impact of antioxidant supplementation on chemotherapeutic efficacy: a systematic review of the evidence from randomized controlled trials. Cancer Treat Rev 2007;33:407–18.
36. Bairati I, Meyer F, Gélinas M, et al. Randomized trial of antioxidant vitamins to prevent acute adverse effects of radiation therapy in head and neck cancer patients. J Clin Oncol 2005;23:5805–13.
37. Lawenda BD, Kelly KM, Ladas EJ, et al. Should supplemental antioxidant administration be avoided during chemotherapy and radiation therapy? J Natl Cancer Inst 2008;100:773–83.
38. Deng G, Lin H, Seidman A, et al. A phase I/II trial of a polysaccharide extract from *Grifola frondosa* (Maitake mushroom) in breast cancer patients: immunological effects. J Cancer Res Clin Oncol 2009;135(9):1215–21.
39. Navarro VJ, Khan I, Bjornsson E, et al. Liver injury from herbal and dietary supplements. Hepatology 2017;65(1):363–73.
40. Meyerhardt JA, Heseltine D, Niedzwiecki D, et al. Impact of physical activity on cancer recurrence and survival in patients with stage III colon cancer: findings from CALGB 89803. J Clin Oncol 2006;24(22):3535–41.
41. Meyerhardt JA, Niedzwiecki D, Hollis D, et al. Association of dietary patterns with cancer recurrence and survival in patients with stage III colon cancer. JAMA 2007;298(7):754–64.
42. Courneya KS, McKenzie DC, Mackey JR, et al. Effects of exercise dose and type during breast cancer chemotherapy: multicenter randomized trial. J Natl Cancer Inst 2013;105(23):1821–32.
43. Courneya KS, Sellar CM, Stevinson C, et al. Randomized controlled trial of the effects of aerobic exercise on physical functioning and quality of life in lymphoma patients. J Clin Oncol 2009;27(27):4605–12.
44. Cole SW, Nagaraja AS, Lutgendorf SK, et al. Sympathetic nervous system regulation of the tumor microenvironment. Nat Rev Cancer 2015;15:563–72.

45. Lutgendorf SK, Sood AK. Biobehavioral factors and cancer progression: physiological pathways and mechanisms. Psychosom Med 2011;73(9):724–30.
46. Stagl JM, Lechner SC, Carver CS, et al. A randomized controlled trial of cognitive-behavioral stress management in breast cancer: survival and recurrence at 11-year follow-up. Breast Cancer Res Treat 2015;154(2):319–28.
47. Lin J, Blalock JA, Chen M, et al. Depressive symptoms and short telomere length are associated with increased mortality in bladder cancer patients. Cancer Epidemiol Biomarkers Prev 2015;24(2):336–43.
48. Cohen L, Cole SW, Sood AK, et al. Depressive symptoms and cortisol rhythmicity predict survival in patients with renal cell carcinoma: role of inflammatory signaling. PLoS One 2012;7(8):e42324.
49. Kushi LH, Doyle C, McCullough M, et al. American Cancer Society guidelines on nutrition and physical activity for cancer prevention: reducing the risk of cancer with healthy food choices and physical activity. CA Cancer J Clin 2012;62:30–67.
50. Deng GE, Frenkel M, Cohen L, et al. Evidence-based clinical practice guidelines for integrative oncology: complementary therapies and botanicals. J Soc Integr Oncol 2009;7:85–120.
51. Greenlee H, Balneaves LG, Carlson LE, et al. Clinical practice guidelines on the use of integrative therapies as supportive care in patients treated for breast cancer. J Natl Cancer Inst Monogr 2014;2014(50):346–58.

Integrative Pain Management

Robert Alan Bonakdar, MD

KEYWORDS

- Pain • Integrative • Nonpharmacologic • Yoga • Acupuncture • Mindfulness
- Neuropathic • Low back

KEY POINTS

- Chronic pain affects more than 100 million Americans at a cost of greater than $635 billion a year. On an individual level, it is often accompanied by mood, sleep, and metabolic dysfunction, which require an integrative approach to fully grasp the patient burden as well as collaborate on a person-centered approach to care.
- Pain care over the last several decades has been largely centered on an acute care model, which has increased diagnostic-, procedural-, and analgesic-based approaches, which has not provided any population level improvement in pain or disability.
- An integrative approach, including offerings such as patient education, acupuncture, mind-body approaches such as yoga and mindfulness as well as lifestyle optimization using diet and exercise has increasing evidence for reducing pain and disability in several common pain scenarios.
- Recent guidelines, including the American College of Physicians Guidelines for low back pain, endorse the incorporation of nonpharmacologic approaches in the comprehensive management of pain.

INTRODUCTION
Definition and Overview

Integrative pain management is a person-centered model of pain care based on the principles and practices of integrative medicine, including a focus on the restoration of function, health, and wellness.[1] This model is guided by evidence and shared decision making between practitioner and patient to use individualized therapeutic options. These options may include a spectrum of biological, interventional, and lifestyle approaches guided by health care professionals with a goal of not only

Disclosure Statement: Lippincott, Oxford University Press: Royalties, related to publications: The H.E.R.B.A.L. Guide: Evidence Based Resources for the Clinician & Integrative Pain Management; Elsevier: Advisory Board, Editorial contributor to PracticeUpdate.com; Thorne Research, Metagenics, American Specialty Health: Consultant, in the area of pain management/physical therapy.

Scripps Center for Integrative Medicine, 10820 North Torrey Pines Road, Maildrop FC2, La Jolla, CA 92037, USA
E-mail address: bonakdar.robert@scrippshealth.org

Med Clin N Am 101 (2017) 987–1004
http://dx.doi.org/10.1016/j.mcna.2017.04.012
0025-7125/17/© 2017 Elsevier Inc. All rights reserved.

medical.theclinics.com

reducing pain but also improving function, quality of life, and self-care. Based on existing practice patterns, integrative pain management attempts to enhance current treatment models by incorporating options, such as nutritional, behavioral, spiritual, and self-management approaches, which are not typically optimized in routine care. The following article focuses on these areas of enhancement.

The Epidemiology of Chronic Pain

Chronic pain is one of the most common conditions encountered by humans worldwide, affecting 20% of the world's population.[2] For many reasons, including an aging population and increases in chronic disease, the prevalence of chronic pain seems to be increasing worldwide. Importantly, chronic pain can occur at any age. It is estimated that 25% to 46% of children and young adults experience chronic pain, most commonly with recurrent headache, and abdominal or musculoskeletal pain.[3,4] Likewise, studies examining end-of-life care of hospitalized patients have noted that the majority suffer from moderate to severe pain.[5]

In the United States, the most recent estimate of pain and its cost was published in the Institute of Medicine 2011 report, *Relieving Pain in America*, and placed the number of adults living with chronic pain between 100 and 116 million.[6] This report also estimated the yearly cost of care for those with pain at $560 to $635 billion. When pain was compared with other common conditions, it exceeded the costs associated with cardiovascular disease, diabetes, and cancer combined (**Fig. 1**).[7]

Burden of Pain and Relevance to Primary Care

In addition to an extreme cost to society, chronic pain places a multifactorial burden on those affected that may often be overlooked. In this scenario, it is vital for primary care clinicians to evaluate the functional, metabolic, and psychological limitations that may emerge in association with pain.

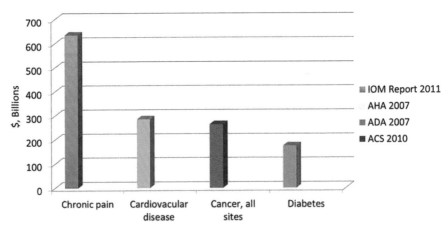

Fig. 1. Cost of chronic conditions, United States. ACS, American Cancer Society. Cancer Facts and Figures 2010; ADA, American Diabetes Association. Economic costs of diabetes in the United States in 2007. Diabetes Care 2008; AHA, American Heart Association figure calculated on Agency for Healthcare Research and Quality. Medical Expenditure Panel Survey 2007; IOM, Institute of Medicine, Relieving Pain in America: A Blueprint for Transforming Prevention, Care, Education, and Research. 2011. (*Data from* Georgi K. Calculating the cost of pain. Chronic Pain Perspect 2011;12:F2.)

Functional Limitation and Distress

Low back pain is a classic example of such a condition. Low back pain is extremely common in that more than 80% of adults in the United States will experience it at some point during their lifetime.[8] However, as low back pain becomes chronic, several additional sequelae often emerge. These sequelae include being 3 times as likely to have limited functional ability and 4 times as likely to suffer psychological distress as those without low back pain.[9] Chronic low back pain is also associated with brain atrophy, with one study noting a 5% to 11% loss in gray matter volume versus controls. This level of decrease is equivalent to the gray matter volume loss from 10 to 20 years of normal aging.[10]

Obesity-Related Pain

Obesity-related pain is a conceptual framework to describe pain and related disability in individuals with obesity and metabolic dysregulation.[11,12] Changes in function, mood, and the brain may in part explain the metabolic ramifications of chronic pain. Stone and Broderick[13] noted in their study of greater than one million Americans a direct correlation between body mass index (BMI) and pain (**Fig. 2**). This association appeared to be heightened in women as well as with increasing age and level of obesity. Specific to low back pain, elevated BMI and fat mass have been positively associated with low back pain episodes, intensity, and level of disability.[14]

In addition to the factors above, this association may also be explained by changes in diet and inflammatory status. In a controlled study, chronic low back pain compared with healthy controls was associated with dietary shifts, including decreased satiety with foods containing sugar and fat with a higher likelihood for overconsumption.[15] These dietary shifts is postulated to be related to alterations in brain circuitry in areas related to pain and satiety. In addition, Briggs and colleagues[16] examined the relationship of C-reactive protein (CRP) and obesity on the prevalence and the odds of reporting low back pain. Participants with elevated CRP had 1.74 greater odds of reporting low back pain. Those who were obese with elevated CRP had 2.87 greater odds of reporting low back pain. Both obesity and higher CRP levels were independently associated with greater pain interference.[17]

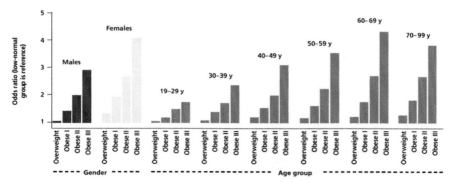

Fig. 2. Odds ratios for pain based on BMI classifications by gender and age groups. BMI classifications: low through normal, less than 25 kg/m²; overweight = 25 kg/m² to less than 30 kg/m²; obese I = 30 to less than 35 kg/m²; obese II = 35 to less than 40 kg/m²; obese III, ≥40 kg/m². Based on a survey of greater than 1 million Americans. (*From* Bonakdar RA. Targeting systemic inflammation in patients with obesity-related pain: obesity-related pain: time for a new approach that targets systemic inflammation. J Fam Pract 2013;62(9 Suppl CHPP):S23; with permission.)

Prevalence of Integrative Therapy Use

Pain is the most common reason medical care is sought as well as the most common reason for seeking integrative treatments.[18] Based on the 2012 National Health Interview Survey (NHIS), back pain, neck pain, joint pain, arthritis, gout, and fibromyalgia were among the top conditions for which integrative approaches were used (**Fig. 3**).[19] In adults specifically with a musculoskeletal pain disorder, more than 40% had used an integrative approach as compared with 24% of those without pain.[19] Certain therapies appear to have especially high utilization in this population. For example, adults with musculoskeletal pain were 2 to 3 times more likely to use dietary supplements and practitioner-based approaches (eg, acupuncture, manipulation) than those without (**Fig. 4**).

Rationale for Integrative Therapies

There have been numerous studies on the reasons patients use integrative therapies for managing their pain. First and foremost is the potential pain relief derived from these therapies. The 2012 NHIS analysis of those with back pain found that 58.1% perceived "a great deal of benefit" from these therapies.[20] Utilization also appears to increase with higher pain severity or concomitant use of conventional therapies. In a survey of primary care pain patients using opioids, respondents who used integrative therapies noted higher pain severity than nonutilizers. Eighty-one percent of utilizers noted that use of integrative therapies was helpful.[21] In addition to pain relief, the use of many integrative therapies has been found to improve function and quality of life.[22]

More discretely, Hsu and colleagues[23] surveyed those with back pain who had participated in integrative therapy trials to determine potential positive outcomes not captured by standard outcome measures. They found themes including increased hope, ability to relax, and body awareness; improvement in physical conditions unrelated to back pain; and increased ability to cope with back pain.

Overview of Chronic Pain Causes

Chronic pain can occur across a spectrum of causes. Chronic pain can be categorized based on areas of potential disruption, including nociceptive, neuropathic, or central

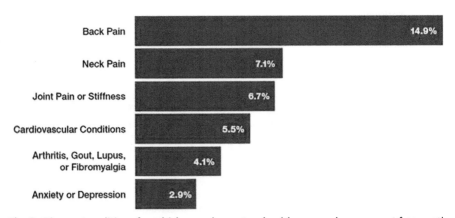

Fig. 3. Diseases/conditions for which complementary health approaches are most frequently used among adults—2012. (*From* NIH. National Center for Complementary and Integrative Health. Use of complementary and integrative health approaches in the United States, 2012. Available at: https://nccih.nih.gov/about/strategic-plans/2016/use-complementary-integrative-health-approaches-2012. Accessed December 12, 2016; with permission.)

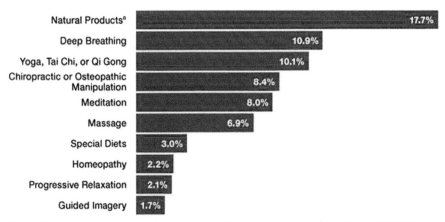

Fig. 4. Ten most common complementary health approaches among adults—2012. [a]Dietary supplements other than vitamins and minerals. (*From* NIH. National Center for Complementary and Integrative Health. Use of complementary and integrative health approaches in the United States, 2012. Available at: https://nccih.nih.gov/about/strategic-plans/2016/use-complementary-integrative-health-approaches-2012. Accessed December 12, 2016; with permission.)

causes (**Fig. 5**). This article focuses on several conditions that occur across this spectrum, including low back pain, neck pain, and central pain states (CPS). Importantly, pain conditions can occur in a continuum such that an initial mechanical low back pain episode (nociceptive) can evolve into sciatica (neuropathic) and potentially extend to a nonlocalized myofascial pain with comorbidities (central). It is thus imperative at all stages of evaluation for primary care clinicians to be aware of the evolution of symptoms, especially behavioral and functional disruption, which requires more comprehensive treatment options to reduce disability.

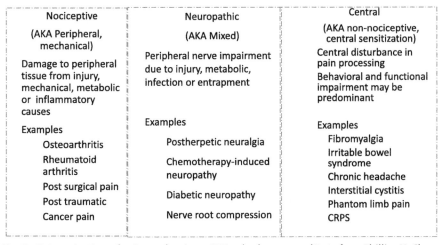

Fig. 5. Categorization of pain mechanisms. AKA, also known as. (*Data from* Phillips K, Clauw DJ. Central pain mechanisms in chronic pain states—maybe it is all in their head. Best Pract Res Clin Rheumatol 2011;25(2):141–54.)

Summary

When assessing pain, it is important to understand the physical and functional limitations that may be imposed. Equally paramount is appreciating and approaching the profound social, psychological, neurologic, and metabolic shifts that occur. This understanding as well as incorporating proper diet, activity, behavioral support, and patient activation as key components of treatment is essential in improving quality of life in those with pain.

LOW BACK PAIN
Pathophysiology

Although low back pain can be categorized by many potential causes, including mechanical, inflammatory, neoplastic, and vascular, more than 85% of cases are nonspecific, that is, no specific underlying cause can be identified.[24]

Evaluation

Although most cases of low back pain will be nonspecific, an important role of the evaluating clinician is to rule out organic causes such as progressive neurologic impairment or infection (red flags) as well as behavioral and functional factors (yellow flags) that can limit recovery and require additional support and treatment. Predictors of disabling chronic low back pain are listed in **Box 1**. These predictors present an important opportunity for primary care clinicians to intervene with several lifestyle and behavioral factors to optimize outcomes. Interestingly, variables such as baseline pain and presence of radiculopathy were less useful for predicting worse outcomes.[25]

In addition to conventional history and physical examination, evaluation should include a biopsychosocial history, which inquires about work, home, social, spiritual, and behavioral status. This discussion can often uncover factors that are contributing to pain persistence or exacerbation. In many cases, patients may not recognize the connection and can benefit from motivational interviewing and coping techniques to enhance their recovery. In addition, there are several questionnaires, such as the Keele STarT Back Screening Tool (see Resources), which can identify those at high risk for worsening or chronic low back pain. Inclusion of this questionnaire as part of stratified primary care management for low back pain has been validated in reducing patient disability and time off work by half, without increasing health care costs.[26]

Box 1
Predictors of disabling chronic low back pain

- Maladaptive pain coping behaviors
  - For instance, fear avoidance, catastrophizing
- Psychiatric comorbidities
  - For instance, depression, anxiety
- Functional impairment
- Poor general health status
  - For instance, obesity, inactivity, smoking, inflammatory or nutrient-deficient diet
- Nonorganic signs
  - For instance, overreaction to stimuli, nonreproducibility of pain, superficial or nonanatomic tenderness

Data from Chou R, Shekelle P. Will this patient develop persistent disabling low back pain? JAMA 2010;303(13):1295–302.

Imaging and Laboratory

In cases where emergent or potential organic causes are not present, immediate radiological evaluation (MRI, computed tomography, or plain radiography) is not warranted. Imaging added to usual care for patients with acute and subacute low back pain does not significantly improve short- or long-term outcomes.[27] Similarly, laboratory evaluation is limited in most cases. Exception would be in cases of suspected autoimmune causes (eg, ankylosing spondylitis) or nutrient depletion (eg, osteoporotic fractures). In cases where metabolic dysfunction and obesity may be contributing to pain, markers such as CRP, lipids, and hemoglobin A1C may be useful to evaluate inflammatory and metabolic status.

Prevention

Likely the most important initial intervention in the treatment of low back pain is education. Education can help dispel myths and reduce fear avoidance beliefs. Fear avoidance behaviors include refraining from physical activity and work because of an inappropriate belief that it will damage or worsen the patient's back condition. In addition, education can assist patients to recognize the potential contribution of mood and lifestyle factors, including sleep, stress, and physical activity. A recent review for preventing back pain found that exercise alone or in combination with education prevented low back pain episodes in the next year by 35% and 45%, respectively. Other interventions, including education alone, back belts, and shoe insoles, did not appear to be preventive.[28]

Treatment

Clinical guidelines for the treatment of low back pain issued in 2017 by the American College of Physicians recommend several nonpharmacologic therapies as first-line treatment.[29] Several of these are discussed here. In addition, emerging evidence for the potential role of nutritional and dietary supplement interventions is presented.

Physical activity

Physical activity and exercise are important to discuss early in treatment because many patients due to fear avoidance reduce their activity rather than increase as tolerated. Encouraging exercise, especially a combination of aerobic and resistance, is critical. Exercise has also been found to have a significant anti-inflammatory effect, especially in the setting of metabolic syndrome.[30] In addition, physical activity can help patients unlearn maladaptive movement patterns and reduce comorbidities such as depression. As with all interventions, individualization is important to enhance compliance and effectiveness. Exercise and physical therapy recommendations for management of low back pain that match the patient's clinical scenario and treatment preferences have been found to provide increased short-term reduction in pain than general activity advice.[31]

Aquatic exercises

Other types of exercise have also been found helpful for low back pain. Aquatic exercise may be an especially effective choice for individuals with advanced deconditioning, pain, or obesity in the setting of low back pain. For example, a 2-month, 5 times per week aquatic therapy treatment program for sedentary adults with chronic low back pain improved pain, disability, quality of life, body composition, and fitness level.[32]

Mindful exercise: tai chi and yoga

Tai chi is a type of gentle martial arts exercise incorporating movements that empha-size stretching, balance, strengthening, and body awareness. It is commonly used as a daily preventive health measure throughout Asia. More recently, it has gained atten-tion as an exercise for helping older participants improve balance, functional mobility, and risk of falls. In the setting of low back pain, a 10-week randomized trial of 160 par-ticipants found that tai chi was more effective than usual care at reducing pain inten-sity and disability.[33]

Yoga

Yoga is a multicomponent practice originating in India more than 2000 years ago with the goal of combining physical, mental, dietary, and spiritual practices. In its modern form, yoga involves the practice of physical postures (asanas), breathing (pranayama), and meditative awareness exercises. As yoga has increased in popularity, it has been evaluated in several pain scenarios, especially low back pain. In a year-long study comparing yoga to usual care, Tilbrook and colleagues[34] found yoga participants had higher pain self-efficacy scores as well as improved back-related function. A sys-tematic review of 10 yoga trials for low back pain noted short- and long-term effects on pain and moderate to strong effects on global improvement and back-specific disability.[35]

Nutrition and supplementation

Weight loss Dietary interventions can have a significant effect on the progression of low back pain. Several mechanisms may explain benefit, including reduction in obesity, inflammation, and nutrient deficiency. Roffey and colleagues[36] evaluated a weight loss program for reducing the severity of low back pain in obese adults. The program used exercise and dietary modification for 6 months with a 12-month follow-up. During the trial, there was significant improvement in pain and disability that was significantly associated with reduction in BMI.

Omega 3 fatty acids Specific nutrient support may be beneficial because of their abil-ity to reduce associated inflammation. Li and colleagues[37] in their PLoS meta-analysis noted that marine-derived n-3 polyunsaturated fatty acids supplementation provided significant reduction of CRP, interleukin-6, and tumor necrosis factor-α (TNF-α). The clinical role of omega-3s in the setting of low back pain is less clear. A 1-month non-randomized trial of 250 participants with low back pain using 1200 to 2400 mg of omega-3 fatty acids noted that 59% of participants were able to discontinue prescrip-tion nonsteroidal anti-inflammatory drugs, and 60% noted overall improvement in pain.[38] Other than in settings where omega-3s are contraindicated (eg, patients on an-ticoagulants), omega 3s should be considered for a trial when low back pain coexists with an elevated inflammatory state.

Curcumin Curcumin is a component of the spice turmeric. Similar to omega 3s, cur-cumin can reduce inflammation when used typically at 1000 mg per day. A meta-analysis of 6 trials of curcumin found that supplementation was associated with a significant reduction in circulating CRP levels.[39] Animal studies have also noted anti-nociceptive properties in several pain models.[40] Clinically, most trials have examined the use of curcumin in osteoarthritis of the knee. Moderately strong evidence exists for curcumin's effectiveness in joint arthritis based on a recent meta-analysis.[41] In this analysis, curcumin caused a significant 2-point reduction in visual analogue score for pain as well as significant improvement in Western Ontario and McMaster Univer-sities Osteoarthritis Index scores. Furthermore, in trials comparing curcumin to pain medication, there was no significant mean difference in reduction of visual analogue scores for pain. In the setting of acute pain, one recent randomized crossover trial examined the effects of curcumin, acetaminophen, and a COX-2 selective, nonsteroidal anti-inflammatory drug. Curcumin at 2 g per day demonstrated similar analgesic ability to the other agents with greater tolerability.[42] Onset of relief from curcumin was delayed compared with the other treatments.

Vitamin D In an observational study of more than 9000 participants, hypovitaminosis D was significantly associated with back pain, pain severity, and higher limitations in daily activities.[43] More recently, a meta-analysis of 7 trials demonstrated moderate evidence of a link between low vitamin D and nonspecific low back pain.[44] In addition, polymorphism of the vitamin D receptor gene has been associated with more frequent and significant levels of lumbar disc disease.[45] Evidence for a therapeutic benefit of vitamin D replacement in low back pain is emerging. An open-label study of 60,000 IU of vitamin D_3 per week in vitamin D–deficient low back pain patients found that 53% and 63% achieved greater than 50% reduction in pain scores at 3 and 6 months, respectively.[46] In a randomized double blind trial, Gendelman and colleagues[47] compared 4000 IU of vitamin D_3 to placebo for patients with chronic musculoskeletal pain, most of whom had spinal pain. Those on vitamin D reported a significantly larger decline in pain scores and use of rescue medication at 3 months. Interestingly, several inflammatory cytokines, including TNF-α and Prostaglandin E2, also significant improved in the vitamin D group compared with placebo.[47] Until there is more definitive evidence of efficacy, it is reasonable to evaluate vitamin D levels in patients with back pain and replete when needed to achieve therapeutic levels.

Magnesium Magnesium deficiency is prevalent in several pain states as well as the American population in general.[48] It is estimated that 68% of Americans do not consume the recommended dietary allowance (RDA) for magnesium. Magnesium deficiency can be associated with inflammation.[49] King and colleagues[49,50] noted that subjects who consumed less than the RDA of magnesium were 1.48 to 1.75 times more likely to have elevated CRP. In addition, those who consumed less than 50% of the RDA and had a BMI greater than 25 were 2.24 times more likely to have elevated CRP. Yousef and Al-deeb[51] performed a trial evaluating the role of magnesium replacement in patients with chronic low back pain. In comparison to placebo, those receiving magnesium over 6 weeks noted reduced pain intensity and improvement in lumbar spine mobility during a 6-month follow-up period.

Mind-Body Therapies

Several mind-body therapies have shown benefit for chronic low back pain. The 2 most researched are cognitive-behavioral therapy (CBT) and mindfulness-based stress reduction (MBSR). CBT and MBSR help patients develop improved awareness, behavioral, and coping strategies for pain. In a trial of nearly 350 adults with chronic low back pain randomized to 8 weeks of MBSR or CBT classes, both demonstrated similar clinically meaningful improvement ($\geq$30%) in functional limitations and pain inconvenience. Effectiveness persisted at 26 to 52 weeks after treatment. Additional mind-body therapies that may be considered include hypnosis and biofeedback. These modalities also appear to provide clinically meaningful reductions in pain intensity with the ability to maintain benefits for 6 months or longer after initial treatment.[52]

Manual and manipulation therapies

Massage therapy is commonly used in various forms as an approach for predominantly reducing the soft tissue abnormalities associated with low back pain.

Systematic reviews of massage have noted only short-term benefit when evaluating massage for low back pain.[53] Specific types of massage, including shiatsu, acupressure, structural, and relaxation, yield similar benefit.[54,55]

Manipulation refers to treatment focused predominately on correcting spinal joint abnormalities using various techniques. These treatments are typically done by osteopathic physicians and chiropractic clinicians. Numerous techniques are used that may be of benefit in the setting of pain. For example, several studies have shown that osteopathic manipulation techniques including craniosacral therapy can be additionally effective in improving pain, lumbar range of motion, and functional disability when added to traditional physical therapy and massage.[56,57] Several systematic reviews of chiropractic spinal manipulation have noted a small but consistent treatment effect similar to that seen with other conservative care options.[58,59] One study that examined the dose response of manipulation found the greatest disability reduction occurred with 12 sessions.[60]

CENTRAL PAIN STATES

CPS represent a collection of syndromes, including pain amplification syndrome, amplified musculoskeletal pain syndrome, central sensitization, and functional chronic pain syndromes. These umbrella terms encompass pain disorders, including fibromyalgia, myofascial pain syndrome, complex regional pain syndrome (CRPS), psychogenic pain, phantom-limb pain, reflex neurovascular dystrophy, irritable bowel syndrome, temporomandibular joint disorder, and chronic daily headache. These disorders are differentiated from nociceptive and neuropathic conditions based on predominant and persistent central sensitization. This is defined by neuronal changes that promote enhanced pain signaling and neurogenic inflammation.[61] Of note, these conditions (eg, fibromyalgia) may not always have identifiable tissue or nerve damage or may overlap with those that do as noted in **Box 1**.

Treatments

Many of the treatments outlined for low back pain have potential benefit in the setting of CPS. However, once CPS has been identified, treatment often requires a more comprehensive rehabilitation approach as compared with non–central pain disorders. CPS often requires a multilayered team approach to reduce the typically high levels of pain, hypersensitivity, and comorbidities.[62] Fortunately, several therapies, including acupuncture, MBSR, and CBT, have demonstrated the ability to positively influence the neuroplastic changes often noted with CPS.[63,64] Other therapies, including several biological and neurostimulation therapies, have emerging benefit in the setting of CPS.

Behavioral Support

Mind-body therapies hold promise in helping to reverse aspects of central sensitization. One of the most studied behavioral interventions, CBT, has recently been shown to reverse aspects of dysfunctional neuronal connectivity that may promote chronic pain.[64] In addition, because of the common negative ramifications of progressive pain on mood and outlook, it is important to incorporate behavioral retraining interventions to reduce disability. For example, a trial on the effects of a tailored positive psychology intervention for chronic pain noted improvements in pain intensity, pain control, pain catastrophizing, pain interference, life satisfaction, positive affect, and depression.[65]

Integrative Therapeutics

In addition to currently available approved pharmaceutical therapies such as anticonvulsants and serotonin norepinephrine reuptake inhibitors, several natural and novel prescription therapies may be considered for CPS (**Table 1**). These therapies have the ability to potentially improve CPS because of actions on N-methyl-D-aspartame glutamate receptors, glial cells, BDNF, neuroinflammation, and oxidative stress.[66]

Vitamin D and Magnesium

As noted previously, vitamin D and magnesium have been shown to be low in chronic pain states. Bagis and colleagues[67] used 300 mg of magnesium citrate alone or in combination with amitriptyline in patients with fibromyalgia. Magnesium alone appeared to improve many pain parameters, especially in those with low magnesium levels. Additional benefit was observed when magnesium was used in combination with amitriptyline.

Coenzyme q10 and Alpha-Lipoic Acid

CPS appears to also create significant oxidative stress, which may coexist with nutrient depletion. The antioxidants coenzyme q10 (Coq10) and alpha-lipoic acid appear to be beneficial in reducing nutrient deficiency and associated oxidative stress while improving pain levels.[68,69]

Omega 3s, Curcumin, and Melatonin

Several natural therapies may have intrinsic central antinociceptive effects. Examples of these are omega-3s, curcumin, and melatonin. In addition to local anti-inflammatory effects, they may modulate central inflammation and pain signaling.[70,71] Of note, the dosage of these therapies, such as with melatonin, may be different than typically used for common non–chronic pain conditions[72] (see **Table 1**).

Table 1
Dosage of selected integrative therapeutics for chronic pain

Therapy	Typical Daily Dosage[a]
Alpha-lipoic acid	600 mg
Coq10	100–300 mg[b]
Curcumin	1–2 G
Magnesium	200–600[b] mg[c]
Melatonin	3–10 mg at bedtime
Omega-3 (EPA/DHA)	1–3 G
Vitamin D_3	1000 iu[b] based on serum levels
Off-label medications	
Ketamine, intranasal	50 mg[b]
LDN	1.5–4.5 mg

[a] Dosages vary based on formulation.
[b] Implies that dosage may increase beyond stated amount based on individual response and tolerability.
[c] Formulations vary and should be based on tolerability. Common formulations that may cause gastrointestinal side effects include citrate, oxide, and sulfate. Typically, chelated formulations (eg, glycinate, malate) tend to have less gastrointestinal side effects.

Low-Dose Naltrexone and Ketamine

The use of currently available therapeutics in new dosages and formulations is gathering support in the setting of CPS. Naltrexone is a currently available prescription therapy approved in the setting of addiction due to its ability to block opiate receptors. Low-dose naltrexone (LDN) refers to dosages typically at 4.5 mg, which instead appear to modulate glial cell hypersensitivity. LDN has several preliminary trials demonstrating benefit in CPS, especially fibromyalgia.[73] Similarly, ketamine has been traditionally used as an intravenous anesthetic with the ability to reduce pain and related memories. More recently, preliminary use as an intranasal formulation has demonstrated the potential to reduce chronic pain and associated depression. This is thought possible because of modulation of central circuitry at nearby areas of the prefrontal cortex (BA24 and BA25), which influence depression and aspects of pain processing.[74]

Topical Applications

Several topical applications may be considered for chronic pain related to CPS. Many of these are topical versions of currently approved oral or intravenous agents such as ketamine and amitriptyline. These agents have local effects while reducing systemic absorption. Over time, they may reduce peripheral hyperstimulation, which is thought to be one mechanism by which peripheral sensitization contributes to CPS. There is moderate evidence of efficacy in reducing pain, especially allodynia in conditions such as CRPS.[75] These treatments are typically made by a compounding pharmacy and may not be covered by insurance. It is recommended that providers work closely with pharmacies with extensive experience compounding pain treatments.[76]

Neurostimulation

Several neurostimulation modalities have emerged for CPS, including high-frequency repetitive transcranial magnetic stimulation (rTMS), transcranial direct current stimulation, supraorbital transcutaneous neurostimulation, auricular/vagal nerve stimulation, and specially applied transcutaneous electrical nerve stimulation.[77,78] Many of these therapies have preliminary evidence of clinic benefit in CPS, such as fibromyalgia. Some therapies, such as rTMS, also have evidence of enhancing brain metabolic activity that may explain potential long-term benefit seen with treatment.[79–81]

SUMMARY

Pain guidelines increasingly recommend incorporation of nonpharmacologic and integrative therapies in the setting of pain.[29,82] In most cases, recommendations start this approach with education, reassurance, and activity in the absence of red flags. After this, an individualized comprehensive approach should be developed that incorporates evidence-based therapies such as those noted for low back pain from the American College of Physicians.[29] The types and intensity of treatment should be determined using clinical presentation and preference, comorbidities, and available screening tools as recommended. Especially attractive among these approaches are mind-body therapies, which provide enhanced benefit over time as a component of self-care. For all therapies incorporated, it is important that they have appropriate interprofessional communication and coordination as well as regular evaluation of progress and ongoing shared decision making to optimize outcomes. This approach is summarized in **Fig. 6**.

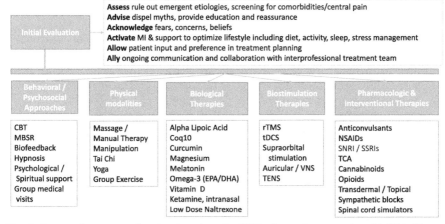

Fig. 6. Integrative approaches to chronic pain. DHA, docosahexanenoic acid; EPA, Eicosa-pentaenoic acid; MI, motivational interviewing; MS, magnetic stimulation; NSAIDs, nonste-roidal anti-inflammatory drugs; SNRI, serotonin norepinephrine reuptake inhibitor; SSRIs, selective serotonin reuptake inhibitor; TCA, tricyclic antidepressants; tDCS, transcranial direct current stimulation; TENS, transcutaneous electrical nerve stimulation; VNS, vagal nerve stimulation.

As the treatment of chronic pain evolves, it is important to note several points:

- Chronic pain, especially CPS, requires a different approach than acute pain states. Increased attention to behavioral and functional comorbidities is required in order to optimize recovery.
- Chronic pain can be accompanied by higher rates of metabolic syndrome, and optimal treatments, such as diet and physical activity, should aim to not only benefit pain but also reduce risk factors for metabolic syndrome and obesity.[83]
- Integrative therapies show promise in enhancing outcomes when combined with conventional care. Providers may evaluate clinical scenarios where a trial of evidence-based treatment reviewed above is worthwhile.[84]
- Screening and self-care tools, as noted below in the resources, should be increasingly incorporated to enhance outcomes and promote patient empower-ment in the management of chronic pain.

RESOURCES

- Questionnaires for triage and monitoring of chronic pain:
  - Keele STarT Back Screening Tool for stratifying care
    - https://www.keele.ac.uk/sbst
- Fibromyalgia Impact Questionnaire
  - http://www.fiqr.info
- Online and self-care modules for chronic pain and fibromyalgia
  - FibroGuide from the University of Michigan
    - https://fibroguide.med.umich.edu/

REFERENCES

1. Bonakdar RA, Sukiennik A, editors. Integrative pain management, Weil integrative medicine series. 1st edition. New York: Oxford University Press; 2016.
2. Goldberg DS, McGee SJ. Pain as a global public health priority. BMC Public Health 2011;11(1):1.
3. Perquin CW, Hazebroek-Kampschreur AA, Hunfeld JA, et al. Pain in children and adolescents: a common experience. Pain 2000;87(1):51–8.
4. King S, Chambers CT, Huguet A, et al. The epidemiology of chronic pain in children and adolescents revisited: a systematic review. Pain 2011;152(12): 2729–38.
5. Connors AF, Dawson NV, Desbiens NA, et al. A controlled trial to improve care for seriously ill hospitalized patients: the study to understand prognoses and preferences for outcomes and risks of treatments (SUPPORT). JAMA 1995;274(20): 1591–8.
6. IOM (Institute of Medicine). Relieving pain in America: a blueprint for transforming prevention, care, education, and research. Washington (DC): The National Academies Press; 2011.
7. Georgi K. Calculating the cost of pain. Chronic Pain Perspect 2011;12:F2. Available at: http://www.chronicpainperspectives.com/the-publication/past-issue-single-view/calculating-the-cost-of-pain/5f1e3ed6046880e062fe28ab1dbcab5f.html. Accessed April 2, 2014.
8. Hoy D, Bain C, Williams G, et al. A systematic review of the global prevalence of low back pain. Arthritis Rheum 2012;64(6):2028–37.
9. National Center for Health Statistics. Health, United States, 2005: with chart book on trends in the health of Americans. Hyattsville (Maryland): US Department of Health and Human Services, Centers for Disease Control and Prevention; 2005.
10. Apkarian AV, Sosa Y, Sonty S, et al. Chronic back pain is associated with decreased prefrontal and thalamic gray matter density. J Neurosci 2004;24(46): 10410–5.
11. Bonakdar RA. Targeting systemic inflammation in patients with obesity-related pain: obesity- related pain: time for a new approach that targets systemic inflammation. J Fam Pract 2013;62(9 Suppl CHPP):S22–9.
12. Romero-Corral A, Somers VK, Sierra-Johnson J, et al. Normal weight obesity—a risk factor for cardiometabolic dysregulation and cardiovascular mortality. Eur Heart J 2010;31:737–46.
13. Stone AA, Broderick JE. Obesity and pain are associated in the United States. Obesity (Silver Spring) 2012;20(7):1491–5.
14. Urquhart DM, Berry P, Wluka AE, et al. Increased fat mass is associated with high levels of low back pain intensity and disability. Spine (Phila Pa 1976) 2011;36(16): 1320–5.
15. Geha P, Dearaujo I, Green B, et al. Decreased food pleasure and disrupted satiety signals in chronic low back pain. Pain 2014;155(4):712–22.
16. Briggs MS, Givens DL, Schmitt LC, et al. Relations of C-reactive protein and obesity to the prevalence and the odds of reporting low back pain. Arch Phys Med Rehabil 2013;94(4):745–52.
17. Eslami V, Katz MJ, White RS, et al. Pain intensity and pain interference in older adults: role of gender, obesity and high-sensitivity C-reactive protein. Gerontology 2016;63(1):3–12.
18. Pain. National Center for Complementary and Integrative Health (NCCIH). Available at: https://nccih.nih.gov/health/pain. Accessed November 26, 2016.

19. Clarke TC, Nahin RL, Barnes PM, et al. Use of complementary health approaches for musculoskeletal pain disorders among adults: United States, 2012. National Health Statistics Reports; no. 98. Hyattsville (MD): National Center for Health Statistics; 2016.

20. Ghildayal N, Johnson PJ, Evans RL, et al. Complementary and alternative medicine use in the US adult low back pain population. Glob Adv Health Med 2016;5(1):69–78.

21. Fleming S, Rabago DP, Mundt MP, et al. CAM therapies among primary care patients using opioid therapy for chronic pain. BMC Complement Altern Med 2007; 7(1):1.

22. Boyd C, Crawford C, Paat CF, et al. The impact of massage therapy on function in pain populations—a systematic review and meta-analysis of randomized controlled trials: part II, cancer pain populations. Pain Med 2016;17(8):1553–68.

23. Hsu C, Bluespruce J, Sherman K, et al. Unanticipated benefits of CAM therapies for back pain: an exploration of patient experiences. J Altern Complement Med 2010;16(2):157–63.

24. Chou R, Qaseem A, Snow V, et al, Clinical Efficacy Assessment Subcommittee of the American College of Physicians, American College of Physicians, American Pain Society Low Back Pain Guidelines Panel. Diagnosis and treatment of low back pain: a joint clinical practice guideline from the American College of Physicians and the American Pain Society. Ann Intern Med 2007;147(7):478–91.

25. Nicholas MK, Linton SJ, Watson PJ, et al, "Decade of the Flags" Working Group. Early identification and management of psychological risk factors ("yellow flags") in patients with low back pain: a reappraisal. Phys Ther 2011;91(5):737–53.

26. Foster NE, Mullis R, Hill JC, et al. Effect of stratified care for low back pain in family practice (IMPaCT Back): a prospective population-based sequential comparison. Ann Fam Med 2014;12(2):102–11.

27. Chou R, Fu R, Carrino JA, et al. Imaging strategies for low-back pain: systematic review and meta-analysis. Lancet 2009;373(9662):463–72.

28. Steffens D, Maher CG, Pereira LS, et al. Prevention of low back pain: a systematic review and meta-analysis. JAMA Intern Med 2016;176(2):199–208.

29. Qaseem A, Wilt TJ, McLean RM, et al, Clinical Guidelines Committee of the American College of Physicians. Noninvasive treatments for acute, subacute, and chronic low back pain: a clinical practice guideline from the American College of Physicians. Ann Intern Med 2017;166(7):514–30.

30. Balducci S, Zanuso S, Nicolucci A, et al. Anti-inflammatory effect of exercise training in subjects with type 2 diabetes and the metabolic syndrome is dependent on exercise modalities and independent of weight loss. Nutr Metab Cardiovasc Dis 2010;20(8):608–17.

31. Hahne AJ, Ford JJ, Hinman RS, et al. Individualized functional restoration as an adjunct to advice for lumbar disc herniation with associated radiculopathy. A preplanned subgroup analysis of a randomized controlled trial. Spine J 2016;17(3): 346–59.

32. Baena-Beato PÁ, Artero EG, Arroyo-Morales M, et al. Aquatic therapy improves pain, disability, quality of life, body composition and fitness in sedentary adults with chronic low back pain. A controlled clinical trial. Clin Rehabil 2014;28(4): 350–60.

33. Hall AM, Maher CG, Lam P, et al. Tai chi exercise for treatment of pain and disability in people with persistent low back pain: a randomized controlled trial. Arthritis Care Res (Hoboken) 2011;63(11):1576–83.

34. Tilbrook HE, Cox H, Hewitt CE, et al. Yoga for chronic low back pain: a randomized trial. Ann Intern Med 2011;155(9):569–78.
35. Cramer H, Lauche R, Haller H, et al. A systematic review and meta-analysis of yoga for low back pain. Clin J pain 2013;29(5):450–60.
36. Roffey DM, Ashdown LC, Dornan HD, et al. Pilot evaluation of a multidisciplinary, medically supervised, nonsurgical weight loss program on the severity of low back pain in obese adults. Spine J 2011;11(3):197–204.
37. Li K, Huang T, Zheng J, et al. Effect of marine-derived n-3 polyunsaturated fatty acids on C-reactive protein, interleukin 6 and tumor necrosis factor α: a meta-analysis. PLoS One 2014;9(2):e88103.
38. Maroon JC, Bost JW. Omega-3 fatty acids (fish oil) as an anti-inflammatory: an alternative to nonsteroidal anti-inflammatory drugs for discogenic pain. Surg Neurol 2006;65(4):326–31.
39. Sahebkar A. Are curcuminoids effective C-reactive protein-lowering agents in clinical practice? Evidence from a meta-analysis. Phytother Res 2014;28(5):633–42.
40. Leamy AW, Shukla P, McAlexander MA, et al. Curcumin ((E,E)-1,7-bis(4-hydroxy-3-methoxyphenyl)-1,6-heptadiene-3,5-dione) activates and desensitizes the nociceptor ion channel TRPA1. Neurosci Lett 2011;503(3):157–62.
41. Daily JW, Yang M, Park S. Efficacy of turmeric extracts and curcumin for alleviating the symptoms of joint arthritis: a systematic review and meta-analysis of randomized clinical trials. J Med Food 2016;19(8):717–29.
42. Di Pierro F, Rapacioli G, Di Maio EA, et al. Comparative evaluation of the pain-relieving properties of a lecithinized formulation of curcumin (Meriva(®)), nimesulide, and acetaminophen. J Pain Res 2013;6:201–5.
43. e Silva AV, Lacativa PG, Russo LA, et al. Association of back pain with hypovitaminosis D in postmenopausal women with low bone mass. BMC Musculoskelet Disord 2013;14:184.
44. Chatterjee R, Hemmings S, Laupheimer MW. The effect of low vitamin D on chronic non-specific low back pain: a systematic review. International Musculoskeletal Medicine 2016;38(2):43–50.
45. Kawaguchi Y, Kanamori M, Ishihara H, et al. The association of lumbar disc disease with vitamin-D receptor gene polymorphism. J Bone Joint Surg Am 2002;84(11):2022–8.
46. Ghai B, Bansal D, Kanukula R, et al. Vitamin D supplementation in patients with chronic low back pain: an open label, single arm clinical trial. Pain Physician 2017;20(1):E99–105.
47. Gendelman O, Itzhaki D, Makarov S, et al. A randomized double-blind placebo-controlled study adding high dose vitamin D to analgesic regimens in patients with musculoskeletal pain. Lupus 2015;24(4–5):483–9.
48. Rosanoff A, Weaver CM, Rude RK. Suboptimal magnesium status in the United States- are the health consequences underestimated? Nutr Rev 2012;70(3):153–64.
49. Nielsen FH. Magnesium, inflammation, and obesity in chronic disease. Nutr Rev 2010;68(6):333–40.
50. King DE, Mainous AG 3rd, Geesey ME, et al. Dietary magnesium and C-reactive protein levels. J Am Coll Nutr 2005;24(3):166–71.
51. Yousef AA, Al-deeb AE. A double-blinded randomised controlled study of the value of sequential intravenous and oral magnesium therapy in patients with chronic low back pain with a neuropathic component. Anaesthesia 2013;68(3):260–6.

52. Tan G, Rintala DH, Jensen MP, et al. A randomized controlled trial of hypnosis compared with biofeedback for adults with chronic low back pain. Eur J Pain 2015;19(2):271–80.
53. Furlan AD, Giraldo M, Baskwill A, et al. Massage for low-back pain. Cochrane Database Syst Rev 2015;(9):CD001929.
54. Hsieh LL, Kuo CH, Lee LH, et al. Treatment of low back pain by acupressure and physical therapy: randomised controlled trial. BMJ 2006;332(7543):696–700.
55. Cherkin DC, Sherman KJ, Kahn J, et al. A comparison of the effects of 2 types of massage and usual care on chronic low back pain: a randomized, controlled trial. Ann Intern Med 2011;155(1):1–9.
56. Ali MF, Selim MN, Elwardany SH, et al. Osteopathic manual therapy versus traditional exercises in the treatment of mechanical low back pain. American Journal of Medicine and Medical Sciences 2015;5(2):63–72.
57. Castro-Sánchez AM, Lara-Palomo IC, Matarán-Penarrocha GA, et al. Benefits of craniosacral therapy in patients with chronic low back pain: a randomized controlled trial. J Altern Complement Med 2016;22(8):650–7.
58. Rubinstein SM, van Middelkoop M, Assendelft WJ, et al. Spinal manipulative therapy for chronic low-back pain. Cochrane Database Syst Rev 2011;(2):CD008112.
59. Goertz CM, Pohlman KA, Vining RD, et al. Patient-centered outcomes of high-velocity, low-amplitude spinal manipulation for low back pain: a systematic review. J Electromyogr Kinesiol 2012;22(5):670–91.
60. Haas M, Vavrek D, Peterson D, et al. Dose-response and efficacy of spinal manipulation for care of chronic low back pain: a randomized controlled trial. Spine J 2014;14(7):1106–16.
61. Nijs J, Meeus M, Versijpt J, et al. Brain-derived neurotrophic factor as a driving force behind neuroplasticity in neuropathic and central sensitization pain: a new therapeutic target? Expert Opin Ther Targets 2015;19(4):565–76.
62. Harris RE. Central pain states: a shift in thinking about chronic pain. J Fam Pract 2011;40:S37.
63. Chassot M, Dussan-Sarria JA, Sehn FC, et al. Electroacupuncture analgesia is associated with increased serum brain-derived neurotrophic factor in chronic tension-type headache: a randomized, sham controlled, crossover trial. BMC Complement Altern Med 2015;15:144.
64. Shpaner M, Kelly C, Lieberman G, et al. Unlearning chronic pain: a randomized controlled trial to investigate changes in intrinsic brain connectivity following Cognitive Behavioral Therapy. Neuroimage Clin 2014;5:365–76.
65. Müller R, Gertz KJ, Molton IR, et al. Effects of a tailored positive psychology intervention on well-being and pain in individuals with chronic pain and a physical disability: a feasibility trial. Clin J Pain 2016;32(1):32–44.
66. Littlejohn G. Neurogenic neuroinflammation in fibromyalgia and complex regional pain syndrome. Nat Rev Rheumatol 2015;11(11):639–48.
67. Bagis S, Karabiber M, As I, et al. Is magnesium citrate treatment effective on pain, clinical parameters and functional status in patients with fibromyalgia? Rheumatol Int 2013;33(1):167–72.
68. Cordero MD, Alcocer-Gómez E, Culic O, et al. NLRP3 inflammasome is activated in fibromyalgia: the effect of coenzyme Q10. Antioxid Redox Signal 2014;20(8):1169–80.
69. Eren Y, Dirik E, Neşelioğlu S, et al. Oxidative stress and decreased thiol level in patients with migraine- cross-sectional study. Acta Neurol Belg 2015;115(4):643–9.

70. Wagner K, Vito S, Inceoglu B, et al. The role of long chain fatty acids and their epoxide metabolites in nociceptive signaling. Prostaglandins Other Lipid Mediat 2014;113-115:2–12.
71. Kulkarni SK, Dhir A. An overview of curcumin in neurological disorders. Indian J Pharm Sci 2010;72(2):149–54.
72. Srinivasan V, Lauterbach EC, Ho KY, et al. Melatonin in antinociception: its therapeutic applications. Curr Neuropharmacol 2012;10(2):167–78.
73. Younger J, Parkitny L, McLain D. The use of low-dose naltrexone (LDN) as a novel anti-inflammatory treatment for chronic pain. Clin Rheumatol 2014;33(4):451–9.
74. Opler LA, Opler MG, Arnsten AF. Ameliorating treatment-refractory depression with intranasal ketamine- potential NMDA receptor actions in the pain circuitry representing mental anguish. CNS Spectrums 2016;21(01):12–22.
75. Finch PM, Knudsen L, Drummond PD. Reduction of allodynia in patients with complex regional pain syndrome: a double-blind placebo-controlled trial of topical ketamine. Pain 2009;146(1–2):18–25.
76. Branvold A, Carvalho M. Pain management therapy: the benefits of compounded transdermal pain medication. J Gen Pract 2014;2014.
77. Massé-Alarie H, Schneider C. Revisiting the corticomotor plasticity in low back pain: challenges and perspectives. Healthcare (Basel) 2016;4(3) [pii:E67].
78. Riederer F, Penning S, Schoenen J. Transcutaneous supraorbital nerve stimulation (t-SNS) with the Cefaly(®) device for migraine prevention: a review of the available data. Pain Ther 2015;4(2):135–47.
79. Knijnik LM, Dussán-Sarria JA, Rozisky JR, et al. Repetitive transcranial magnetic stimulation for fibromyalgia: systematic review and meta-analysis. Pain Pract 2016;16(3):294–304.
80. Napadow V, Edwards RR, Cahalan CM, et al. Evoked pain analgesia in chronic pelvic pain patients using respiratory-gated auricular vagal afferent nerve stimulation. Pain Med 2012;13(6):777–89.
81. Boyer L, Dousset A, Roussel P, et al. rTMS in fibromyalgia: a randomized trial evaluating QoL and its brain metabolic substrate. Neurology 2014;82(14):1231–8.
82. Maher C, Underwood M, Buchbinder R. Non-specific low back pain. Lancet 2017;389(10070):736–47.
83. Paoli A, Moro T, Bosco G, et al. Effects of n-3 polyunsaturated fatty acids (ω-3) supplementation on some cardiovascular risk factors with a ketogenic Mediterranean diet. Mar Drugs 2015;13(2):996–1009.
84. Kizhakkeveettil A, Rose K, Kadar GE. Integrative therapies for low back pain that include complementary and alternative medicine care: a systematic review. Glob Adv Health Med 2014;3(5):49–64.

Integrative Medicine for Geriatric and Palliative Care

Mikhail Kogan, MD[a],*, Stephanie Cheng, MD[b], Seema Rao, MD[c],
Sharon DeMocker, MD[d], Mariatu Koroma Nelson, MD[e,1]

KEYWORDS

- Geriatrics • Palliative care • Osteoporosis • Falls • Frailty

KEY POINTS

- US health care for elderly with chronic illnesses is expensive and not fully effective in part because lifestyle interventions are underutilized.
- Common geriatric syndromes, such as falls, frailty, and others, are often overtreated with medical interventions, whereas nonpharmacologic integrative modalities are underutilized.
- Evidenced integrative approaches for falls, osteoporosis, and end-of-life syndromes are available and recommended for comprehensive quality care.

INTRODUCTION

Societies worldwide are challenged by the ongoing growth in health care expenditures and the changing patterns in the demand for medical services.[1] Contemporary health care systems face difficulties in solving these challenges, because they have originally been designed to solve single-episode, acute short-term diseases.[2] Worsening this situation, ongoing specialization and technological improvements have led to fragmentation of care delivery and resulted in a substantial increase in health care expenditures. This negatively affects the provision of integrated long-term care and support for the chronically ill and for elderly people with complex care needs.[3]

Disclosure Statement: The authors have nothing to disclose.
[a] Center for Integrative Medicine, George Washington University, School of Medicine, 908 New Hampshire Avenue, Suite 200, Washington, DC 20037, USA; [b] Division of Geriatrics, Department of Medicine, University of California, 3333 California Street, Suite 380, Box 1265, San Francisco, CA 94143, USA; [c] 11686 Wannacut Place, San Diego, CA 92131, USA; [d] War Related Illness & Injury Study Center, VA Medical Center, 50 Irving Street Northwest, MS 127, Washington, DC 20422, USA; [e] Geriatric Medicine, Virginia Hospital Center, Arlington, VA, USA
[1] Present address: 3440 South Jefferson Street, Falls Church, VA 22041.
* Corresponding author.
E-mail address: mkogan@mfa.gwu.edu

Med Clin N Am 101 (2017) 1005–1029
http://dx.doi.org/10.1016/j.mcna.2017.04.013
0025-7125/17/© 2017 Elsevier Inc. All rights reserved.

Epidemiologic research shows that in the United States approximately 80% of all persons aged ≥65 years have at least one chronic condition and 50% have 2 or more.[4,5] Chronic illness and appropriate management is an increasingly important issue because many aspects of disability and mortality among older adults may be preventable through a change in lifestyle behaviors. Studies show that lifestyle factors (ie, tobacco use, poor diet, and physical inactivity) directly contribute to the leading causes of death (ie, heart disease, malignancy, cerebrovascular disease, and chronic lower respiratory disease) in aging adults.[6]

FALLS AND FRAILTY

A fall is considered to have occurred when a person comes to rest inadvertently on the ground or lower level. Falls are one of the most common geriatric syndromes threatening the independence of older persons. Between 30% and 40% of community-dwelling adults older than 65 years fall each year, and the rates are higher for nursing home residents. Falls are associated with increased morbidity, mortality, and nursing home placement.[7] Adjusted for inflation, the direct medical costs for fall injuries are $31 billion annually.[8] Falls are symptomatic of underlying clinical deficits, and a multidisciplinary approach is essential in identifying the risk factors and appropriate treatments for these patients.[9]

Frailty in the elderly carries an increased risk of falls that can lead to fractures, dependency, and disability. Frailty is defined as a clinically recognizable state of older adults with increased vulnerability, resulting from age-associated declines in physiologic reserve and function across multiple-organ systems. Frailty occurs in 7% to 12% of community-dwelling adults. Prevalence of frailty increases from 3.9% in the 65- to 74-year-old age group to 25% in the 85-year-old and older age group.[10]

Frailty can be *primary*, resulting from aging, or *secondary*, associated with diseases such as cancer, chronic obstructive pulmonary disease (COPD), heart failure, and HIV/AIDS. Frailty syndrome is diagnosed based on the presence of 3 or more of 5 phenotypic components: weight loss (>10 pounds in 1 year), weakness (measured by grip strength), slow walking speed (time to walk 15 feet), low physical activity (expends <270 kcal/wk), and patient-reported exhaustion.[11] Many patients may present without the full syndromic definition of frailty. Clinicians caring for the elderly need to be aware of the syndrome because early intervention can improve outcomes and prevent falls. Adults at least 70 years old should be screened for frailty syndrome. Frailty can be assessed in several different ways: presence of 3 of the above criteria (preferred method), use of the FRAIL scale[12] (http://www.albertahealthservices.ca/assets/about/scn/ahs-scn-bjh-hf-frail-scale.pdf), and the Clinical Global Impression of Change in Physical Frailty.[13] The FRAIL scale is interview-based, quick, and sensitive in the clinical setting.

Pathophysiology and Risk Factors for Falls

Although fall-related injuries are not a common cause of death in older adults, fall-related complications are the leading cause of death in adults ≥65 years old. **Box 1** lists risk factors for falls.

Sarcopenia, defined as a decrease in muscle power and muscle mass,[17] is an important cause of frailty leading to falls. Physical inactivity, poor nutrition, and age-related changes in hormones and cytokine levels are important risk factors for muscle loss.[17] Estrogens prevent loss of muscle mass.[18] However, trials have not shown increases in muscle mass after hormone replacement therapy.[19] Testosterone levels decline with age, and low levels of testosterone are associated with loss of muscle

---

Box 1
Risk factors for falls

Age and gender: Advanced age, female gender

Past history: History of falls (can be associated with fear of falling), recent hospitalization

Musculoskeletal: Arthritis, gait problems, foot disorders, inability to get out of a chair, balance problems, pain, sarcopenia, and frailty

Cognition: Cognitive impairment, psychotropic medications (sedatives, antidepressants, and antipsychotics), inability to follow instructions

Central and peripheral nervous system: Stroke, Parkinson disease, decreased cerebral perfusion, decreased sensation, and proprioception

Environmental: Environmental hazards, dim lighting, uneven floors, slippery surfaces, stairs without handrails

Cardiovascular: Hypotension, syncope (eg, due to arrhythmia)

Special senses: Visual impairment, disorders of vestibular system

Others: Improper footwear, reckless wheelchair use, hypovitaminosis D

Data from Refs.[14–16]

---

mass.[20,21] Dehydroepiandrostenedione (DHEA), an anabolic steroid, decreases dramatically with age.[22] Several studies have reported the association between low 1,25-OH vitamin D and sarcopenia, decreased balance, and increased risk of falls.[23,24] Poor protein intake or general malnutrition can predispose to loss of muscle strength and mass. High levels of interleukin-6 and C-reactive protein are associated with an increased risk for loss of muscle strength.[25]

Assessment and Management of Falls

The following section and **Box 2** provide an outline for assessment and management strategies. This assessment is followed by discussion on interventions to improve muscle strength, muscle mass, coordination, and balance. History taking and assessment should include physical, cognitive, and functional assessments. Determination of risk factors for falls and frailty should be made. To assess risk of falls, balance and gait can be usefully evaluated routinely with the Get Up and Go test and the Tinetti Balance and Gait test.[26] The "Get Up and Go" test requires the patient to get up from a chair and return to a seated position in the chair after walking 3 m and turning around. It can be scored qualitatively on a scale from I (normal) to 5 (severely impaired) or quantitatively by timing each step.[26] The Tinetti Balance and Gait test is a standardized evaluation of mobility and stability and conveys a picture of the degree of difficulty a patient is experiencing with balance and ambulation.[26,27] Balance and gait are assessed and scored individually in a 16-item test.[26] For more extensive evaluation of gait and balance, other tests can be included, such as the Functional Reach Test, Berg Balance Test, and Performance Oriented Mobility Assessment.[28]

Muscle Strength, Muscle Mass, Coordination, and Balance

Interventions to improve muscle strength, muscle mass, coordination, and balance, such as exercise and proper nutrition, can improve outcomes for frailty and reduce the risk of falls. Interventions can be generally categorized into diet, exercise, supplements, and use of hormones.

Box 2
Management strategies for prevention of falls

- Modification of home environment after assessment by a health care professional can reduce risk of falling. These include lower bedrails, floor mats, nonslip tiles in the shower, and removal of unnecessary barriers to prevent falls.

- Discontinue, minimize, or taper psychoactive medications. Pay special attention to dose and drug interactions.

- Discontinue or minimize other medications. A prescribing modification program that includes a medication review checklist and pharmacist feedback can help reduce the risk of falling. A good understanding of general principles of pharmacology and therapeutics, dose modification, and possible interactions, especially in the geriatric population is essential.

- Manage postural hypotension.

- Manage foot problems and footwear. For example, footwear should have a high amount of surface area contact with the floor. Footwear with high heels and decreased surface area can increase risk of falls.

- Manage heart rate and rhythm abnormalities.

- Treat vision impairment. American Geriatrics Society recommends cautioning older adults with multifocal lenses to be more attentive to falling while walking, particularly on stairs.

- Educate cognitively intact patients, significant others, and caregivers on risk of falls and consequences, proper footwear, home hazard, and importance of regular exercise.

- Implement interventions aimed at improving muscle mass and strength, balance, and coordination.

Data from Refs.[16,27,29]

Diet

Many experts have recommended increasing the protein intake in the elderly to more than 0.8 g/kg/d.[30,31] A large amount of amino acid supplementation in one meal is more effective than intermittent protein intake. Protein supplementation with essential amino acids, especially leucine, will help maximize the anabolic effect.[17,32] Administering easily digestible protein or predigested protein is an interesting approach to maximizing postprandial protein anabolism.[33,34] In clinical practice, the authors often use high-quality whey protein, which provides an excellent balance of essential amino acids. In addition, it supports glutathione production, which positively affects oxidative stress and decreases inflammation.[35] Soy protein and isoflavone-enriched soy protein may also be helpful by counteracting chronic inflammation through regulation of the nuclear transcription factor κB signaling pathway and cytokine production.[35] Consumption of fatty fish rich in omega-3 fatty acids or fish oil supplements confer an anti-inflammatory effect by reducing proinflammatory cytokines involved in sarcopenia.[36] Redox modulators such as carotenoids may be important factors influencing loss of muscle strength and functional limitation.[37,38] Higher carotenoid and α-tocopherol status were independently associated with higher strength measures among older women living in the community.[37] Dietary sources for carotenoids include carrots, sweet potatoes, dark leafy greens, and tomatoes. Sources for α-tocopherol include spinach, broccoli, asparagus, pumpkin, seeds, and nuts, such as almonds, hazelnuts, pine nuts, Brazil nuts, and pistachios. The Mediterranean diet has been shown to reduce the risk of frailty (and thus risk of falls) over 6 years in community-dwelling adults ≥65 years.[39]

Exercise Resistance strength training has shown consistent benefits in improving and preventing decline in muscle strength and function.[16,17] Aerobic activities, such as walking, increase maximal oxygen consumption and improve muscle quality, neuromuscular adaptation, and muscle function.[17] Promoting an active lifestyle is of paramount importance because inactivity is an important contributor to loss of muscle mass and strength.[17]

Tai chi has the potential to reduce risk of falls in the elderly,[40] improve aerobic capacity,[41] and balance confidence in older adults.[42] Lower-extremity stretching exercises enhance balance in the elderly population and thereby can reduce the number of falls.[43] Yoga may also be beneficial in improving mobility and reducing fear of falling.[44] Simple yoga exercises, such as Tadasana (The Mountain Pose), Dronasana (The Bowel Pose), Uttana Vakrasana (The Spinal Twist Posture), Marjarasana (The Cat Stretch Pose), Ardha Shalabhasana (The Half-locust Pose), and Hastapadasana (Forward Bend Pose) can help in muscle stretching and improve muscle function (for specific instructions on the poses and technique, see www.yogicwayoflife.com and http://docslide.us/documents/lsm-lesson-18.html). Training with a professional instructor for yoga or tai chi is recommended for geriatric patients and especially for those who are new to these practices. Meditation and yogic pranayama (breathing exercises) help mindfulness and awareness for coordination and balance.

Supplements Vitamin D supplementation is universally accepted as one way of decreasing risk of falls and fractures. A Cochrane meta-analysis concluded that vitamin D supplementation did not reduce the risk of falls among community dwellers overall, but it did reduce the risk in those with low vitamin D levels at baseline (relative risk 0.70).[45] Vitamin D supplements of at least 800 to 1000 IU/d should be provided to older adults residing in long-term care settings with proven or suspected vitamin D insufficiency, abnormal gait, or imbalance, or who are otherwise at risk of falls.[46,47] Levels of 25-OH vitamin D should be measured in all older individuals and levels should be maintained higher than 30 ng/mL.[46,47]

Probiotics promote gastrointestinal (GI) microbiota that improve immune function and reduce inflammation.[48] Curcumin (found in the Indian curry yellow spice turmeric) has rich anti-inflammatory properties. Curcumin modulates the inflammatory response by downregulating production of inflammatory cytokines[49,50] involved in sarcopenia. Curcumin can be provided as food (1 tablespoon turmeric per day). Adding oil and black pepper during cooking enhances bioavailability. Curcumin can also be obtained through supplements, including the most researched product Meriva, which is available from several manufacturers. Typical dose is 500 to 1000 mg/d and is well tolerated.

Hormones A recent meta-analysis indicated that androgen treatment in the elderly moderately improved muscle strength.[51] However, despite growing evidence, testosterone or DHEA is not recommended for routine use to improve muscle strength and mass. Hormone replacement therapy in postmenopausal women has an unfavorable safety profile[52] and is therefore not recommended to improve muscle mass or strength.

Table 1 provides a summary of integrative approaches to prevent decline and improve muscle strength and coordination.

In the community, home-care, acute-care, and long-term care settings, screening for fall and injury risk should be performed during general annual physical examinations or routine health care visits using any standardized risk assessment tool such

Table 1
Integrative approaches to preventing decline and improving muscle strength and coordination

Diet	Mediterranean diet, anti-inflammatory diet (include fatty fish, more vegetables and fruits), increase carotenoid intake, soy
Exercise	Promote mobility, walking, resistance training, yoga, tai chi, comprehensive fall prevention programs
Supplements	Fish oil, vitamin D, whey protein, soy protein, and soy isoflavones, amino acid supplementation; anti-inflammatory herbs like curcumin, if general inflammation is present or suspected; role of vitamin E is not clear
Androgens/ testosterone	Only if deficiency state is present after careful assessment of risks; not recommended for routine use

as the Tinetti screening tool.[26–28] For patients who screen positive, referral to fall-injury prevention programs for focused fall-injury risk assessment and management is recommended. Providers should familiarize themselves with local geriatric fall prevention resources and American Geriatrics Society recommendations.[16]

OSTEOPOROSIS
Pathophysiology

Osteoporosis occurs when replacement of bone is slower than the rate of bone loss.[53] The prevalence of osteoporosis is 40% and 13% in women and men ≥50 years old, respectively.[54] In 2005, annual cost for osteoporosis-related fractures was $17 billion. It is estimated by 2025 the incidence and cost of osteoporotic fractures will increase by almost 50%.[55] Several factors play a role in the pathophysiology of osteoporosis: dysregulation of sex hormones, thyroid function, and nutritional factors are particularly notable. Chronic inflammation has also been proposed to be a contributing factor.[56] A comprehensive review of risk factors, screening, and treatment is beyond the scope of this article, but can be found in the American Association of Clinical Endocrinologists Medical Guidelines for Clinical Practice.[57]

Osteoporosis by itself it does not cause any symptoms. Often its first clinical manifestation is a fall-related fracture. Risk of spontaneous fractures in patients with osteopenia is less than 0.5%, but the risk increases to nearly 30% in patients with severe osteoporosis.[58]

Screening and diagnosis

Dual energy X-ray absorption (DXA) of a biologically relevant site, such as lumbar spine, forearm, and hip, is the only accepted screening test for osteoporosis. DXA assesses bone mineral density (BMD). The US Preventive Services Task Force recommends osteoporosis screening for women ≥65 years old and in younger women whose risk for fracture is greater than or equal to the fracture risk for a 65-year-old white woman with no other risk factors. For men, the Task Force concludes that there is insufficient evidence to make a recommendation. Furthermore, it is less clear at what age screening should be started if multiple risk factors are present.[59]

The World Health Organization (WHO) defines osteopenia as a DXA T-score of −1.0 SD to −2.5 SD as compared with Caucasian women aged 20 to 29 years. Osteoporosis is defined as a T-score ≤ −2.6 SD.[60] The fracture prediction assessment tool (FRAX) is the most commonly used assessment tool and estimates 10-year fracture probability with and without use of BMD. FRAX variations are based on country-specific data. Generally speaking, FRAX tends to underestimate true risk mostly because of not including individually important risk factors. The FRAX tool can easily be found online (http://www.shef.ac.uk/FRAX/tool.jsp?locationValue=9) and can be bookmarked by clinicians for easy access.

Bone markers Many practitioners use a variety of serum and urine markers of bone metabolism, mostly for treatment monitoring. Two most commonly used are serum C-terminal telopeptide collagen type 1 (CTx) and procollagen type 1 N-terminal propeptide (P1NP). CTx is a marker for bone resorption, and P1NP is a marker for bone formation. It is recommended that the test be performed at baseline before starting osteoporosis therapy and again 3 to 6 months later.[61]

Vitamin D A vitamin D level less than 20 ng/mL is a well-known contributor to osteoporosis. The target therapeutic level is 30 to 50 ng/mL.[53]

Prevention and treatment
Basic lifestyle recommendations for prevention and treatment of osteoporosis are similar, important, and reviewed in later discussion.

Diet

Given the link between inflammation and osteoporosis, anti-inflammatory dietary approaches may be helpful. Foods high in Ω-3 fatty acids are typically part of anti-inflammatory diets, including Mediterranean and others. High Ω-3 diets are associated with higher BMD and lower risk of osteoporosis, with the converse being true as well.[62–65] Studies have failed to link high animal protein diets to an increased risk of osteoporosis.[66] Furthermore, vegetarian diets low in protein have not been linked to lower BMD. However, vegans do have a higher risk of osteoporosis and lower BMD. This appears to be due to lower bioavailable calcium intake as a result of no dairy in the diet.[67]

Soy-based protein containing isoflavones is an excellent choice for a dietary plant-based protein source. It has been shown to improve calcium retention, stimulate bone formation, and suppress bone loss in animals and humans.[68] Large numbers of controlled and epidemiologic studies have been conducted assessing use of isoflavones from food and supplements for prevention and treatment of osteoporosis.[69] The data are heterogeneous, but growing evidence suggests soy may be a useful adjunctive dietary approach. Theoretic concerns about risks of thyroid dysregulation, and uterine and breast cancer have been largely disproven.[70] Many Asian diets are high in soy and often can provide as much as 200 mg of isoflavones per day. The authors recommend organic soy foods such as tofu, miso soup, soy milk, and others.

Exercise

A 2011 *Cochrane Review* found a small but likely important impact of exercise on BMD. Most effective was non-weight-bearing exercise, such as progressive resistance strength training for the legs.[71] This appears to contradict the common practice of recommending weight-bearing exercises. Of interest are a few less well-known methods shown to be effective in randomized controlled trials:

- Use of low-frequency vibratory plates has been shown in a randomized control trial to be effective in reducing the risk of fracture.[72] Plates for whole body vibration are available commercially varying from a few hundred to thousands of dollars and can also be found in fitness facilities.
- At least 12 minutes of daily yoga helps in prevention of osteoporosis.[73]

- Wayne and colleagues[74] conducted a systematic review of the effect of tai chi on BMD. They found that tai chi may be an effective, safe, and practical intervention for maintaining BMD in postmenopausal women.

Supplements

Adequate calcium intake

The recommended daily amount of total calcium intake increases to 1200 mg when women turn 50 and men turn 70. Intake should be no more than 2000 mg a day.[53] Several observational studies have linked supplemental calcium greater than 1000 mg daily to an increased risk of cardiovascular events. The association is not well established, and at least one review suggests there is no evidence to justify decreasing use of calcium supplements.[75] Assessing dietary intake of calcium for geriatric patients is important. Most people who are able to consume high-calcium foods (eg, dairy products, dark green leafy vegetables, canned salmon or sardines with bones, soy products, calcium-fortified cereals and orange juice) should be able to meet their calcium requirements from food alone.[53] For patients who are not able to consume sufficient dietary calcium, until future large well-designed randomized trials suggest otherwise, the authors recommend 600 to 1000 mg of calcium per day in divided doses. There are no clear data that any specific form of calcium is better than another. Thus, cost and tolerability should direct specific recommendations.

Vitamin D

All geriatric patients should be supplemented with vitamin D of at least 800 IU per day.[76] Patients who are vitamin D deficient should first have their deficiency treated, which often requires much higher doses (eg, 50,000 IU per week for 8 weeks). After that, a long-term individual maintenance dose should be established and maintained. Although vitamin D skin production from sun decreases in the elderly, it never fully stops. Thus, sun exposure can be a contributor to vitamin D stores, but must be balanced of course against an increased risk of skin cancer.[77]

Vitamin K

Although Vitamin K1 is best known for its role in blood clotting, it also plays an important role in muscle and bone metabolism. Vitamin K1 is an important cofactor in the conversion of osteocalcin into an active form to stimulate bone mineralization. In a 2-year randomized controlled trial, adding vitamin K1 to vitamin D and calcium led to increased BMD.[78] Vitamin K2 exists in several forms, including menoquinone-4 (MK4). Vitamin K2 is not available from food, and most of it is manufactured by normal gut microbes. A review of several human studies recommends supplementing with 45 mg of MK4 for all postmenopausal women with existing osteoporosis.[79,80] **Table 2** summarizes additional supplements, vitamins, and herbs.

Of note, strontium ranelate 2000 mg/d is approved for the treatment of osteoporosis in Europe but not in the United States. However, in 2014 the European Medicine Agency (EMA) published a report describing an increased risk of cardiovascular events[86] and thus restricted its use to only those patients who have no other treatment options. Strontium is widely available in the United States as a dietary supplement, typically in the citrate form. Given the EMA report, the authors strongly recommend avoiding any supplemental strontium except for trace amounts (typically <30 mg/d, which is the US Pharmacopeia orally permitted daily dose).

Given that a high proportion of elderly patients take multivitamins, one practical way of assuring adequate intake of many specific nutrients critical for prevention and treatment of osteoporosis is switching from a regular to bone-specific multivitamin. There are a number of products on the market that provide adequate doses of vitamin D,

Table 2
Common dietary supplements used for osteoporosis

Name	Mechanism of Action	Daily Dosing	Side Effects	References
Vitamin D	Increases GI and renal tubular calcium absorption	600–800 IU or more if deficient	Very high dose can cause diarrhea	76,77
Vitamin C	Essential collagen formation cofactor. High intake associated with lower bone loss in both elderly women and men	250–3000 mg	Diarrhea with high doses	81,82
Zinc	Enhances calcium absorption and vitamin D metabolism. High doses may negatively affect bone health	5–30 mg	Well tolerated at typical doses; prolonged high dose >50 mg/d can cause copper deficiency	83
Magnesium	Magnesium deficiency has been linked to increased risk of osteoporosis	100–500 mg; doses depend on the type and preparations	Magnesium can cause diarrhea if taken orally Caution advised in renal disease; high doses can increase bone loss	84,85
Manganese	Role is not clear, but both deficiency and toxicity are known to cause loss of bone	2–10 mg	Overdose of manganese can cause neurologic symptoms and has been described; high-dose supplementation should be avoided	83
Copper	Copper deficiency can block normal collagen production; dietary copper intake should be adequate	0.5–1 mg	Inorganic copper intake from supplements has been linked to increased risk of Alzheimer dementia	83
Vitamins K1, K2, and MK4	Important for conversion of osteocalcin into an active form to stimulate bone mineralization	MK4 45 mg	None reported; K1 should not be used in patients on anticoagulation	See text
Ω-3 fatty acids	EPA enhances calcium absorption and stimulates bone formation; high Ω6:Ω3 ratio associated with lower BMD	1–3 g of EPA/DHA Avoid using >4 g/d	"Fishy" aftertaste, bloating; high dose may increase risk of bleeding	See text
Soy Isoflavones	See text	50–300 mg of extract	Well tolerated; no increased risk of uterine cancer demonstrated	68–70

Abbreviations: DHA, Docosahexaenoic acid; EPA, Eicosapentaenoic acid.

calcium, vitamin C, magnesium, vitamin K1 and K2 as well as other important trace minerals such as manganese, boron, and silica. The authors recommend avoiding exceeding recommended daily allowances for copper and keeping the daily dose of manganese to less than 10 mg. Most bone-specific multivitamins have trace amounts of strontium (<25 mg), which is too low to be concerned about cardiac risk. In clinical practice, the authors often supplement with additional vitamin K2 because most commercially available bone-specific multivitamins provide less than 45 mg of MK4, best-evidenced dosage.

For a summary of common dietary supplements used for osteoporosis, purported mechanism, dosing, effectiveness, and adverse effects, please see **Table 2**.

Medications

Several medications beyond the commonly used bisphosphonates are US Food and Drug Administration (FDA) approved for the treatment of osteoporosis and are summarized in **Table 3**.

INTEGRATIVE PALLIATIVE CARE
Introduction

Integrative medicine and palliative care share much common ground. In both spheres, the patient is at the center of treatment decisions, and there is a focus on improving function and quality of life, while addressing the full range of mind, body, and spiritual needs.

Palliative medicine originated with the hospice movement in the 1960s and has recently been recognized as a distinct subspecialty by the American Board of Medical Specialties in 2006. Palliative care is defined according to the WHO as "an approach that improves the quality of life of patients and their families facing the problem associated with life-threatening illness, through the prevention and relief of suffering by means of early identification and impeccable assessment and treatment of pain and other problems, physical, psychosocial and spiritual."[87] Between 2015 and 2030, the number of persons aged 60 years or over is projected to grow by 56%, from 901 million to 1.4 billion, so the need for palliative care is likely to grow in tandem with this dramatic increase.[88]

Integrative medicine also focuses on developing a therapeutic partnership between the patient and their provider, blending the best of evidence-based mainstream and complementary treatments. This holistic approach is designed to treat the person not just the disease. Although a primary focus of palliative care is the relief of suffering, integrative medicine makes use of all appropriate therapies to achieve optimal health and healing as well as relieve suffering.

With this shared focus on compassionate care of the whole person, it is natural that integrative medicine and palliative care would work well together, combining the best elements of care to optimize symptom management and quality of life for patients.

Integrative Approaches to Palliative Symptom Management

Although symptoms vary from patient to patient depending on their disease processes, there are some commonly experienced symptoms toward the end of life and in those who are seriously ill. An integrative approach to the most common symptoms is presented.

Pain

See Robert Alan Bonakdar's article, "Integrative Pain Management," in this issue.

Table 3
Medications

Name	Type of Medication	Mechanism of action	Dosing	Possible Side Effects
Alendronate Risedronate Ibandronate	Bisphosphonates	Bind to hydroxyapatite in bone mineral and their inhibitory effects on mature osteoclasts	70 mg oral/wk 35 mg oral/wk or 5 mg daily 150 mg oral/mo or 3 mg IV every 3 mo+	Esophageal cancer, osteonecrosis of the jaw and femur fractures
Zoledronic acid			5 mg IV annually	Acute renal failure, myalgia, bone pain
Raloxifene	Hormone therapy	Selective estrogen receptor modulator that decreases bone resorption	60 mg oral daily	Deep vein thrombosis, stroke, breast cancer, and hot flashes
Estrogens	Hormone therapy	Decreases bone resorption	Individual dosing	Deep vein thrombosis, stroke, breast cancer, and hot flashes
Denosumab	Biological (monoclonal antibodies)	Monoclonal antibody directed against the receptor activator of the nuclear factor-kappa B ligand, which is essential for osteoclast activation	10 mg injection every 6 mo	Myalgia, eczema, skin infections, hypocalcemia; contraindicated in patients with hypocalcemia
Teriparatide	Recombinant parathyroid hormone	Stimulates osteoblast function	20 µg injection daily	Should be used for 2 y Hypercalcemia, Paget disease, osteosarcoma
Miacalcin	Calcitonin	Decreases osteoclast activity	200 IU daily intranasal	Rhinitis, irritation of nasal mucosa

Nausea and Vomiting

Nausea and vomiting are frequent complaints associated with cancer and its related therapies as well as other disease processes, especially toward the end of life. A thorough history and physical examination are essential as cause, and therefore, treatment can vary significantly. Nausea is mediated through the GI lining, vestibular system, cerebral cortex, and chemoreceptor trigger zone in the medulla oblongata. Common causes of nausea are dysmotility, obstruction, medication side effects, brain metastases, and vestibular apparatus irritation. Often overlooked, constipation is a common cause of nausea and vomiting and can be easily addressed.

Pharmaceuticals

Pharmacologic antiemetic agents abound and target a variety of receptors (including serotonin, dopamine, histamine, acetylcholine, neurokinin). **Table 4** lists typical first-line antiemetics for various common clinical scenarios. **Table 5** lists mechanism, dose, and side effects for commonly used antiemetics.

Nutrition/Botanicals

- Ginger has been shown to help with nausea in a variety of settings, including postoperative,[89] HIV/antiretroviral-induced,[90] and motion sickness. Ginger may also reduce chemotherapy-induced nausea, but data thus far have been conflicting.[91] A systematic review found 5 of 7 studies reported favorable results. Mixed results may be due to the varying dosages and formulations used in different studies.[92] Results from mixed-model analyses showed that all concentrations of ginger significantly reduced the incidence of acute, but not delayed, nausea, with 0.5 and 1.0 g being the most effective.[93]
  - Dosage: 500 to 1000 mg ginger root extract every 4–6 hours as needed, or 1 teaspoon eaten or 5 g of crystallized ginger every 2 to 3 hours as needed. Ginger tea can also be consumed.
  - Precautions/side effects: Avoid in thrombocytopenia given possible anticoagulant effects. Excessive doses can cause heartburn.

Medical marijuana Cannabis has been shown to help alleviate nausea and vomiting. A recent *Cochrane Review* analyzed 23 randomized controlled trials of cannabinoids compared with placebo or with other antiemetic drugs. Patients were more likely to report a complete absence of nausea and vomiting with cannabis than with placebo, and there was little discernible difference between the effectiveness of cannabinoids and prochlorperazine, metoclopramide, domperidone, or chlorpromazine. However, none of the trials involved the agents now most widely used—the serotonin 5-HT3 antagonists.[94] Cannabis contains several potentially therapeutic cannabinoids, including Δ^9-tetrahydrocannabinol (THC), the most psychoactive cannabinoid in the plant, and cannabidiol.

- Dosage
  - Dronabinol: 2.5 to 10 mg 3 or 4 times daily
  - Nabilone: 1 to 2 mg twice a day (maximum 6 mg divided in 3 doses daily)
  - Cannabis also available as a tincture, a transdermal patch, and other forms (to be applied topically, inhaled or ingested), from individual dispensaries, or can be edible.
- Precautions/side effects: Dry mouth, fatigue, dizziness, agitation, and poor memory. Side effects are significantly more common and more severe with high-dose pure THC products. Severe delirium has been reported from both nabilone and

Table 4
Clinical scenarios, mechanisms, and pharmacologic therapy for nausea and vomiting at the end of life

Clinical Scenario	Mechanism of Nausea and Vomiting	Typical First-Line Antiemetics
Opioid-induced nausea and vomiting	Stimulation of CTZ (D2) Gastroparesis (D2) Constipation (H1, muscarinic acetylcholine receptor) Sensitization of labyrinth (H1, muscarinic acetylcholine receptor)	Metoclopramide, haloperidol, prochlorperazine
Chemotherapy-induced nausea and vomiting	5HT3 released in gut, stimulating peripheral pathways Stimulation of CTZ (D2, 5HT3, NK1) Anxiety	5HT3 antagonists (such as ondansetron), dexamethasone, aprepitant
Malignant bowel obstruction	Stimulation of CTZ (D2) Stimulation of peripheral pathways (H1, muscarinic acetylcholine receptor)	Metoclopramide (if incomplete obstruction), haloperidol, dexamethasone, hyoscyamine, nasogastric tube, venting gastrostomy tube
Impaired GI tract mobility of advanced cancer	Gastroparesis (D2)	Metoclopramide
Radiation-associated nausea and vomiting	Stimulation of peripheral pathways via 5HT3 released from enterochromaffin cells in GI tract	5HT3 antagonists
Brain tumor	Increased ICP or meningeal irritation activate meningeal mechanoreceptors, which stimulate the vomiting center	Dexamethasone
Motion-associated nausea and vomiting	Stimulation via vestibulocochlear nerve (muscarinic acetylcholine receptor, H1)	Scopolamine, diphenhydramine, promethazine

Abbreviations: 5HT3, 5-hydroxytryptamine type 3 receptor; CTZ, chemoreceptor trigger zone; D2, dopamine type 2 receptor; H1, histamine type 1 receptor; ICP, intracranial pressure; NK1, neurokinin type 1 receptor.

Adapted from Wood GJ, Shega JW, Lynch B, et al. Management of intractable nausea and vomiting in patients at the end of life: "I was feeling nauseous all of the time... nothing was working". JAMA 2007;298(10):1201; with permission.

dronabinol. Most patients prefer the botanic form of cannabis for a variety of reasons, mostly because of the smallest chance of side effects and the easiest control of the dosage.

Acupuncture/Acupressure

Several studies show the benefit of acupuncture and acupressure for nausea and vomiting.[95] The use of acupressure, in the form of a wristband, popularly found under the name Sea-Band, has been used for chemotherapy-related nausea (and other

Table 5
Antiemetics: mechanism, dose, and adverse effects

Antiemetic	Presumed Primary Receptor Site of Action	Dosage/Route	Major Adverse Effects
Metoclopramide	D2 (primarily in GI tract) or 5HT3 (only at high doses)	5–20 mg PO, SC, or IV before every meal and before bed	Dystonia, akathisia, esophageal spasm, colic in GI tract and obstruction
Haloperidol	D2 (primarily in CTZ)	0.5–4 mg PO, SC, or IV every 6 h	Dystonia, akathisia
Prochlorperazine	D2 (primarily in CTZ)	5–10 mg PO or IV every 6 h or 25 mg rectally every 6 h	Dystonia, akathisia, sedation
Promethazine	H1, muscarinic acetylcholine receptor or D2 (primarily in CTZ)	12.5–25 mg PO or IV every 6 h or 25 mg rectally every 6 h	Dystonia, akathisia, sedation
Diphenhydramine	H1	25–50 mg PO, IV, or SC every 6 h	Sedation, dry mouth, urinary retention
Scopolamine	Muscarinic acetylcholine receptor	1.5 mg transdermal patch every 3 d	Dry mouth, blurred vision, ileus, urinary retention, confusion
Hyoscyamine	Muscarinic acetylcholine receptor	0.125–0.25 mg SL or PO every 4 h or 0.25–0.5 mg SC or IV every 4 h	Dry mouth, blurred vision, ileus, urinary retention, confusion
Ondansetron[a]	5HT3	4–8 mg PO or IV every 4–8 h	Headache, fatigue, constipation
Mirtazapine	5HT3	15–45 mg PO every night	Somnolence at low dose, dry mouth, increased appetite

Abbreviations: PO, oral; IV, Intravenous; SC, subcutaneous.

[a] Ondansetron is included as an example of 5HT3 antagonists because it was the first agent of this class and adopted in many hospital formularies. Its inclusion is not meant to indicate superiority over other members of the class, such as dolasetron, granisetron, and palonosetron.

Adapted from Wood GJ, Shega JW, Lynch B, et al. Management of intractable nausea and vomiting in patients at the end of life: "I was feeling nauseous all of the time... nothing was working". JAMA 2007;298(10):1202; with permission.

causes of nausea) with good effect.[96,97] Acu-stimulation bands like ReliefBand are also available.

Constipation

Constipation is a common and distressing symptom in the seriously ill. Fecal impaction is more common in older adults and can lead to urinary retention. Constipation is prevalent toward the end of life and involves a complex interaction of anatomic, neurologic, and iatrogenic factors.[98] Palliative medicine patients are at especially high risk due to the following factors:

- Low intake of food, fluid, and fiber
- Impaired mobility
- Opioid analgesics and other drugs that impair gut motility
- Complicating medical conditions, such as bowel obstruction or hemorrhoids[99]

Dehydration can lead to constipation, so taking in adequate fluid is important. Drinking 8 to 12 glasses of water daily is recommended if possible. In addition, flaxseed meal or oil (1 tablespoon on cereal or mixed in water/juice/smoothie 3 times a day) can help.[100,101] No data support the use of one laxative over another. In the palliative care population, the mainstay of constipation treatment is to start with a bowel stimulant (eg, senna) and escalate dose as needed. Osmotic agents (eg, polyethylene glycol, milk of magnesia) may be added if necessary. Suppositories, enemas, or manual disimpaction may also be required. A rectal examination should be performed to rule out fecal impaction and a KUB (kidney, ureters, and bladder radiograph) should be considered to rule out obstruction. A stool softener and/or laxative should be started prophylactically and given regularly with the start of any opioid. In general, bulk-forming fiber agents (eg, psyllium, methylcellulose) have little role in palliative care because of their tendency to form impactions when patients stop drinking adequate amounts of fluids. There are limited data supporting the use of newer small intestinal secretagogues (eg, lubiprostone and linaclotide) at the end of life. Various therapies are summarized in **Table 6**.

Dyspnea

Dyspnea is defined as "a subjective feeling of breathing discomfort."[96] Dyspnea is experienced by almost all terminally ill patients at some point. There are several possible causes, and dyspnea is often multifactorial. Common causes include infection, fluid overload, malignancy, muscle weakness, COPD, and anxiety. If possible, address any underlying (and potentially reversible) causes first. If dyspnea still remains after disease-focused treatment, focus then on treating dyspnea with palliative measures.

Behavioral
Positioning can impact a patient's sensation of breathing comfort. Many patients find that sitting up can bring greater ease of breathing. Increasing air movement by opening a window or placing a fan in front of a patient's face can improve symptoms.[102] In addition, increasing or decreasing humidity by using a humidifier or air conditioner, respectively, can be helpful. Breathing exercises, guided imagery, and hypnotherapy can also help reduce anxiety, which often contributes to dyspnea. In addition, discontinuing intravenous fluids in imminently dying patients is appropriate.

Pharmaceuticals
Opiates are the mainstay of medical treatment of dyspnea at the end of life as well as dyspnea refractory to disease-focused treatments. **Table 7** lists opioid dosage recommendations.

Treatment with other medications can be helpful: anticholinergics for secretions (eg, scopolamine transdermal patch, atropine drops, glycopyrrolate intravenous/subcutaneous [IV/SC], or hyoscyamine tablets); benzodiazepines (eg, lorazepam) for anxiety; bronchodilators, corticosteroids, and diuretics for their disease-modifying effects.

Supplemental oxygen
Widespread use of oxygen is not recommended for relief of dyspnea, even in the dying phase.[103] However, a therapeutic trial of oxygen supplementation in hypoxemic patients may be helpful. For nonhypoxemic patients, although no data support supplemental oxygen use, some patients may report relief. Use of oxygen in hypoxemic and nonhypoxemic dying patients should therefore be based on symptom relief, not pulse oximetry. Patients generally prefer nasal cannula, but masks or face tents can also be used.

Table 6
Prevention and treatment of constipation

Medication	Dosage and Frequency	Comments
Stool softener (detergent laxative)		
Docusate sodium (capsules/tablets or liquid)	Starting dose: 100 mg PO twice daily or 200 mg; titrate dose up to 2 or 3 times daily, max. 600 mg daily	Generally well tolerated and safe; usually insufficient if used alone
Stimulants		
Senna	1 tablet PO daily; titrate up to 4 tablets PO twice daily	Useful when added to docusate; can cause cramping; can worsen colic in bowel obstruction
Bisacodyl	Start with 1 (5 mg) tablet PO daily; titrate to 3 tablets twice daily; suppository 10 mg PR daily PRN	Can worsen colic in bowel obstruction; suppository causes more cramping than glycerin suppository; can cause more cramping than senna
Osmotic agents		
Glycerin suppository	1 PR daily PRN	Acts as both lubricant and osmotic agent; generally well tolerated, but rarely adequate alone
Sorbitol	15–60 mL PO 2 to 4 times daily	Sweet taste can be unpleasant; can cause bloating
Lactulose (10 g/15 mL)	15–60 mL PO 2 or 3 times daily	More expensive than sorbitol but with similar efficacy and side effects
Polyethylene glycol	17 g powder dissolved in liquid PO 1 to 3 times daily	Tasteless; often well tolerated; available over the counter
Magnesium hydroxide	15–30 mL daily PRN	Can cause cramping; avoid in renal failure as magnesium accumulation could be toxic
Magnesium citrate	200–400 mg powder daily in divided doses; 195–300 mL oral solution given once or in divided doses	Can cause cramping; avoid in renal failure as magnesium accumulation could be toxic
Enemas		
Warm "tap" water	Can repeat daily or twice daily	Administration can soften stool before manual disimpaction
Saline or sodium phosphate	NA	*Use Is Not Recommended*: High electrolyte load may cause dehydration, renal failure, exacerbation of hepatic or cardiac failure; risk highest in pediatric and older patients
Mineral oil	118 mL as a single dose	Oral intake should be avoided due to risk of severe pneumonitis if aspirated; PR administration can soften stools before manual disimpaction

(continued on next page)

Table 6
(continued)

Medication	Dosage and Frequency	Comments
Milk and molasses (or corn syrup)	1:1 whole milk to molasses ratio (<300 mL total)	Combines both osmotic and colonic stimulant
Soap suds	NA	*Not Recommended*: colon irritant, risk of bowel-wall damage with large dose or repeated use
Other agents		
Prune juice	120–240 mL PO 1 or 2 times daily	Combines both soluble fiber and stimulant; a recognized traditional approach; good adjuvant
Metoclopramide	10–20 mg PO every 6 h	Promotility agent; contraindicated in complete bowel obstruction; potential for tardive dyskinesia (FDA black box warning); avoid prolonged use
Methylnaltrexone	0.15 mg/kg of body weight (up to 12 mg) SC injection every other day	Rule out bowel obstruction before use; requires SC injection; usually produces bowel movement within 30 min; peripheral μ-opioid receptor antagonist; effectively treats opioid-induced constipation without reversing analgesia or precipitating withdrawal; expensive, generally used as rescue therapy in refractory cases
Lubiprostone	8–24 μg PO twice daily with food	Chloride channel activator; FDA approved for constipation-predominant irritable bowel syndrome and chronic idiopathic constipation; may cause nausea

Abbreviations: PR, rectal; PRN, as needed.
Adapted from Quill TE, Bower KA, Holloway RG, et al. Primer of palliative care. 6th edition. Chicago (IL): American Academy of Hospice and Palliative Medicine; 2014. p. 82–3; with permission.

Fatigue

Fatigue is one of the most common end-of-life symptoms across all disease states. Prevalence estimates of fatigue range from 48% to as high as 97%.[96] Reported prevalence rates are highest among those with cancer. However, patients with chronic or end-stage renal, hepatic, pulmonary, or cardiac disease, HIV, or neurologic disease also frequently experience fatigue, which has been associated with poorer quality of life.[104,105] Fatigue has been defined as "a subjective feeling of tiredness, weakness, or lack of energy" and may have both physical and cognitive dimensions.[96] Fatigue is frequently multifactorial, and as always, a thorough history and physical examination are essential to diagnosing underlying factors. In many cases, patients experience primary fatigue (related directly to disease mechanism) in addition to secondary fatigue

Table 7
Opioid dosing for management of dyspnea

Opioid Tolerance	Dosage
Opioid naive	5 mg PO morphine equivalent as single dose; if tolerated, can administer every 4 h around the clock, hold for sedation; an additional dose every hour in between scheduled doses can be made available PRN for severe dyspnea
Older adults, CO_2 retainers, or patients with renal impairment	Consider reducing starting dose by half; avoid use of morphine in renal disease
If current opioid dosage is inadequate	Titrate by increments of 25% to 50% to effect
Dyspnea with exertion or movement	Give 30 min before activity
If acutely dyspneic or actively dying	Use IV morphine bolus (2–5 mg or 10% of daily dosage) every 5–10 min PRN, titrate to effect (decline of self-reported dyspnea on 10-point scale); consider starting a continuous infusion based on the dosage needed to improve the patient's symptoms For patients who cannot self-report, an improvement of nonverbal signs of distress or a decline in elevated respiratory rate toward the normal range may be used as surrogate markers of dyspnea
If on stable opioid dosage	Consider a trial of scheduled short-acting opioid or long-acting opioid as baseline, with immediate-release opioid PRN in between

Abbreviation: CO_2, carbon dioxide.
From Brown DJF. Palliative care. Clin Med 2006;6:135; with permission.

(related to non-disease-specific factors that are often reversible, eg, medications, untreated pain, infection, sleep apnea). There are limited data to guide treatment of fatigue at end of life, and most research to date has focused on stimulants; however, results have been mixed.

In cases of primary fatigue, several nonpharmacologic approaches may be helpful. Educating patients about sleep hygiene can help improve sleep quality and decrease daytime fatigue. Meta-analyses evaluating the effect of various exercise programs on fatigue in patients with cancer have found that physical exercise improved fatigue.[106] However, it is unclear what the optimal exercise intensity and duration are. Given that functional status may be limited in the seriously ill, an individualized exercise plan is recommended based on each individual's capabilities. There is evidence that gentle or chair yoga can improve symptoms of fatigue in cancer[107,108] and end-stage renal disease.[109] Studies suggest that massage, acupuncture, and reiki may also play a beneficial role in reducing fatigue in patients with cancer.[110–112] Meditation can improve fatigue in several conditions, including heart failure and cancer.[113–115] Hypnosis in combination with cognitive behavioral therapy has been shown to help fatigue in patients with breast cancer and may help fatigue in other patient populations.[116]

SUMMARY

Integrative Medicine blends the best evidence-based practices of mainstream and complementary medicine to provide effective, patient-centered care. This holistic focus on the patient, rather than the disease, is particularly well suited to the many complex conditions commonly seen in chronically ill and aging populations.

Focusing on simple preventive measures, diet, and lifestyle changes can optimize function and quality of life, while actually being more cost-effective than conventional forms of care. By using the least toxic intervention that effectively improves symptoms or function, many of the common side effects of polypharmacy or complications of more invasive treatments can be avoided. Although much more research is needed to elucidate best integrative geriatric practices, the rapidly growing geriatric population creates a large impetus to provide the type of care described in this article.[117] The authors hope that more clinical, training, and research programs in integrative geriatrics will be developed in the near future to address these specific needs of the worldwide growing aging population.

ACKNOWLEDGMENTS

The authors would like to acknowledge Bianca Palushaj, MS2 at George Washington University School of Medicine, for her assistance with this article.

REFERENCES

1. Spoorenberg SLW, Uittenbroek RJ, Middel B, et al. Embrace, a model for integrated elderly care: study protocol of a randomized controlled trial on the effectiveness regarding patient outcomes, service use, costs, and quality of care. BMC Geriatr 2013;13(1):62.
2. World Health Organization. Innovative care for chronic conditions: building blocks for action. Geneva (Switzerland); 2002.
3. Smith M, Saunders R, Stuckhardt L, et al, editors. Medicine I of. Best care at lower cost: the path to continuously learning health care in America. Washington, DC: The National Academies Press; 2012.
4. Marengoni A, Angleman S, Melis R, et al. Aging with multimorbidity: a systematic review of the literature. Ageing Res Rev 2011;10(4):430–9.
5. Vogeli C, Shields AE, Lee TA, et al. Multiple chronic conditions: prevalence, health consequences, and implications for quality, care management, and costs. J Gen Intern Med 2007;22(Suppl 3):391–5.
6. Spalding MC, Sebesta SC. Geriatric screening and preventive care. Am Fam Physician 2008;78(2):206–15.
7. Rao SS. Prevention of falls in older patients. Am Fam Physician 2005;72(1):81–8.
8. Vellas BJ, Wayne SJ, Romero LJ, et al. Fear of falling and restriction of mobility in elderly fallers. Age Ageing 1997;26:189–93.
9. Lin JT, Lane JM. Falls in the elderly population. Phys Med Rehabil Clin N Am 2005;16(1):109–28.
10. Fried LP, Ferrucci L, Darer J, et al. Untangling the concepts of disability, frailty, and comorbidity: implications for improved targeting and care. J Gerontol A Biol Sci Med Sci 2004;59:255–63.
11. Fried LP, Tangen CM, Walston J, et al. Frailty in older adults: evidence for a phenotype. J Gerontol Med Sci 2001;56A:M146–56.
12. Abellan van Kan G, Rolland Y, Houles M, et al. The assessment of frailty in older adults. Clin Geriatr Med 2010;26(2):275–86.
13. Studenski S, Hayes RP, Leibowitz RQ, et al. Clinical global impression of change in physical frailty: development of a measure based on clinical judgment. J Am Geriatr Soc 2004;52(9):1560–6.

14. Institute of Medicine (US) Division of Health Promotion and Disease Prevention, Berg RL, Cassells JS, editors. The second fifty years: promoting health and preventing disability. Washington, DC: National Academies Press (US); 1992. p. 15. Falls in older persons: risk factors and prevention. Available at: https://www.ncbi.nlm.nih.gov/books/NBK235613/. Accessed April 25, 2017.

15. Rubenstein LZ. Falls in older people: epidemiology, risk factors and strategies for prevention. Age Ageing 2006;35(Suppl 2):ii37–41.

16. American Geriatrics Society and British Geriatrics Society. Summary of the Updated American Geriatrics Society/British Geriatrics Society clinical practice guideline for prevention of falls in older persons. J Am Geriatr Soc 2011;59(1): 148–57. Available at: http://geriatricscareonline.org/ProductAbstract/updated-american-geriatrics-societybritish-geriatrics-society-clinical-practice-guideline-for-prevention-of-falls-in-older-persons-and-recommendations/CL014.

17. Rolland Y, Czerwinski S, Abellan Van Kan G, et al. Sarcopenia: its assessment, etiology, pathogenesis, consequences and future perspectives. J Nutr Health Aging 2008;12(7):433–50.

18. Dionne IJ, Kinaman KA, Poehlman ET. Sarcopenia and muscle function during menopause and hormone-replacement therapy. J Nutr Health Aging 2000; 4(3):156–61.

19. Jacobsen DE, Samson MM, Kezic S, et al. Postmenopausal HRT and tibolone in relation to muscle strength and body composition. Maturitas 2007;58(1):7–18.

20. Morley JE, Kaiser FE, Perry HM 3rd, et al. Longitudinal changes in testosterone, luteinizing hormone, and follicle stimulating hormone in healthy older men. Metabolism 1997;46(4):410–3.

21. Bhasin S, Woodhouse SL, Storer TW. Proof of the effect of testosterone on skeletal muscle. J Endocrinol 2001;170:27–38.

22. Genazzani AD, Lanzoni C, Genazzani AR. Might DHEA be considered a beneficial replacement therapy in the elderly? Drugs Aging 2007;24(3):173–85.

23. Szulc P, Duboeuf F, Marchand F, et al. Hormonal and lifestyle determinants of appendicular skeletal muscle mass in men: the MINOS study. Am J Clin Nutr 2004;80(2):496–503.

24. Bischoff-Ferrari HA, Dawson-Hughes B, Willett WC, et al. Effect of vitamin D on falls: a meta-analysis. JAMA 2004;291(16):1999–2006.

25. Schaap LA, Pluijm SM, Deeg DJ, et al. Inflammatory markers and loss of muscle mass (sarcopenia) and strength. Am J Med 2006;119(6):526.e9-17.

26. Vaught SL. Gait, balance, and fall prevention. Ochsner J 2001;3(2):94–7.

27. Tinetti ME. Performance-oriented assessment of mobility problems in elderly patients. J Am Geriatr Soc 1986;34:119–26.

28. Persad CC, Cook S, Giordani B. Assessing falls in the elderly: should we use simple screening tests or a comprehensive fall risk evaluation? Eur J Phys Rehabil Med 2010;46(2):249–59.

29. Lukaszyk C, Harvey L, Sherrington C, et al. Risk factors, incidence, consequences and prevention strategies for falls and fall-injury within older indigenous populations: a systematic review. Aust N Z J Public Health 2016;40(6): 564–8.

30. Campbell WW, Evans WJ. Protein requirements of elderly people. Eur J Clin Nutr 1996;50(Suppl 1):S180–3.

31. Campbell WW, Trappe TA, Wolfe RR, et al. The recommended dietary allowance for protein may not be adequate for older people to maintain skeletal muscle. J Gerontol A Biol Sci Med Sci 2001;56(6):M373–80.

32. Arnal MA, Mosoni L, Boirie Y, et al. Protein pulse feeding improves protein retention in elderly women. Am J Clin Nutr 1999;69(6):1202–8.
33. Boirie Y, Dangin M, Gachon P, et al. Slow and fast dietary proteins differently modulate postprandial protein accretion. Proc Natl Acad Sci U S A 1997; 94(26):14930–5.
34. Dangin M, Boirie Y, Guillet C, et al. Influence of the protein digestion rate on protein turnover in young and elderly subjects. J Nutr 2002;132(10):3228S–33S.
35. Draganidis D, Karagounis LG, Athanailidis I, et al. Inflammaging and skeletal muscle: can protein intake make a difference? J Nutr 2016;146(10):1940–52.
36. Robinson SM, Jameson KA, Batelaan SF, et al. Diet and its relationship with grip strength in community-dwelling older men and women: the Hertfordshire cohort study. J Am Geriatr Soc 2008;56(1):84–90.
37. Semba RD, Lauretani F, Ferrucci L. Carotenoids as protection against sarcopenia in older adults. Arch Biochem Biophys 2007;458(2):141–5.
38. Semba RD, Blaum C, Guralnik JM, et al. Carotenoid and vitamin E status are associated with indicators of sarcopenia among older women living in the community. Aging Clin Exp Res 2003;15:482–7.
39. Talegawkar SA, Bandinelli S, Bandeen-Roche K, et al. A higher adherence to a Mediterranean-style diet is inversely associated with the development of frailty in community-dwelling elderly men and women. J Nutr 2012;142(12):2161–6.
40. Taylor-Piliae RE. The effectiveness of Tai Chi exercise in improving aerobic capacity: an updated meta-analysis. Med Sport Sci 2008;52:40–53.
41. Leung DP, Chan CK, Tsang HW, et al. Tai chi as an intervention to improve balance and reduce falls in older adults: a systematic and meta-analytical review. Altern Ther Health Med 2011;17(1):40–8.
42. Liu H, Frank A. Tai chi as a balance improvement exercise for older adults: a systematic review. J Geriatr Phys Ther 2010;33(3):103–9.
43. Reddy RS, Alahmari KA. Effect of lower extremity stretching exercises on balance in geriatric population. Int J Health Sci (Qassim) 2016;10(3):389–95.
44. Galantino ML, Green L, DeCesari JA, et al. Safety and feasibility of modified chair-yoga on functional outcome among elderly at risk for falls. Int J Yoga 2012;5(2):146–50.
45. American Geriatrics Society. Recommendations abstracted from the American Geriatrics Society consensus statement on vitamin D for prevention of falls and their consequences. J Am Geriatr Soc 2014;62(1):147–52.
46. Gillespie L, Robertson M, Gillespie W, et al. Interventions for preventing falls in older people living in the community. Cochrane Database Syst Rev 2012;(9):CD007146.
47. Drinka PJ, Krause PF, Nest LJ, et al. Determinants of vitamin D levels in nursing home residents. J Am Med Dir Assoc 2007;8(2):76–9.
48. Li D, Wang P, Wang P, et al. The gut microbiota: a treasure for human health. Biotechnol Adv 2016;34(7):1210–24.
49. Goel A, Kunnumakkara AB, Aggarwal BB. Curcumin as "Curecumin": from kitchen to clinic. Biochem Pharmacol 2008;75:787–809.
50. Abe Y, Hashimoto S, Horie T. Curcumin inhibition of inflammatory cytokine production by human peripheral blood monocytes and alveolar macrophages. Pharmacol Res 1999;39:41–7.
51. Ottenbacher KJ, Ottenbacher ME, Ottenbacher AJ, et al. Androgen treatment and muscle strength in elderly men: a meta-analysis. J Am Geriatr Soc 2006; 54(11):1666–73.

52. Rossouw JE, Anderson GL, Prentice RL, et al. Risks and benefits of estrogen plus progestin in healthy postmenopausal women: principal results from the Women's Health Initiative randomized controlled trial. JAMA 2002;288:321–33.

53. MedlinePlus Osteoprosis US National Library of Medicine. Available at: https://medlineplus.gov/osteoporosis.html. Accessed April 25, 2017.

54. Looker AC, Borrud LG, Dawson-Hughes B, et al. Osteoporosis or low bone mass at the femur neck or lumbar spine in older adults: United States, 2005-2008. NCHS Data Brief 2012;(93):1–8. Available at: http://www.ncbi.nlm.nih.gov/pubmed/22617299.

55. Burge R, Dawson-Hughes B, Solomon DH, et al. Incidence and economic burden of osteoporosis-related fractures in the United States, 2005–2025. J Bone Miner Res 2007;22(3):465–75.

56. Straub RH, Cutolo M, Pacifici R. Evolutionary medicine and bone loss in chronic inflammatory diseases-a theory of inflammation-related osteopenia. Semin Arthritis Rheum 2015;45(2):220–8.

57. Watts NB, Bilezikian JP, Camacho PM, et al. American Association of Clinical Endocrinologists medical guidelines for clinical practice for the diagnosis and treatment of postmenopausal osteoporosis: executive summary of recommendations. Endocr Pract 2010;16(6):1016–9.

58. Viceconti M, Taddei F, Cristofolini L, et al. Are spontaneous fractures possible? An example of clinical application for personalised, multiscale neuro-musculo-skeletal modelling. J Biomech 2012;45(3):421–6.

59. US Preventive Task Force Osteoporosis Screening DEXA. Available at: https://www.uspreventiveservicestaskforce.org/Page/Document/UpdateSummaryFinal/osteoporosis-screening. Accessed April 25, 2017.

60. WHO Osteoporosis Review. Available at: http://www.who.int/chp/topics/Osteoporosis.pdf.

61. Bauer D, Krege J, Lane N, et al. National bone health alliance bone turnover marker project: current practices and the need for US harmonization, standardization, and common reference ranges. Osteoporos Int 2012;23(10):2425–33.

62. Chen Y, Ho SC, Lam SS. Higher sea fish intake is associated with greater bone mass and lower osteoporosis risk in postmenopausal Chinese women. Osteoporos Int 2010;21(6):939–46.

63. Weiss LA, Barrett-Connor E, Von Mühlen D. Ratio of n-6 to n-3 fatty acids and bone mineral density in older adults: the rancho bernardo study. Am J Clin Nutr 2005;81(4):934–8.

64. Pizzorno J, Frassetto LA, Katzinger J. Diet-induced acidosis: is it real and clinically relevant? Br J Nutr 2010;103(8):1185–94. Available at: http://journals.cambridge.org/abstract_S0007114509993047.

65. Buclin T, Cosma M, Appenzeller M, et al. Diet acids and alkalis influence calcium retention in bone. Osteoporos Int 2001;12(6):493–9.

66. Calvez J, Poupin N, Chesneau C, et al. Protein intake, calcium balance and health consequences. Eur J Clin Nutr 2012;66(3):281–95.

67. Burckhardt P. The role of low acid load in vegetarian diet on bone health: a narrative review. Swiss Med Wkly 2016;146:w14277.

68. Pawlowski JW, Martin BR, McCabe GP, et al. Impact of equol-producing capacity and soy-isoflavone profiles of supplements on bone calcium retention in postmenopausal women: a randomized crossover trial[1,2]. Am J Clin Nutr 2015;102(3):695–703.

69. Zheng X, Lee S-K, Chun OK. Soy isoflavones and osteoporotic bone loss: a review with an emphasis on modulation of bone remodeling. J Med Food 2016; 19(1):1–14. Available at: http://www.ncbi.nlm.nih.gov/pubmed/26670451.

70. Alekel DL, Genschel U, Koehler KJ, et al. Soy isoflavones for reducing bone loss study. Menopause 2015;22(2):185–97.

71. Bonaiuti D, Shea B, Iovine R, et al. Exercise for preventing and treating osteoporosis in postmenopausal women. Cochrane Database Syst Rev 2002;(3):CD000333.

72. Gusi N, Raimundo A, Leal A. Low-frequency vibratory exercise reduces the risk of bone fracture more than walking: a randomized controlled trial. BMC Musculoskelet Disord 2006;7(1):92. Available at: http://www.biomedcentral.com/1471-2474/7/92.

73. Lu YH, Rosner B, Chang G, et al. Twelve-minute daily yoga regimen reverses osteoporotic bone loss. Top Geriatr Rehabil 2015;32(2):81–7. Available at: www.topicsingeriatricrehabilitation.com.

74. Wayne PM, Kiel DP, Krebs DE, et al. The effects of Tai Chi on bone mineral density in postmenopausal women: a systematic review. Arch Phys Med Rehabil 2007;88(5):673–80.

75. Rautiainen S, Wang L, Manson JE, et al. The role of calcium in the prevention of cardiovascular disease-a review of observational studies and randomized clinical trials. Curr Atheroscler Rep 2013;15(11):362.

76. NIH Vitamin D recommendation. Available at: https://ods.od.nih.gov/factsheets/VitaminD-HealthProfessional/.

77. Holick MF, Chen TC, Lu Z, et al. Vitamin D and skin physiology: a D-lightful story. J Bone Miner Res 2007;22(Suppl 2):V28–33.

78. Bolton-Smith C, McMurdo MET, Paterson CR, et al. Two-year randomized controlled trial of vitamin K1 (phylloquinone) and vitamin D3 plus calcium on the bone health of older women. J Bone Miner Res 2007;22(4):509–19.

79. Villa JKD, Diaz MAN, Pizziolo VR, et al. Effect of vitamin K in bone metabolism and vascular calcification: a review of mechanisms of action and evidences. Crit Rev Food Sci Nutr 2016. http://dx.doi.org/10.1080/10408398.2016.1211616.

80. Inaba N, Sato T, Yamashita T. Low-dose daily intake of vitamin K_2 (menaquinone-7) improves osteocalcin gamma-carboxylation: a double-blind, randomized controlled trials. J Nutr Sci Vitaminol (Tokyo) 2015;61(6):471–80.

81. Morton DJ, Barrett-Connor EL, Schneider DL. Vitamin C supplement use and bone mineral density in postmenopausal women. J Bone Miner Res 2001; 16(1):135–40.

82. Sahni S, Hannan MT, Gagnon D, et al. High vitamin C intake is associated with lower 4-year bone loss in elderly men. J Nutr 2008;138(10):1931–8. Available at: http://www.pubmedcentral.nih.gov/articlerender.fcgi?artid=2752366&tool=pmcentrez&rendertype=abstract.

83. Price CT, Langford JR, Liporace FA. Essential nutrients for bone health and a review of their availability in the average north american diet. Open Orthop J 2012; 6:143–9.

84. Castiglioni S, Cazzaniga A, Albisetti W, et al. Magnesium and osteoporosis: current state of knowledge and future research directions. Nutrients 2013;5(8): 3022–33.

85. Jugdaohsingh R. Silicon and bone health. J Nutr Health Aging 2007;11(2): 99–110.

86. Strontium renelate UK Gov safety concern. Available at: https://www.gov.uk/drug-safety-update/strontium-ranelate-cardiovascular-risk. Accessed April 25, 2017.

87. WHO Definition of Palliative Care. World Health Organization Website. 2016. Available at: http://www.who.int/cancer/palliative/definition/en/. Accessed October 30, 2016.

88. UN human rights of older persons resolution. United Nations Website. 2016. Available at: http://www.un.org/ga/search/view_doc.asp?symbol=A/HRC/33/l.9. Accessed October 30, 2016.

89. Mandal P, Das A, Majumdar S, et al. The efficacy of ginger added to ondansetron for preventing postoperative nausea and vomiting in ambulatory surgery. Pharmacognosy Res 2014;6(1):52–7.

90. Dabaghzadeh F, Khalili H, Dashti-Khavidaki S, et al. Ginger for prevention of antiretroviral-induced nausea and vomiting: a randomized clinical trial. Expert Opin Drug Saf 2014;13(7):859–66.

91. Marx W, McCarthy AL, Ried K, et al. Can ginger ameliorate chemotherapy-induced nausea? Protocol of a randomized double blind, placebo-controlled trial. BMC Complement Altern Med 2014;14(1):134.

92. Marx WM, Teleni L, McCarthy AL, et al. Ginger (Zingiber officinale) and chemotherapy-induced nausea and vomiting: a systematic literature review. Nutr Rev 2013;71(4):245–54.

93. Ryan JL, Heckler CE, Roscoe JA, et al. Ginger (Zingiber officinale) reduces acute chemotherapy-induced nausea: a URCC CCOP study of 576 patients. Support Care Cancer 2012;20(7):1479–89.

94. Smith LA, Azariah F, Lavender VTC, et al. Cannabinoids for nausea and vomiting in adults with cancer receiving chemotherapy. Cochrane Database Syst Rev 2015;(11):CD009464.

95. Rithirangsriroj K, Manchana T, Akkayagorn L. Efficacy of acupuncture in prevention of delayed chemotherapy induced nausea and vomiting in gynecologic cancer patients. Gynecol Oncol 2015;136(1):82–6.

96. Molassiotis A, Helin AM, Dabbour R, et al. The effects of P6 acupressure in the prophylaxis of chemotherapy-related nausea and vomiting in breast cancer patients. Complement Ther Med 2007;15(1):3–12.

97. Taspinar A, Sirin A. Effect of acupressure on chemotherapy-induced nausea and vomiting in gynecologic cancer patients in Turkey. Eur J Oncol Nurs 2010;14(1):49–54.

98. Sykes N. The pathogenesis of constipation. J Support Oncol 2006;4(5):213–8.

99. Quill TE, Bower KA, Holloway RG, et al. Primer of palliative care. 6th edition. Chicago(IL): American Academy of Hospice and Palliative Medicine; 2014.

100. Ramos CI, de Lima AF, Grilli DG, et al. The short-term effects of olive oil and flaxseed oil for the treatment of constipation in hemodialysis patients. J Ren Nutr 2015;25(1):50–6.

101. Aliasghari F, et al. Application of laxative foods in prevention and treatment of constipation. MOJ Food Process Technol 2016;2(4):00045.

102. Galbraith S, Fagan P, Perkins P, et al. Does the use of a handheld fan improve chronic dyspnea? A randomized, controlled, crossover trial. J Pain Symptom Manag 2010;39(5):831–8.

103. Campbell ML, Yarandi H, Dove-Medows E. Oxygen is nonbeneficial for most patients who are near death. J Pain Symptom Manage 2013;45:517.

104. Walke LM, Gallo WT, Tinetti ME, et al. The burden of symptoms among community-dwelling older persons with advanced chronic disease. Arch Intern Med 2004;164(21):2321–4.
105. Horigan AE. Fatigue in hemodialysis patients: a review of current knowledge. J Pain Symptom Manage 2012;44(5):715–24.
106. Tomlinson D, Diorio C, Beyene J, et al. Effect of exercise on cancer-related fatigue: a meta-analysis. Am J Phys Med Rehabil 2014;93(8):675–86.
107. Buffart LM, van Uffelen JG, Riphagen II, et al. Physical and psychosocial benefits of yoga in cancer patients and survivors, a systematic review and meta-analysis of randomized controlled trials. BMC Cancer 2012;12:559.
108. Pachman DR, Barton DL, Swetz KM, et al. Troublesome symptoms in cancer survivors: fatigue, insomnia, neuropathy, and pain. J Clin Oncol 2012;30(30): 3687–96.
109. Yurtkuran M, Alp A, Dilek K. A modified yoga-based exercise program in hemodialysis patients: a randomized controlled study. Complement Therap Med 2007;15(3):164–71.
110. Lau CHY, Wu X, Chung VCH, et al. Acupuncture and related therapies for symptom management in palliative cancer care: systematic review and meta-analysis. Medicine 2016;95(9):e2901.
111. Boyd C, Crawford C, Paat CF, et al. The impact of massage therapy on function in pain populations—A systematic review and meta-analysis of randomized controlled trials: part II, cancer pain populations. Pain Med 2016;17(8):1553–68.
112. Fleisher KA, Mackenzie ER, Frankel ES, et al. Integrative reiki for cancer patients a program evaluation. Integr Cancer Ther 2014;13(1):62–7.
113. Carlson LE, Garland SN. Impact of mindfulness-based stress reduction (MBSR) on sleep, mood, stress and fatigue symptoms in cancer outpatients. Int J Behav Med 2005;12(4):278–85.
114. Kwekkeboom KL, Bratzke LC. A systematic review of relaxation, meditation, and guided imagery strategies for symptom management in heart failure. J Cardiovasc Nurs 2016;31(5):457–68.
115. Kim YH, Kim HJ, Do Ahn S, et al. Effects of meditation on anxiety, depression, fatigue, and quality of life of women undergoing radiation therapy for breast cancer. Complement therapies Med 2013;21(4):379–87.
116. Witt CM, Cardoso MJ. Complementary and integrative medicine for breast cancer patients–Evidence based practical recommendations. Breast 2016;26: 37–44.
117. Geriatric Complementary and Alternative Medicines (CAM) Market Research Report Forecast to 2016 – 2024. Available at: http://www.openpr.com/news/416350/Geriatric-Complementary-and-Alternative-Medicines-CAM-Market-Research-Report-Forecast-to-2016-2024.html. Accessed April 25, 2017.

In Pursuit of the Fourth Aim in Health Care
The Joy of Practice

Katherine A. Gergen Barnett, MD

KEYWORDS

- Physician burnout • Quadruple aim • Wellness • Value-based care
- Accountable Care Organizations

KEY POINTS

- In today's health care system where there are increased demands for health care provider productivity, increased pay for performance metrics, decreased reimbursements, and ever-increasing demands of electronic medical records, providers are at risk for high rates of burnout.
- Provider burnout has tremendous downstream consequences on providers, patients, and the well-being of the larger health care system.
- A handful of successful interventions has been deployed to date, mostly focused on burnout on the individual level.
- Larger systems changes need to be made to reduce burnout and capture the joy of practice.
- The Accountable Care Organizations future of medicine (from volume to value) might be part of the solution.

INTRODUCTION

In 2008, Don Berwick and his colleagues[1] published a seminal article on health care delivery entitled, "The Triple Aim: Care, Health, and Cost," where they posited that "improving the US health care system requires simultaneous pursuit of three aims: improving the experience of care, improving the health of populations, and reducing per capita costs of health care." This approach to optimizing health care, dubbed the "Triple Aim," became an important motto for many individuals working within the quickly changing landscape of health care. Although the Triple Aim was masterful in addressing patient outcomes and cost containments, it did not, however, take into account a very important player in health care: the health care practitioner.

Disclosure Statement: Nothing to disclose.
Department of Family Medicine, Boston Medical Center, 1 Boston Medical Center Place, Dowling 5th Floor, Boston, MA 02118, USA
E-mail address: Katherine.gergen-barnett@bmc.org

Med Clin N Am 101 (2017) 1031–1040
http://dx.doi.org/10.1016/j.mcna.2017.04.014
0025-7125/17/© 2017 Elsevier Inc. All rights reserved.

medical.theclinics.com

Bodenheimer and Sinsky[2] artfully synthesized this gap in their paper entitled, "From Triple to Quadruple Aim: Care of the Patient Requires Care of the Provider," published in 2014. In this important account of the "missing aim," the investigators stated that in visiting many practices since the inception of the Triple Aim, they heard many comments from the staff and clinicians that the increased stress in health care served as a barrier to the implementation of the Triple Aim and made them wonder: "might there be a fourth aim—improving the work life of health care clinicians and staff—that, like the patient experience and cost reduction aims, must be achieved in order to succeed in improving population health? Should the Triple Aim become the Quadruple Aim?"

In today's health care system where there are increased demands for health care provider productivity, increased pay for performance metrics, decreased reimbursements, and ever-increasing demands of electronic medical records (EMRs), providers are at risk for high rates of burnout. Indeed, recent studies have indicated that greater than 50% of US physicians are now experiencing burnout and that burnout is rising dramatically faster among physicians than in any other US professional field.[3] These high rates of burnout have a large number of downstream consequences, for both the providers and for the patients that they serve. Thus, it has become imperative for the future of health care that we actively pursue the fourth aim of health care, the care of the provider. How can we instill the "Joy of Practice" into medicine again?

This article reviews what constitutes burnout, the postulated roots of burnout, interventions that have successfully been used to mitigate burnout among health care providers, and what larger system changes need to be addressed to get to the Joy of Practice. The Joy of Practice is so critical to the future of health care that rather than just being a Fourth Aim, it is the primary seat of health care delivery, from which all other aims of health care must stem (**Fig. 1**).

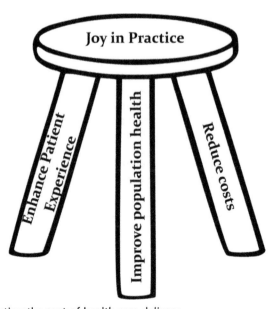

Fig. 1. Joy in practice: the seat of health care delivery.

WHAT IS BURNOUT?

Although burnout may be easily recognized, either personally or in a colleague, Christina Maslach Professor of Psychology at the University of California at Berkeley and creator of the now gold standard Maslach Burnout Inventory, defines burnout as an "erosion of the soul caused by deterioration of one's values, dignity, and spirit".[4] In Maslach's Burnout Inventory Model, she goes on to postulate that there are 3 components of burnout: (1) emotional exhaustion or loss of passion for one's work; (2) depersonalization or treating patients as objects; and (3) the sense that your work is no longer meaningful. (See **Fig. 2** for a colleague's artistic rendition of the three stages of burnout).

With the demands on providers continuing to climb, there is an increased rate of burnout among physicians. Shanafelt, a researcher based at Mayo Clinic and a practicing hematologist, has published several important articles on burnout, citing that one-third to one-half of physicians meet burnout criteria, as measured by Maslach's Burnout Inventory.[5,6] Furthermore, these studies revealed that physicians in specialties at the front line of care access (eg, emergency medicine, general internal medicine, and family medicine) are at greatest risk and that physicians work longer hours and have greater struggles with work-life integration than other US workers.[5,6] Interestingly, higher levels of education and professional degrees seem to act as a protective factor against burnout outside of medicine, whereas a degree in medicine (MD or DO) increases the risk.[6] Other studies show that women physicians are 1.6 times more likely as men to report burnout with lack of control over work hours and schedules being cited as the strongest predictors of burnout.[7]

The increasing rate of burnout among physicians is alarming. Shanafelt and colleagues[3] went on to survey the changing landscape from 2011 to 2014. Using Maslach's Burnout Inventory, they found that although 45.5% of the 3310 physicians surveyed in 2011 showed at least one symptom of burnout, these rates escalated to 54.4% in the 3680 physicians surveyed in 2014. Although burnout had increased significantly among physicians in this study, burnout rates among other working US adults remained steady. There are other studies to suggest that burnout is not unique to just physicians, but is shared by other members of the health care workforce. One survey showed that 34% of nurses working in the hospital and 37% of those working in the nursing home report burnout as compared with 22% of nurses working in other settings.[8]

What Are the Costs of Burnout?

Extensive literature has cited both the professional and the personal impact of burnout among providers. Professionally, physician burnout has been associated with

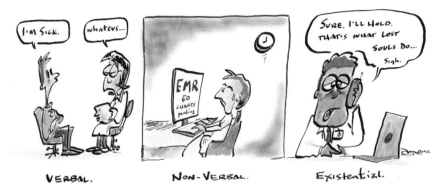

Fig. 2. Flags of impending burnout. (*Courtesy of* Jack Maypole, MD, Boston, MA.)

decreased patient satisfaction, increased medical errors, and increased litigation.[9,10] Personally, burnout among physicians has been linked to increased rates of depression and substance abuse, decreased quality of interpersonal relationships, and increased rates of early retirement.[11–13]

Replacing physicians who retire early or leave the practice because of burnout is an expensive proposition, with estimates of more than 250,000 dollars per physician.[14] High rates of burnout among practicing primary care physicians have also been related to a major decrease in the last 20 years in the percentage of graduates entering careers in primary care.[15–17] The decreased number of medical students entering primary care paired with the growing number of physicians retiring early or leaving primary care leads to a significant decline in access of care for patients.[18,19] This decline in access to primary care is occurring at the same time that the Affordable Care Act (ACA) has increased the number of people with insurance by 20 million, creating more of a need for primary care access than ever.

ROOTS OF BURNOUT

The causes of physician burnout are multivariate and complex. As alluded to before, many have posited the burnout crisis to come from the increased demands on physicians: increased demand of number of patients to be seen, increased communication to physicians through e-mails, EMRs, increased metrics to meet, and decreased autonomy.

Although the causes are complex, some postulate that EMRs may partly be at the root of much of the increased burnout among health care providers. Seen as a means to improve patient care, efficiencies, and communication, EMRs became very popular among federal policymakers, and in 2009, as much as 27 billion dollars were invested in getting hospitals off paper and onto EMRs. Since then, up to 80% of medical practices are now on EMRs (from 15%), and those who do not use them face a risk of financial penalties. However, the rise of EMRs may have led to unintended consequences.

In a survey done of 6375 physicians from all different specialties in the United States, 84.5% responded that they use EMRs. Of those using EMRs, 44% reported that they were dissatisfied or very dissatisfied with them. Forty-one percent disagreed or strongly disagreed with the notion that EMRs improved patient care.[20] Perhaps not surprisingly, younger physicians expressed greater satisfaction with EMRs than did older doctors: 46% of those younger than 40 responded that they were satisfied with their EMR systems compared with 34% of those 60 and older.[20]

One of the very things that the EMR was supposed to address, efficiency, failed to come to fruition among the physicians interviewed. In fact, 63% of physicians responded that EMRs fail to improve efficiency.[12] Many physicians surveyed complained that EMRs added to the amount of time that they spent charting, and when controlling for all other variables, the survey showed that burnout (as measured by Maslach's Burnout Inventory) was 30% more likely in those using an EMR for patient orders.

These results were supported by another recently and artfully done study, which was published in the *Annals of Medicine* in 2016. In this study, 57 US physicians in multiple specialties, including Family Medicine, Internal Medicine, Cardiology, and Orthopedics, were observed for 430 hours and 21 physicians also completed after-hours diaries. The time study revealed that during the day, physicians spent an average of 27.0% of their time on direct clinical face time with patients and 49.2% of their time on EHR and desk work. While in the room with patients, physicians spent 37.0% of their time on the EMR and desk work and only 52.9% of the time on direct clinical face time. Of the 21 physicians who completed after-hours diaries, all reported up to 2 hours of after-hours work each night, devoted mostly to EMR tasks.

The investigators concluded that "for every hour physicians provide direct clinical face time to patients, nearly 2 additional hours is spent on EHR and desk work within the clinic day. Outside office hours, physicians spend another 1 to 2 hours of personal time each night doing additional computer and other clerical work."[21]

These studies confirm much of what many physicians on the front lines experience personally day to day. Addressing the shortcomings of the EMR, while deeply important on the quest toward reclaiming the Joy of Practice, is complicated and calls for greater technological innovations that are yet still on the horizon. What are some of the steps that have been taken to mitigate burnout, on the individual provider level as well as the institutional level, that are well within our reach today?

IN SEARCH OF JOY

Loss of a sense of control in the face of increasing demands and stressors is at the base of much of the burnout literature, pointing some scholars to work toward resiliency training or mindfulness as an antidote. As written by one scholar in resiliency training for physicians: "Resilience is the capacity to respond to stress in a healthy way such that goals are achieved at minimal psychological and physical cost; resilient individuals 'bounce back' after challenges while also growing stronger."[22]

In one study by Krasner and colleagues[23] at the University of Rochester, 70 primary care physicians participated in a course that included "mindfulness meditation, self-awareness exercises, narratives about meaningful clinical experiences, appreciative interviews, didactic material, and discussion." The study had both an 8-week intensive phase (2.5 hours per week and a 7-hour retreat) and a 10-month maintenance phase (2.5 h/mo). Over the course of the program and follow-up, participants demonstrated improvements in mindfulness, which was in turn correlated with statistically significant improvements in total mood disturbance and burnout.

Siedsma and Emlet[24] explored whether a briefer intervention just could be effective. They had 74 practicing physicians in the Department of Medicine at Mayo Clinic involved in 19 biweekly facilitated physician discussion groups incorporating elements of mindfulness, reflection, shared experience, and small-group learning for 9 months. Physicians were given protected time (1 hour of paid time every other week) by the institution. The study assessed for meaning in work, empowerment and engagement in work, burnout, symptoms of depression, quality of life, and job satisfaction using validated metrics. The intervention statistically improved the meaning and engagement in work while also reducing depersonalization, results that were sustained even 12 months after the study.

Another frontier of work is looking at some of the innate risk of physicians and physicians in training and developing workshops to "inoculate" providers from these kinds of risks. In their important thought piece, Nedrow and her colleagues[25] posit that "physician burnout, often defined as emotional exhaustion, ineffectiveness, and depersonalization, may be linked to four values characteristic of physicians and reinforced in medical training: service, excellence, curative competence, and compassion. Although each one is a virtuous strength and source of pride for physicians, each possesses a destructive 'dark side,' deprivation, invincibility, omnipotence, and isolation." They address each of the dark sides of the 4 value characteristics and offer a set of skills and exercises, such as reframing, gratitude, mindful self-compassion and awareness, generous listening, silence, and community building in order to mitigate their potential negative impacts and help prevent burnout. Programs offering training in such skill sets are potentially very valuable in both residency and medical school, and the investigators point to one such existent program being offered in medical school at Oregon Health and Science University, entitled Integrative Self-Care Initiative for Students. Nedrow and her colleagues end by offering physicians questions that may help them feel "unstuck" in their day to day: What did I learn today? Would I do anything differently? What 3 things am I grateful for today? What inspired me? How did I talk to myself today? Did I take myself too seriously? Did anything surprise me?

Although the results of the above studies show significant benefit of such resiliency and mindfulness programs on provider burnout, the interventions work on the individual alone and do not change the system, thereby leaving the effects as potentially unsustainable.

SYSTEMS CHANGE

In order to address the roots of burnout, one could argue that the roots of transformation begin while physicians are in training. The *Journal of the American Medical Association* recently published a systematic review of medical students internationally that estimates the prevalence of depression or depressive symptoms among medical students to be 27.2%. The prevalence of suicidal ideation was 11.1%. Lead author, Rotenstein, and her colleagues[26] posit that these high rates stem from institutional issues, including the notion that unless you work hard there is something "wrong with you" because it has long been the culture of medical education and training to be pushed to physical and mental limits. They go on to say that medical schools do not always do a good job addressing the emotional life of students, leaving depressive symptoms as something to be treated rather than something that should be addressed.

There are, however, some bright spots developing in the medical school curriculum, one of which is an elective medical school course called the "Healer's Art." Started by Dr Rachel Naomi Remen as a small gathering among friends and medical colleagues more than 20 years ago, the elective is now offered annually at more than 70 schools in the United States and 7 schools internationally. More than 1600 students take the course every year and more than 13,000 have gone through it. The Healer's Art is a 15-hour elective for first- and second-year medical students that is conducted over the course of 5 evenings, each evening with a theme including honoring loss, grief, awe in medicine, and the care of the soul. The course is conducted such that students are in groups with attending physicians and there is no hierarchy.[27] Although the format of the course is seemingly simple, many students throughout the years have seen a course such as Healer's Art as the antidote for the "hidden curriculum" of medical school where "doubts and grief are forbidden."[28] Drawing on the age-old core values of medicine such as meaning, loss, awe, and service, the Healer's Art helps students connect to why they went into medicine and is seen by many as a kind of immunization to the later assaults of medical training. As put by Remen, "When doctors learn to read the affective domain, they are shocked to discover that they have gone right past experiences of profound meaning without seeing them. They say, 'I was colorblind.' Medicine offers you a front-row seat on life. Meaning is all around you. When you can see it, it gives you a sense of gratitude for the opportunity to do this work."[28]

It is courses like Healers Art, ones that shift the cultural domain of medical school education and allow people to connect more to their emotional well-being, that serve as a piece of the puzzle in reducing burnout and depression.

CLINICAL PRACTICES

Medical school education, however, is only one small piece of that puzzle. Within the clinical setting, there have been several institutional interventions that show some promise in reducing burnout. The American Medical Association recently gathered data and published a list of concrete ways that clinics can be working on reducing burnout, which include work flow redesign, communication interventions, and targeted quality improvement projects.[29]

The workflow redesign contains many important ideas, which all move in the direction of increasing the interprofessional engagement of care for the patient while taking the individual burden off of the physician. For many clinics, this may mean strengthening the relationship between physician and medical assistant, having nonphysician staff entering more patient data into the EMR, and increasing the amount of work done in previsit huddles.[29]

Communication interventions include daily huddles among team members to discuss complex patients and care coordination, colocation of team members such as physicians, nurses, and medical assistants, and regular team meetings where providers have the opportunity to discuss complex cases.[29] Finally, creating processes whereby physician wellness data can be regularly collected and presented serves as a springboard for open discussion about future interventions.

The suggestions from the American Medical Association report build nicely upon an earlier article by Linzer and colleagues[30] entitled, "Ten Bold Steps to Prevent Burnout." Linzer added that practices could implement mindfulness programs, improve EMRs, increase physician work flexibility by hiring floats and allowing more control over hours, maintain manageable panel sizes for providers, provide opportunities for providers to reconnect to meaning at work, and underscore the importance of provider self-care.

These suggestions are laudable and taken together would make a tremendous impact on burnout. Although some of these steps, such as obtaining regular quality metrics on well-being, colocation of teams, and regular team meetings- are obtainable today, many require significant leadership investment: both on a local and on a national level.

Indeed, leadership has shown some inspiring examples. At the Cleveland Clinic, CEO Cosgrove has instituted several innovations to address burnout. These innovations include items to reduce stress from the EMR such as card readers so that providers save precious time by not having to repeatedly log in and out, increased IT support, EMR customization, primary care scribes, voice recognition software, and iPhones with apps to help chart. The Cleveland Clinic also includes infrastructural support for wellness including more flexibility to be a part-time physician, lectures on delivering bad news and communication skills, employee programs for mindfulness, access to a state-of-the-art gym, and a "Code Lavender" program for any employee in distress. Finally, the Cleveland Clinic supports monthly social events, well-being days, and required annual physicals for its employees.[13]

Sinsky and Sinsky[31] have built an innovative model of care called the Collaborative Care Model whereby the nurse stays with the patient from the beginning to end of the appointment and obtains vitals, performs medication reconciliation, gathers information, helps set the patient agenda, and begins to record the history. The physician's role is to then flesh out any necessary additional history, perform the examination, and help create the plan. After the plan is made, the nurse stays with the patient and helps reinforce instructions and will call the patient between visits as needed. In this model, the care is 3-way with the "explicit goal to increase the percentage of the visit during which the physician provides undivided attention to the patient." The Collaborative Care Model has had initial data to suggest improved patient, nursing, and physician satisfaction.

The Cleveland Clinic and the Collaborative Care Model are only two examples of sites doing innovative work to reduce burnout. There are many clinics across the country making innovative changes, both big and small, to try and address provider burnout. However, as has been explored, there are roots to the cause of burnout that run deep, and therefore, some of the causes of burnout may not be addressed without a real shift in the way care is delivered.

FROM VOLUME TO VALUE?

The Affordable Care Act, an act that totaled a dizzying 16,000 pages, brought with it 700 new quality metrics through Centers for Medicare and Medicaid Services. It also created a road map for a new system of care called Accountable Care Organizations, whereby keeping populations healthy will be the new way to do business. Physicians will no longer be paid by the number of patients seen (volume) but rather by the quality of care (value) that they provide. There are many who see this as good for the future of the care of the patient and for the bottom line. Some could also argue that this may be a big move in the right direction for reducing physician burnout, if done well.

Keeping patients well requires tremendous teamwork. In addition to the engagement of the provider and the patient, it requires the work of the nurses, medical assistants, care managers, pharmacists, behavioral health specialists, patient navigators, and community health workers. These members of the health care team are part of the patient's Patient Centered Medical Home. To truly keep the patient well means that a patient needs to be kept well in the community by using such resources as community centers, neighborhood gyms, safe streets for working, and healthy food vendors. The list goes on.

The health care delivery system thus becomes a matrix and is no longer a dyad or even a triad. This move will require a tremendous amount of communication among many players and a chance to build up the interprofessional nature of where health care delivery is going. The movement toward value-based population health may push medical institutions to begin to redefine whether it is to be a physician, from an "all knowing being" (set up for tremendous fear of failure) to one part of a larger team. Focusing on the outcome of health and prevention may also in turn push medical education institutions to begin to teach more about health and wellness to its learners and, in turn, provide opportunities for learners to experience what wellness feels like.

These changes, although helpful, will not be sufficient in driving physician wellness. Programs must be supported with time and money from legislation and institutions. It is known, however, that physician burnout is dangerous to patients, dangerous to the profession, and extremely detrimental for the financial bottom line.

It is time to take on the mantle of "The Fourth Aim: The Joy of Practice." As we gather for the journey forward, we will need to bring our own tools for wellness, because the road will be long. In the end, however, this journey is critical to the wellness of us all.

REFERENCES

1. Berwick DM, Nolan TW, Whittington J. The triple aim: care, health, and cost. Health Aff (Millwood) 2008;27(3):759–69.
2. Bodenheimer T, Sinsky C. From triple to quadruple aim: care of the patient requires care of the provider. Ann Fam Med 2014;12:573–6.
3. Shanafelt TD, Hasan O, Dyrbye LN, et al. Changes in burnout and satisfaction with work-life balance in physicians and the general US working population between 2011 and 2014. Mayo Clin Proc 2015;90:1600–13.

4. Maslach C, Jackson S, Leiter M. Maslach burnout inventory manual. 3rd edition. Palo Alto (CA): Consulting Psychologists Press; 1996.

5. Shanafelt TD, West CP, Sloan JA, et al. Career fit and burnout among academic faculty. Arch Intern Med 2009;169:990–5.

6. Shanafelt TD, Boone S, Tan L, et al. Burnout and satisfaction with work-life balance among US physicians relative to the general US population. Arch Intern Med 2012;172(18):1377–85.

7. McMurray JE, Linzer M, Konrad TR, et al, SGIM Career Satisfaction Study Group. The work lives of women physicians: results from the physician work life study. J Gen Intern Med 2000;15:372–80.

8. McHugh MD, Kutney-Lee A, Cimiotti JP, et al. Nurses' widespread job dissatisfaction, burnout, and frustration with health benefits signal problems for patient care. Health Aff (Millwood) 2011;30(2):202–10.

9. Shanafelt TD, Balch CM, Bechamps G, et al. Burnout and medical errors among American surgeons. Ann Surg 2010;251:995–1000.

10. Fahrenkopf AM, Sectish TC, Barger LK, et al. Rates of medication errors among depressed and burnt out residents: prospective cohort study. BMJ 2008;336: 488–91.

11. Brown SD, Goske MJ, Johnson CM. Beyond substance abuse: stress, burnout, and depression as causes of physician impairment and disruptive behavior. J Am Coll Radiol 2009;6:479–85.

12. Dyrbye LN, Thomas MR, Massie FS, et al. Burnout and suicidal ideation among US medical students. Ann Intern Med 2008;149:334–41.

13. Cosgrove, T: Doctors in distress: the burnout crisis. Oral Presentation to American College of Surgeons. The Franklin Martin Lecture, delivered 10/17/2016.

14. Buchbinder SB, Wilson M, Melick CF, et al. Estimates of costs of primary care physician turnover. Am J Manag Care 1999;5(11):1431–8.

15. Dorsey ER, Jarjoura D, Rutecki GW. Influence of controllable lifestyle on recent trends in specialty choice by US medical students. JAMA 2003;290(9):1173–8.

16. Landon BE, Reschovsky JD, Pham HH, et al. Leaving medicine: the consequences of physician dissatisfaction. Med Care 2006;44(3):234–42.

17. Rubin DB. Saving primary care. Am J Med 2007;120(1):99–102.

18. Bodenheimer T. Primary care–will it survive? N Engl J Med 2006;355(9):861–4.

19. Treadway K. The future of primary care: sustaining relationships. N Engl J Med 2008;359(25):2086–8.

20. Shanafelt T, Dyrbye L, Sinsky C, et al. Relationship between clerical burden and characteristics of the electronic environment with physician burnout and professional satisfaction. Mayo Clin Proc 2016;91:836–48.

21. Sinsky C, Colligan L, Li L, et al. Allocation of physician time in ambulatory practice: a time and motion study in 4 specialties. Ann Intern Med 2016;165:753–61.

22. Epstein RM, Krasner MS. Physician resilience: what it means, why it matters, and how to promote it. Acad Med 2013;88(3):301–3.

23. Krasner MS, Epstein RM, Beckman H, et al. Association of an educational program in mindful communication with burnout, empathy, and attitudes among primary care physicians. JAMA 2009;302:1284–93.

24. Siedsma M, Emlet L. Physician burnout: can we make a difference together? Crit Care 2015;19:273.

25. Nedrow A, Steckler N, Hardman J. Physician resilience and burnout: can you make the switch? Fam Pract Manag 2013;20:25–30.

26. Rotenstein LS, Ramos MA, Torre M, et al. Prevalence of depression, depressive symptoms, and suicidal ideation among medical students: a systematic review and meta-analysis. JAMA 2016;316(21):2214–36.

27. The healers art overview. Available at: www.rishiprograms.org/programs/medical-educators-students/. Accessed March 9, 2017.

28. Borenstein D. Medicine's search for meaning. The New York Times 2013. Available at: opinionator.blogs.nytimes.com/2013/09/18/medicines-search-for-meaning.

29. Linzer M, Guzman-Corrales L, Poplau S. Preventing physician burnout: improve patient satisfaction, quality outcomes and provider recruitment and retention. AMA steps forward. Available at: https://www.stepsforward.org/modules/physician-burnout. Accessed December 16, 2016.

30. Linzer M, Levine R, Meltzer D, et al. 10 bold steps to prevent burnout in general internal medicine. J Gen Intern Med 2014;29(1):18–20.

31. Sinsky C, Sinky T. Collaborative care model: nurse-physician partnerships in primary care. Available at: https://static1.squarespace.com/static/527a6f47e4b06d382162aed0/t/52c0e87ee4b05b3d6c410f56/1388374142772/Collaborative+Care+Model.pdf. Accessed December 15, 2016.

Moving?

Make sure your subscription moves with you!

To notify us of your new address, find your **Clinics Account Number** (located on your mailing label above your name), and contact customer service at:

Email: journalscustomerservice-usa@elsevier.com

800-654-2452 (subscribers in the U.S. & Canada)
314-447-8871 (subscribers outside of the U.S. & Canada)

Fax number: 314-447-8029

Elsevier Health Sciences Division
Subscription Customer Service
3251 Riverport Lane
Maryland Heights, MO 63043

*To ensure uninterrupted delivery of your subscription, please notify us at least 4 weeks in advance of move.

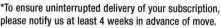

Printed and bound by CPI Group (UK) Ltd, Croydon, CR0 4YY

07/10/2024

01040503-0020